# Stress-Related Disorders

*Edited by Emilio Ovuga*

Published in London, United Kingdom

Stress-Related Disorders
http://dx.doi.org/10.5772/intechopen.94807
Edited by Emilio Ovuga

Contributors
Lee A. Baugh, Jamie L. Scholl, Taylor J. Bosch, Eric T. Graack, Michaela S. Ahrenholtz, Jeannette C.G. Lely, Rolf J. Kleber, Glen Bates, Tony McHugh, Nevzat Tarhan, Muhsin Konuk, Mesut Karahan, Öznur Özge Özcan, Gökben Hızlı Sayar, Sibel Ozturk Ayvaz, Nurper Ulkuer, Hazal Ayas, Feride Zeynep Güder, Sherry H. Stewart, Pablo Romero-Sanchiz, Sarah DeGrace, Catherine Standage, Panagiota Xaplanteri, Takahiro A. Kato, Enomoto Shingo, Emilio Ovuga, Henry Oboke, Anne Abio, Felix Kaducu-Ocaka, Morten Sodemann, Ask Elklit, Leena S. Bagadia, Arun More, Swati Mittal, Smriti Sinha, Shilpi Bhat, Imen Ghorbel, Mariem Chaâbane, Awatef Elwej, Fatma Ghorbel-Koubaa, Najiba Zeghal



First published in London, United Kingdom, 2022 by IntechOpen
IntechOpen is the global imprint of INTECHOPEN LIMITED, registered in England and Wales, registration number: 11086078, 5 Princes Gate Court, London, SW7 2QJ, United Kingdom

British Library Cataloguing-in-Publication Data
A catalogue record for this book is available from the British Library

Additional hard and PDF copies can be obtained from orders@intechopen.com

Stress-Related Disorders
Edited by Emilio Ovuga
p. cm.
Print ISBN 978-1-80355-363-4
Online ISBN 978-1-80355-364-1
eBook (PDF) ISBN 978-1-80355-365-8

# Meet the editor

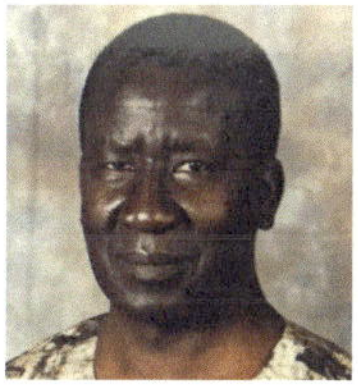

Emilio Baliki Liociri Ovuga, Ph.D., MD, is a retired professor of psychiatry and former dean of the Medical School at Gulu University, Uganda, and professor at the International Institute of Medicine and Science (IIMS), California, USA. He is also a suicidologist, psychiatric epidemiologist, and forensic psychiatrist. He obtained his medical degree and master's degree in Psychiatry at Makerere University, Uganda. He obtained a Ph.D. in Suicidology and Psychiatric Epidemiology from Karolinska Institutet, Sweden. He was the founding chairperson of the Forum of Research Ethics Committees in Uganda (FRECU) and founder and chairperson of the Gulu University Research Ethics Committee (GUREC). He is the executive president of the Society for Advancement of Science in Africa (SASA) and chief executive officer of Bomvitae Agro Industries Limited (BAIL), an agricultural research enterprise in the Adjumani District of Uganda. Dr. Ovuga is also a member of the Special Working Group (SWG) for the decriminalization of suicide of the International Association for the Prevention of Suicide (IASP). Dr. Ovuga is a suicidologist, psychiatric epidemiologist, and forensic psychiatrist. As a practitioner in suicide prevention, Dr. Ovuga has implemented suicide prevention programs in the Adjumani, Gulu, and Amuru Districts in post-conflict Northern Uganda by training and working with lay community representatives to deliver first aid counseling services to individuals in psychological distress. Emilio Ovuga obtained Ph.D. in Suicidology and Psychiatric Epidemiology from Karolinska Institutet. He is a book editor and a guest editor and reviewer for several scientific journals. In his retirement, he continues to mentor upcoming researchers and remains interested in research and the development and implementation of community-based health and social services.

# Contents

# Preface

Stress, as referred to in this book, means the experience of single or multiple events beyond what an average human being can withstand or bear. This form of stress is also known as traumatic stress. Such an event might entail actual or threatened death or severe injury or maiming of one's own body or the body of other individuals. Traumatic stress may also arise in response to viewing photographs of scenes of traumatic events. A considerable body of literature exists about traumatic stress, and it continues to grow as more and more research delves into the subject to provide additional understanding of the nature of human suffering because of exposure to traumatic incidents. This book discusses some of the current understanding of the disorders associated with traumatic stress. It includes eleven chapters.

In Chapter 1, Dr. Stewart Sherry provides a literature review of the current knowledge in the field. In Chapter 2, Dr. Baugh Lee et al. discuss the biomarkers that researchers and clinicians alike will need in dealing with the complex phenomenon of traumatic stress. The knowledge of biomarkers is likely to help researchers direct attention to further inquiries in future research. Likewise, information on biomarkers will help clinicians to carry out novel clinical investigations to enhance the rapid diagnosis and understanding of stress-related disorders. Of relevance of the knowledge of biomarkers is the potential use of biomarkers in decisions on what interventions will work in the short-term, medium-term, and long-term.

Using information from animal studies and postmortem data in Chapter 3, Dr. Shingo Enomoto and Takahiro A. Kato discuss the interesting and complex roles of microglia activation, proliferation, and neuro-inflammation in the genesis of mental disorders and pain in traumatic stress. In Chapter 4, Dr. Leena S. Bagadia and Arun More discuss the role of anger in the genesis and maintenance of hypertension. Along the same lines in Chapter 5, Tony McHugh and Glen Bates provide insight into the role of anger and imagery in the maintenance of stress-related disorders. In Chapter 6, Dr. Ghorbel et al. show how oxidative stress at the mitochondrial level might be involved in the etiology and maintenance of cardiovascular diseases.

In Chapter 7, Dr. Xaplanteri Panagiota provides compelling information against the practice of "mobbing" that medical residents experience during their training. Mobbing, which is a form of professional bullying in the training of students, is also used to make junior hospital staff feel belittled, ignorant, and inferior in the workplace. While mobbing might encourage learning, albeit, under uncomfortable circumstances, the practice makes healthcare providers resentful and vengeful toward other colleagues of lower rank.

Chapter 8 by Professor Tarhan Nevzat et al. provide a candid discussion of ontology and neurobiology as well as a variety of new diagnostic procedures in traumatic stresses from the adverse effects of childhood experiences (ACEs), genomics, epigenomics, and neuroimaging and positron emission computerised tomography (PECT). The chapter also addresses the concept of "toxic stress" and cybercrimes as new and emerging forms of traumatic stress. Prof. Nevzat's discussion is particularly relevant given the rising tide of crimes committed online.

In Chapter 9, Jeannette C.G. Lely and Rolf J. Kleber discuss the problem of traumatic stress in later life. Individuals aged 70 years and older face a variety of challenges that people accept as normal processes of aging. People in this age group might have no jobs and incomes, might be lonely, might have a variety of somatic conditions (such as cancer, chronic pulmonary disorders, and cardiovascular disorders), and might suffer from dementia or depression in addition to the ever-present realization of their mortality. Under these conditions, traumatic stress disorders in later life deserve attention from every caregiver.

In Chapter 10, Dr. Mittal Swati et al. discuss the mental health impacts of the COVID-19 pandemic. Since the emergence of the pandemic, several thousand publications based on research and anecdotal observations have appeared in the scientific literature. The unique thing about COVID-19 is that it struck the world suddenly and many health experts did not quite know how to respond to it. The world has lost many lives either directly from the physical effects of the virus or the mental health complications of the pandemic. Dr. Swati's contribution to the mental health effects of the COVID-19 pandemic is therefore timely.

Finally, in Chapter 11, Professor Ovuga et al. provide data on the mental health wellness of lay counselors in situations of chronic and prolonged mass trauma. Professor Ovuga and his colleagues demonstrate from personal experience that lay counselors must be mentally sound to support their colleagues well.

**Emilio Ovuga**
Gulu University,
Gulu, Uganda

International Institute of Medicine and Science (IIMS),
USA

Section 1

# Current State of Understanding

Chapter 1

# A Scoping Review of the Literature on Trauma Cue-Induced Drug Craving in Substance Users with Trauma Histories or PTSD

*Sarah DeGrace, Pablo Romero-Sanchiz, Catherine Standage and Sherry H. Stewart*

## Abstract

Among trauma-exposed individuals, substances may be used as a means of obtaining symptom relief following exposure to trauma reminders. Repeated pairing of trauma cues with substance use may lead to the development of classically conditioned craving to trauma cues. Conditioned craving following cue exposure can be studied in-lab using the cue-reactivity paradigm. To map cue-reactivity research conducted with trauma-exposed substance users, we aimed to synthesize research which studied our population of interest, used a cue-reactivity paradigm, and measured craving as an outcome. Three databases were searched using relevant keywords. Twenty-eight studies met our criteria. Four key 19 themes are discussed in our review of these scoped studies—(1) craving as an outcome; (2) methodological subtypes across paradigms; (3) affect as an additional outcome or as a mediator of cue-induced craving; and (4) cue-reactivity paradigms as an intervention outcome assessment tool. Overall, there is strong evidence for cue-reactivity paradigms as a useful means of eliciting craving in response to trauma cues. Our scoping review suggests the need for a meta-analysis to determine the magnitude of the trauma cue-induced craving effect in substance users with trauma histories, and to determine significant moderators (e.g., PTSD symptom severity) and mediators of this effect (e.g., negative affect).

**Keywords:** cue-reactivity, substance use, posttraumatic stress disorder, trauma, craving

## 1. Introduction

Posttraumatic stress disorder (PTSD) is an often debilitating mental disorder that may occur following trauma exposure [1]. PTSD is characterized by four diagnostic clusters—(1) the re-experiencing the traumatic event (e.g., recurrent memories, dreams, or flashbacks); (2) symptoms of avoidance (e.g., efforts to evade trauma reminders); (3) arousal (e.g., hypervigilance, sleep disruptions); and (4) negative cognitions and mood (e.g., self-blame) [1]. Substance use disorder (SUD) is another psychiatric disorder characterized by 11 possible symptoms which involve negative consequences arising from one's substance use and inability to control one's substance use [1]. In the last version of the *Diagnostic and Statistical Manual of Mental Disorders* (the DSM-5; [1]), craving, the often intrusive desire to use the substance, was added as one of the 11 symptoms characterizing a SUD [1].

PTSD often co-occurs with SUD. Research has documented high rates of comorbidity between PTSD and alcohol use disorder (AUD) [2], cannabis use disorder (CUD) [3, 4], and other SUDs [5]. The prognosis of comorbid PTSD-SUD is worse than either disorder alone [6] with comorbid PTSD-SUD leading to greater functional impairment in comparison to those with only PTSD or a SUD [7].

It has been suggested that PTSD and SUD are likely functionally related to one another [8] in comorbid individuals. While the precise underlying mechanisms are not well understood, there are several learning theories that may help explain the high rates of substance misuse in people with trauma histories and help us understand the high comorbidity of PTSD with SUD. The first is the two-factor learning theory which was originally developed by Mowrer to explain the acquisition and maintenance of phobias [9] and which has more recently been applied by Stasiewicz [10] to the acquisition and maintenance of SUDs. Two-factor learning theory applies a combination of classical conditioning and operant conditioning mechanisms to the development and maintenance phases of these disorders, respectively. Applying this theory to the co-occurrence of PTSD and SUDs in traumatized individuals, trauma-relevant cues that were paired with the original traumatic experience (e.g., loud noises of gunfire paired with witnessing a comrade fatally injured in wartime) are thought to come to elicit negative affect through the process of classical conditioning [10]. Future exposures to the trauma cue alone (e.g., loud noises alone) motivate avoidance/escape behavior, including substance misuse, to reduce the associated negative affect and thereby experience relief [10]. Avoidance/escape behaviors like substance misuse are thus negatively reinforced in individuals with trauma histories/PTSD as they remove the aversive experience of negative affect. Therefore, substance misuse is maintained as a self-medication type of coping response through operant conditioning processes where behavior is repeated when it is followed by desirable consequences, in this case, relief from negative affect.

Another theory that is relevant to understanding the links of trauma/PTSD with SUD involves the role of classical conditioning in the development of conditioned craving—a strong urge to use the substance in response to exposure to the conditioned cues. It has long been known that drug-related stimuli that are frequently paired with drug-taking can come to elicit a conditioned craving response through the process of classical conditioning [11]. For example, a needle and other drug use paraphernalia that are frequently paired with heroin use can come to elicit craving when presented alone, for an injection drug user. Similarly, for a substance user with a trauma history/PTSD, the frequent pairing of trauma cues (e.g., intrusive memories of the trauma, exposure to external trauma reminders) with substance use, as explained by the two-factor learning theory above [10], can come to create strong associations between trauma cues and substance use [12]. The result is that such trauma cues can become conditioned stimuli that elicit a conditioned craving response when presented on their own [13]. For example, if a young woman with sexual assault-related PTSD drinks alcohol each time she has an intrusive memory about her sexual assault, such trauma cues can come to elicit a strong craving for a drink, which may motivate her alcohol seeking and maintain her alcohol use.

The study of the above putative mechanisms under controlled, laboratory conditions is crucial for a better understanding of the intertwined relationships between trauma/PTSD and substance misuse. Specifically, the use of cue-reactivity paradigms allows researchers to examine how substance-related and trauma cues may come to elicit craving and/or negative affective responses through the conditioning processes described above.

The cue-reactivity paradigm is broadly defined as a lab-based method in which participants are exposed to a set of stimuli meant to elicit a "reactivity" response—that is, a change from baseline in response to the stimulus [14]. In the context of addictions research, stimuli may be substance-related cues, such as a syringe or other drug-related paraphernalia for an injection drug user [15]; these stimuli serve as analogs for real-life stimuli which may evoke a craving response outside of the lab. Indeed, research in this area has shown that relevant drug-related cues presented in the lab can elicit a heightened craving response among substance users [16, 17]. More recently, cue-reactivity paradigms have been used to study conditioned craving as a possible mechanism underlying the relationship between trauma/PTSD and SUD [18, 19]. Indeed, extant research has shown that in-lab exposure to cues representing trauma reminders (e.g., a video of a violent crime) activates both substance-related craving responses as well as increased negative affect [20].

Craving has been measured in a number of ways in substance- and trauma-related cue-reactivity research, including with subjective self-report measures, such as the Desire for Drug Questionnaire [21], and measures specific to the substances used, such as the Alcohol Urge Questionnaire [22] and the Marijuana Craving Questionnaire [23]. Craving has also been measured more objectively in cue-reactivity studies, albeit less commonly than via self-report. Specifically, physiological measures, such as salivary flow and heart rate monitoring, are often used as a more objective proxy measure of craving [24]. Craving has also been further differentiated into reward-related craving (i.e., a desire for reward or stimulation from a substance) and relief-related craving (i.e., a desire for a reduction in tension or negative affect from using a substance) using certain self-report measures [23].

While cue exposure paradigms are homogenous in their goal to elicit some form of reactivity (e.g., change from baseline in craving or emotional state in response to the stimulus), the types of cues and paradigms used in this area of research have varied widely. For example, cues may be standardized across participants in the study or may be personalized to the individual's own trauma history details; cues may be presented through the use of script-driven imagery (i.e., audio recordings, such as a retelling of a traumatic event) or *in vivo* (i.e., physical objects, such as drug paraphernalia); and cues maybe a photo or video stimuli (i.e., a video of an assault).

Indeed, it is evident that cue-reactivity paradigms vary widely in design, are used in an expansive variety of contexts and with a wide range of populations, with many different outcomes used to capture cue-reactivity effects. Thus, in this chapter, we intend to scope the extant cue-reactivity literature in the context of PTSD-SUD comorbidity research to identify patterns and variations in methodology, measures, and outcomes used in this growing field.

### 1.1 Aims and objectives

Our first aim was to examine how cue-reactivity paradigms have been used in samples of substance users with trauma histories. Specifically, we were interested in how these studies lead to a further understanding of the mechanisms underlying comorbid PTSD-SUD. Second, we intended to examine the different types of cues used within the cue-reactivity paradigm as well as the specific effects, strengths, and weaknesses of variations in paradigm design. Specifically, we compared the merit of personalized vs. non-personalized cues, as well as other cue variations, in PTSD-SUD cue-reactivity research (e.g., *in vivo*, imagery-based). Third, we sought to assess the use of several measures of reactivity that have been examined using the cue-reactivity paradigm (i.e., craving [subjective, objective], negative affect) used in PTSD-SUD research. Lastly, we examined the types of participants who have been studied using a cue-reactivity methodology (e.g., trauma-exposed vs. suffering from PTSD).

## 2. Method

The present scoping review followed preferred reporting items for systematic reviews and meta-analyses (PRISMA) guidelines appropriate for a scoping review. Specifically, we used the PRISMA Scoping Review checklist [25].

### 2.1 Inclusion and exclusion criteria

Studies were included if they used an experimental design if they utilized a cue-reactivity paradigm and if self-reported craving was assessed following the cue-reactivity paradigm. Furthermore, the population of interest had to include individuals who had experienced a traumatic event consistent with Criterion A of a DSM-5 PTSD diagnosis [1]. Alternatively, PTSD symptoms must have been assessed for each participant. Additionally, it was required that participants report on their substance use.

We excluded studies that were not written in English, or if humans were not the research participants. We did not exclude gray literature. Specifically, we included theses and dissertations to gather the full scope of research in this area and to reduce publication bias.

### 2.2 Literature search

The databases PsycInfo, PubMed, and PTSDPubs were searched to identify studies of interest. Each search was conducted using a Boolean search logic and relevant keywords: ("PTSD" OR "post traumatic stress disorder" OR "posttraumatic stress disorder" OR "post-traumatic stress disorder" OR "trauma") AND ("cue" OR "cue exposure" OR "cue-reactivity" OR "conditioned response" OR "stimuli") AND ("substance" OR "substances" OR "alcohol" OR "drug" OR "drugs" OR "cocaine" OR "cannabis" OR "marijuana" OR "opioids" OR "opiates" OR "tobacco" OR "nicotine") AND ("craving" OR "urge"). There were no search restrictions based on year of publication or language.[1]

## 3. Results

### 3.1 Screening of search results

One hundred fifty-eight studies were initially imported into Covidence, a literature screening software. After duplicates were removed by Covidence, 128 studies remained. Abstracts of all studies were screened by two independent raters (SDG and

---

[1] Non-English language studies were captured in our search and were excluded if an English translation could not be found.

CS) who removed all irrelevant studies; a moderate rate of agreement of 74% was achieved [26]. A third screener (PRS) aided in resolving any conflicts between the two raters. A total of 28 studies met our final inclusion criteria (**Figure 1**).

### 3.2 Data extraction

The data were extracted into a spreadsheet, including information on the study sample, sample characteristics, outcome measures, cue-reactivity methodology, hypotheses/aims, outcomes of interest, and general findings. A quality assessment and risk of bias assessment were not conducted, as these are not typical in scoping reviews [27]. The extracted data were then synthesized into common categories by the first author to further examine themes in the scoped research.

### 3.3 Summary of included studies

#### *3.3.1 Cue-reactivity Paradigm*

Script-driven imagery cues were the most common cue paradigm used in the present sample of studies (n = 20). These were often paired with a substance-related

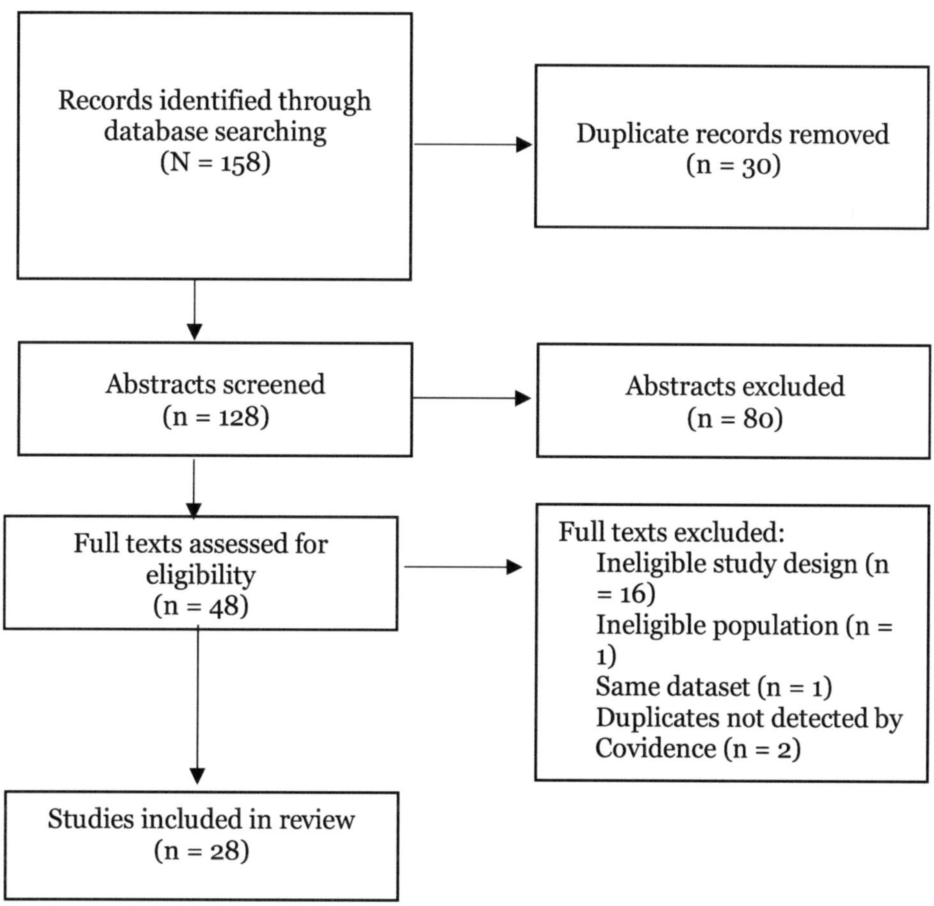


**Figure 1.**
*PRISMA flowchart of literature search and screening.*

*in vivo* cue (n = 9), with substance-related *in vivo* cues used independently only in two studies (n = 2). One study used a semi-structured interview as a cue (n = 1) where participants described their most traumatic experience verbally. Standardized video cues were employed in n = 2 studies. Photographic cues were used in the n = 1 study which took place in an fMRI environment. Three (n = 3) studies utilized photographic cues as part of what we are calling "task-based" cue-reactivity paradigms, that is, cognitive tasks that included substance or trauma-related stimuli. Specifically, Garland and colleagues [28] used an Emotional Regulation Task as a cue exposure paradigm where participants sorted and viewed negative images. Kaag et al. [29] also utilized a sorting task as a cue exposure where participants sorted cocaine and neutral photos. Finally, Beckham and colleagues [30] used the Stroop color-naming task [31] with combat-related words as a cue exposure. Overall, 22 studies employed only personalized cues, five studies employed only standardized cues, and one study [32] employed both personalized cues and standardized cues.

### *3.3.2 Craving and other reactivity measures*

All studies used subjective self-report measures of craving as a measure of reactivity (n = 28); this was an inclusion criterion for this scoping review. However, many did include objective craving measures in addition to subjective measures (i.e., salivation, heart rate; n = 9). Other reactivity measures assessed included affect (n = 14), subjective stress (n = 6), objective stress (i.e., cortisol; n = 3), attentional/memory tasks (n = 3), and neural activation (n = 3).

### *3.3.3 Substances*

Types of substances used/misused by participants in the study were alcohol (n = 17), cocaine (n = 6), nicotine (n = 3), heroin (n = 1), opioids (n = 1), and any substance (n = 4). It is important to note that some studies (n = 4) allowed for combinations of specific drugs (i.e., individuals who use alcohol and/or cocaine were recruited for one study).

### *3.3.4 Cue type*

Studies identified in the present scoping review employed the use of several types of cues. Specifically, neutral cues (n = 24; e.g., brushing your teeth), trauma cues (n = 23; e.g., a physical assault), substance cues (n = 14; i.e., cannabis paraphernalia), stress cues (n = 5; a presentation at work), and social cues (n = 1; speaking with a friend; [33]) were used. The average number of cue types used per study was 2.36 (SD = .731).

### *3.3.5 Comparator*

The majority of studies utilized pre-cue baseline as a comparator for their measures of reactivity (n = 22); a minority only compared reactivity data across cue types (i.e., comparing neutral vs. trauma responses; n = 6). However, many studies used a combination of comparators by comparing to baseline data and across cue types as well (n = 12).

While we have summarized the key components of included studies here, a full summary of each study across the coded variables of interest is available in Appendix A.

### 3.4 Population considerations

Populations of interest were largely adults who were assessed for PTSD symptoms/diagnoses and/or trauma history, and substance use. Participants across studies were more often male (*M* = 61.5%, SD = 24.6), with n = 5 studies recruiting only males [29, 30, 34–36] and one study recruiting only females [28]. Four studies included only veterans [30, 36–38], and 12 included only patients in treatment for SUD ([39]; n = 10), PTSD (n = 1), or both (n = 1). Four studies examined emerging adult college students specifically [13, 40–42] and one study recruited low-income, inner-city adults [43].

All studies included participants with either PTSD (n = 14) or those who had been exposed to a lifetime trauma (n = 10), or both with PTSD and/or trauma histories assessed continuously (n = 4). PTSD was assessed but not required for some studies, with others requiring trauma exposure but not a PTSD diagnosis (see [44, 45]). To assess for PTSD, most studies used some form of a validated structured interview (n = 25), such as the MINI [46], the SCID-5-RV [47], and the Clinician-Administered PTSD Scale [48]. Those studies examining trauma-exposed individuals typically administered a questionnaire to assess trauma history (n = 3), such as the Trauma History Questionnaire [49] or the Life Events Checklist [50], as well as continuous measures of PTSD symptoms, such as the PTSD Checklist for DSM-5 [51].

Substance use among the study populations was similarly measured. Specifically, the majority of studies (n = 18) required an SUD as inclusion criteria [18, 52], with some using inpatients receiving treatment for PTSD, SUD, or both (n = 12; [32, 53]). Fewer studies required less extreme forms of substance use, such as occasional drinking (n = 6) (see [13, 54]) and other cut-off points for use of various substances (n = 3; [55]). To assess for the presence of a SUD, most studies (n = 18) used structured interviews, such as the C-DIS IV [56] or the SCID-5-RV [47], but others used shorter self-report measures, such as the Alcohol Use Disorders Identification Test (AUDIT; n = 10) [57].

### 3.5 The cue-reactivity paradigm.

#### *3.5.1 Personalized vs. standardized cues*

Many of the studies employed personalized cues within their cue-reactivity paradigms, either through interviews where they obtained information about a participant's worst traumatic experience and transcribed the interview into an imagery-based cue [58] or utilized the participants' preferred substance as part of an *in vivo* cue [59]. The vast majority of these studies found significant reactivity results in their research, specifically noting that trauma, substance, and/or stress-related cues elicited greater craving responses (i.e., greater change from baseline) compared to neutral cues (n = 24 of 28). Even interviews in which the participant described their worst traumatic experience functioned well as a personalized cue for eliciting reactivity on craving measures [36]. Photo, video, or task-based cues were standardized rather than personalized [28, 54] although one study did take into account participants' preferred substances when selecting substance-related video cues [60]. Studies utilizing standardized cues did find cue-reactivity effects on their outcomes, with some caveats. For example, Trautmann and colleagues [54] found craving increased in response to their trauma film cues only among females. Other studies using standardized, non-personalized cues that used control groups found cue-reactivity effects (craving and neural activation, respectively) only in substance-using [29] and trauma-exposed [60] experimental groups vs. non-using/non-exposed controls.

### *3.5.2 Task-based cues*

Studies that utilized photographic cues as part of task-based cue paradigms found to support that their paradigms functioned as effective cue-reactivity paradigms, even though craving was not the primary outcome of interest. For example, Garland and colleagues [28] showed participants trauma-related images and asked them to either simply view the photos or reappraise the photos by reinterpreting the photo's meaning to regulate their emotions in reaction to the photo. Following this task, relief craving increased; this increase was associated with the number of adverse childhood experiences to which participants reported having been exposed. Similarly, Beckham et al. [30] utilized a Stroop color-naming attentional [31] task with trauma-related words with a veteran sample of cigarette smokers. Results demonstrated trauma words, relative to neutral words, led to greater cigarette craving as well as more withdrawal symptoms.

## 3.6 Subjective and physiological craving

One of our inclusion criteria was the measurement of craving following a cue-reactivity paradigm. Accordingly, all studies included a measure of craving, with all studies including a measure of subjective craving. Many studies measured craving using a Visual Analog Scale (VAS) or various Likert-type rating scales. Among those who examined craving changes from baseline by cue type, subjective craving responses were highest following trauma-related cues compared to substance, stress, and/or neutral cues (n = 9). Studies that did not use trauma cues found substance-related cues elicited greater craving compared to neutral cues (n = 3). In those studies that used trauma cues, substance cues, and neutral cues (n = 9), typically trauma cues elicited the greatest craving, followed by substance cues, and then neutral cues. Interestingly, studies, where trauma imagery cues were paired with *in vivo* substance cues (n = 5), found craving was higher for these combined cues compared to trauma imagery cues alone, as well as compared to neutral imagery and *in vivo* substance cue combinations [18, 58].

While our inclusion criteria did not specifically require an objective assessment of craving, the frequent use of salivation, heart rate, and other measures of physiological reactivity warrants a brief summary of this work. Most studies that included physiological/objective craving measures did so by measuring salivary flow (n = 5). Coffey et al. [18] found a significant increase in salivation following trauma and alcohol cues relative to neutral cues. Nosen et al. [59] found an increase in salivation following alcohol *in vivo* cues as well, and this increase was greatest when paired with trauma imagery cues. Two intervention studies examined craving pre- and post-treatment and found a significant decrease in salivation during trauma cue exposure at post-treatment compared to pre-treatment [53, 61]. Interestingly, one study did not find any significant effect of trauma cue imagery and *in vivo* alcohol cue exposure on salivary flow among depressed individuals, but did among those with PTSD [41]. Finally, one study which used heart rate as an objective measure of craving found *in vivo* alcohol cues significantly increased heart rate relative to neutral water cues among males with comorbid PTSD-AUD [35].

### 3.7 Treatment outcome studies

Seven studies examined outcomes of pharmacological or psychotherapeutic treatment in clinical populations, utilizing cue reactivity as a secondary outcome measure or adjunct to symptom measures. Two studies examined the effectiveness of pharmaceuticals as a treatment for comorbid PTSD-SUD. Specifically, in a pre-clinical lab-based study, Stauffer et al. [35] examined the use of intranasal oxytocin (20 IU and 40 IU) vs. placebo in males with comorbid PTSD-AUD. Each participant took part in each condition across three counterbalanced sessions. Following drug or placebo administration, participants were exposed to *in vivo* cues of their preferred alcoholic beverage and water. Both heart rate and subjective craving response increased the following alcohol *in vivo* cue exposure relative to neutral *in vivo* (water) cues, but neither dose of oxytocin reduced cue-induced heart rate nor subjective craving responses relative to placebo. Similarly, Kwako et al. [32] combined the Trier Social Stress Test [62] with personalized *in vivo* alcohol cues and conducted separate sessions involving guided imagery scripts of stress, alcohol, and neutral cues. All experimental cues increased subjective craving responses and blood cortisol when compared to the neutral cues. However, they found no effect of the neurokinin-1 receptor antagonist aprepitant (125 mg/day) vs. placebo on subjective craving in response to stress or alcohol vs. neutral cues; however, participants who received the aprepitant had reduced cortisol levels during the presentation of the stress cue.

Five studies examined the effects of several psychotherapeutic interventions on cue-elicited craving as well as distress, PTSD symptoms, and resilience. Coffey and colleagues [18] examined the effects of trauma-based imaginal exposure vs. relaxation using a cue-reactivity paradigm to assess trauma cue-reactivity (i.e., craving), showing a decrease in craving to the trauma-alcohol cue combination only among those enrolled in prolonged exposure (PE) therapy but not among those in the relaxation condition. However, craving following the trauma-only cue decreased relative to baseline among both intervention groups. Similarly, two studies [53, 61] assessed the merits of PE therapy in comparison to a health/lifestyle therapy using a craving to a cue-reactivity paradigm as an outcome measure; one study [53] found both healthy lifestyle (control) and trauma cue-exposure treatments led to a decrease in craving responses to trauma imagery and *in vivo* substance cues compared to pre-treatment baseline responses. While the other study [61] only included those enrolled in the trauma cue-exposure group in analyses, they too found a decrease in cue-induced craving when exposed to trauma and substance cues from pre- to post-treatment. Additionally, a study [36] that examined trauma cue exposure during cognitive processing therapy, a form of cognitive behavior therapy, in veterans with comorbid PTSD-SUD, also found a decrease in trauma cue-induced craving from pre- to post-treatment, the magnitude of which was associated with a degree of increase in resilience and degree of decrease in PTSD symptoms. Finally, one study [37] used *in vivo* cues as part of the COPE (Concurrent Treatment of PTSD and Substance Use Disorders Using Prolonged Exposure) therapeutic intervention. Specifically, Badour et al. combined PE therapy to trauma cues with CBT for substance disorders and *in vivo* substance cue presentations. They examined cue-induced craving at each *in vivo* substance cue exposure session. Craving significantly decreased across sessions, and this decrease was associated with a concurrent decrease in PTSD symptom severity and distress.

### 3.8 Neural activation

Three studies combined fMRI and a cue-reactivity paradigm. One study [34] examined neural activation during the presentation of stress, neutral, and substance-related cues among cocaine-dependent individuals with and without childhood maltreatment histories. The degree of craving to the stress cues predicted activation of the rostral anterior cingulate cortex to a lesser extent in the participants with maltreatment histories. The authors interpreted this to suggest that childhood maltreatment interferes with a key mechanism for resolving conflict and responding adaptively to stress [34]. Conversely, the degree of craving to the substance-related cues was associated with activation of the supplemental motor area and the visual cortex to a greater extent in those with maltreatment histories. The authors interpreted this latter finding to suggest that childhood maltreatment enhances the anticipatory reward response to substance cue exposure [34]. Further, during substance cue presentation, another study [35] found childhood trauma histories among substance users were significantly associated with increased activation of the frontal striatal circuit and the amygdala. However, a third study [32] did not find any psychological correlates of neural activation during the presentation of substance-related vs. neutral stimuli in a sample of adults with comorbid PTSD-AUD. It is difficult to know if this failure to observe an effect of cue exposure on neural activation was due to an ineffective manipulation since craving responses were not measured.

### 3.9 Affect

Fourteen studies included a measure of effect as part of their evaluation of cue-reactivity. Eleven of such studies examined both positive and negative affect, and three examined negative affects only. The Positive and Negative Affect Schedule or PANAS [63] was overwhelmingly used as the standardized measure of this variable (n = 10), although other measures were used as well, such as the Affect Grid [64] (n = 2). Among the majority of studies (n = 9), negative affect increased following stress and trauma-related cues [38]. In those studies which also examined positive affect, positive affect tended to decrease following stress and trauma-related cues [42, 33] but this was not always consistent. For example, Coffey et al. [39] did not find any statistically significant differences in positive affect across cue types. Interestingly, one study reported that substance-related cue exposure increased both positive and negative affect, and this ambivalent response was associated with the strongest substance cravings [55].

## 4. Discussion

The primary aim of this scoping review was to map the use of cue-reactivity paradigms in PTSD-SUD research among substance users with trauma histories and/or PTSD. Specifically, we sought to summarize the characteristics of the samples, examine outcomes measured followed the cue-reactivity paradigm (e.g., subjective/objective craving, negative affect), and map how such paradigms vary across the literature on several dimensions (e.g., cue type, personalization/standardization, cue presentation). Furthermore, we aimed to assess the consequences of methodological differences in cue-reactivity research. While prior literature has summarized cue-reactivity methodology in substance use research [65] and one group has briefly summarized cue-reactivity research in a comorbid PTSD-AUD population as part of a broader review of mechanisms involved in this form of comorbidity [66], we aimed to map the use of cue-reactivity paradigms in a way which could lead to further understanding of conditioned craving as a mechanism in the maintenance of comorbid PTSD-SUD. Specifically, our systematic scoping of the literature identified 28 studies that assessed craving following a cue-reactivity paradigm in a population of substance users with trauma histories and/or PTSD.

Our scoping review revealed wide variations in methodologies used to examine cue-induced craving. Specifically, characteristics of study samples, the methodological details of the cue-reactivity paradigm, and the types of outcomes assessed, all varied broadly. We have identified four themes in the studies through our scoping of the literature that may help elucidate commonalities and important distinctions across the identified studies—(1) increases in craving following trauma cue presentation; (2) the use of methodological subtypes of cue-reactivity paradigms; (3) affect as an outcome and possible mediator of craving in cue-reactivity research; and (4) the cue-reactivity paradigm as an adjunct outcome measure in intervention research.

From the above literature review, it is evident that craving has been repeatedly shown to increase following exposure to certain cues in substance users with trauma histories and/or PTSD. In particular, trauma cues tend to elicit the greatest increase from baseline in craving responses when compared to substance-related and neutral cues. This was true across studies using both personalized [43] and standardized cues [54]. However, this effect was typically magnified when a combination of trauma-related imagery and *in vivo* substances cues were paired together [45, 53]. The latter finding supports the notion that "cue chains" may be an effective means of bolstering cue-reactivity responses [67]. Indeed, while direct comparison across all studies is made difficult due to variable methodologies across studies, it appears that trauma cues, and in particular, trauma and substance cue combinations elicit strong craving responses among individuals with trauma histories who use substances. This effect was evident across different substances used by the populations of interest (e.g., alcohol, cocaine, nicotine). Several studies found that such effects were the strongest among those with higher PTSD symptom severity [45, 52] or those with the greatest cumulative trauma exposure [28]. Moreover, studies with control groups, such as healthy non-drug using controls [29] and those without trauma histories [34] were unable to find any significant change in craving with cue exposure among control groups, suggesting a lack of a conditioned cue-induced craving response among controls and specificity of these cue-reactivity effects to "experimental" groups (e.g., cocaine users with childhood trauma histories [34]). These findings are consistent with predictions that would be made on the basis of the conditioning theories presented at the outset of this chapter. Specifically, it is only those with trauma histories/PTSD who would have opportunities to learn to use substances to reduce the negative affect conditioned to trauma cues (two-factor learning theory; [10]) and to develop conditioned craving responses to trauma cues (via classical conditioning; [12]). Theoretically, such cue-induced craving effects could lead to substance seeking and consumption in response to exposure to real-world trauma reminders—both via intrusive traumatic memories and exposure to external reminders of the trauma—thereby contributing to SUD development, maintenance, or exacerbation in those with trauma histories and/or PTSD.

Second, the cue-reactivity methodologies used in the studies identified through our scoping review tended to vary widely. While the majority of studies utilized imagery-based audio cues to elicit cue-reactivity craving responses, some used combinations of imagery-based trauma and substance-related *in vivo* cues to understand how to cue combinations may further bolster craving responses [39, 40]. These combined cues serve as an in-lab analog of real-world exposure to a trauma reminder simultaneous with exposure to substance-related cues, such as when an individual with PTSD experiences an intrusive memory about their trauma within proximity of substance-related cues like a bottle of alcohol. Less commonly, standardized cues (e.g., standardized trauma-related videos) were used to elicit cue reactivity craving responses [54]. While such standardized cues often did elicit an increase in craving responses relative to the pre-exposure baseline, there were typically caveats to such effects which may indicate a less robust elicitation of craving given the use of non-personalized cues. For example, one study [54] found an increase in craving following a standardized trauma film only in females, which could perhaps be attributed to the fact that the film subject was also female. Generally, a more consistent craving response was found in studies that utilized personalized cues. Additionally, several studies used cue-reactivity paradigms involving tasks that were being used for other purposes (e.g., Stroop color-naming task [31] to assess attentional bias) but that contained relevant trauma or substance cues, allowing for a secondary test of cue-induced craving [28–30]. Indeed, combining a craving assessment with a cognitive task containing relevant cue exposures may be useful in simultaneously assessing outcomes directly related to the cognitive task and assessing cue-induced craving. For example, this was accomplished by Garland and colleagues [28] who aimed to assess participants' ability to regulate emotions related to trauma-related images on their emotional regulation task which simultaneously served as a cue reactivity craving assessment.

Third, while we did not systematically aim to include effect as an outcome in the present scoping review, we decided to cover this outcome as many of the studies included in the review (50%) did include a measure of effect as an additional outcome alongside craving. Our findings elucidated the importance of effect in helping explain the relationship between trauma cue-reactivity and craving. To elaborate, negative affect has quite consistently been shown to increase following trauma cue exposure [44, 59]. This is consistent with suggestions that conditioned *relief* craving may be an important motivator of continued substance use in those with trauma histories who use substances. Relief craving involves the urge to use substances to reduce negative affective states—the very mood states that are triggered when those with trauma histories are faced with trauma reminders. This is consistent with Stasiewicz and Maisto's application of the two-factor avoidance theory to substance use [10]. They suggested that trauma reminders can be classically conditioned to elicit fear themselves, which motivates avoidance responses such as substance abuse to escape the aversive emotional state. Through this two-factor learning process, an individual may become motivated to reduce the negative affect triggered through trauma cue exposure and to crave the relief that can be achieved through substance use. This theory is partially supported by the results of the present scoping review. Specifically, one study [61] found trauma cue-induced craving decreased following prolonged exposure treatment, and this decrease was associated with a concurrent decrease in negative emotional responses to trauma stimuli. While causality cannot be determined from these data, perhaps a decrease in trauma cue-induced negative affective responses may be responsible for the decreases in trauma cue-induced substance cravings following prolonged exposure treatment. The present scoping review found no studies which tested the links of cue-induced craving with cue-induced emotional responses; further, only one study [28] alluded to the distinction between reward and relief craving. We suggest that the roles of both cue-induced negative and positive affect in eliciting reward and relief craving should be explored further in future research.

Finally, it is important to note that seven studies utilized cue-reactivity paradigms as an additional outcome in trauma and/or substance-related therapeutic interventions. Notably, neither of the two pharmacological studies found an effect of the respective medications (oxytocin and neurokinin-1 receptor antagonist aprepitant) relative to placebo as a means of reducing either PTSD symptoms or stress cue- or substance cue-induced craving (see [32, 35]). Conversely, all studies examining the efficacy of PE therapy for PTSD or PTSD-SUD found that trauma cue-induced craving, as well as other forms of cue-reactivity (e.g., salivation, distress), decreased over time in those who received PE when compared to patients who received a control intervention [36, 37, 39, 53, 61]. Indeed, behavioral interventions seem to be more efficacious than pharmacological interventions in reducing reactivity to both trauma and substance-related cues among trauma-exposed substance users, at least for the few pharmacotherapies that have been investigated with this paradigm thus far, and at least in comparison to PE therapy. Furthermore, the use of cue-reactivity paradigms as a secondary outcome in randomized controlled trials of therapeutic interventions speaks to the multifaceted functionality of the cue-reactivity paradigm in the PTSD/trauma-exposed population, offering a mechanism-based outcome that informs beyond the decrease of symptoms.

## 5. Limitations and future directions

First, it is important to note that no formal examination of the study quality of the included literature was completed, as this step is not typical for scoping reviews [27]. It should also be noted that our choice to include unpublished theses and dissertations in the present review may have led to the inclusion of some studies with poor methodological quality, although it does help ensure that our conclusions are not hampered by publication bias.

To further assess the studies included in the present scoping review, we recommend a formal analysis of methodological quality be completed in the future to better understand how methodological variations in cue-reactivity may influence relevant outcomes. Additionally, the use of cue-reactivity paradigms as secondary outcomes in the context of behavioral and pharmacological intervention trials is an interesting research direction that should be studied further, as this may lead to important implications for understanding the breadth of response to the use of psychotherapeutic or pharmacological interventions in this population, and may point to potential mechanisms of action. We also recommend that a formal systematic review and meta-analysis be conducted to quantify the magnitude of trauma cue-induced craving responses in this population, and to identify significant moderators of this response in terms of sample characteristics (e.g., percentage of the sample with PTSD), and methodological variables (e.g., personalized vs. standardized cues). Providing that relevant data could be obtained from published papers or authors, novel techniques, such as two-step meta-analytic structural equation modeling (TS-MASEM; [68]) could also be employed to examine theorized mediational pathways (e.g., that trauma cue exposure leads to activation of negative affect which in turn activates craving). Finally, meta-analyses could also quantify the degree of reduction in trauma cue-induced craving that is achieved with various forms of treatment for PTSD, SUD, and their comorbidity, and its relations to treatment efficacy (i.e., symptom reduction).

## 6. Conclusion

Our scoping review maps the use of cue-reactivity paradigms across the trauma-exposed, substance-using population with and without PTSD, and summarizes methodological variations in cue-reactivity paradigms across this body of literature, as well as the results of identified studies. Cue-reactivity paradigms have proven efficacious in eliciting cue-induced craving responses in populations of trauma-exposed individuals who use substances. Cue-reactivity research may help increase understanding of the learning processes that are involved in the development, maintenance, or exacerbation of a SUD among trauma-exposed individuals with and without PTSD who use substances. Furthermore, cue-reactivity paradigms may be used as an important means of assessing whether behavioral and/or pharmacological treatments for PTSD and/or SUD have had an impact on the ability of trauma cues to elicit a conditioned craving response in this population.

## Appendix A

| First author (year) | Sample characteristics and context | Cue reactivity paradigm and method | Outcome(s) of interest | Craving measure | Relevant findings |
|---|---|---|---|---|---|
| Elton et al. [34] | 38 cocaine-dependent males with (n = 20) and without (n = 18) childhood maltreatment histories. | Script-driven imagery. All participants listened to a personalized neutral, stress, and cocaine-related audio cue whilst in an fMRI scanner. | Brain region activation, anxiety, and subjective craving response. | Cue-induced cocaine craving was measured using the visual analog scale (VAS) from 0 to 10. | Stress-Neutral: The interaction between maltreatment severity and craving responses was associated with activation of the left premotor cortex and right cerebellum. Substance-Neutral: The interaction between maltreatment severity and craving responses was associated with activation of the bilateral occipital cortex, caudal pre-supplementary motor area [SMA], and cuneus. Findings suggest that childhood maltreatment |

| First author (year) | Sample characteristics and context | Cue reactivity paradigm and method | Outcome(s) of interest | Craving measure | Relevant findings |
|---|---|---|---|---|---|
| | | | | | alters neural correlates of cue-induced substance craving. |
| Dutton [33] | 46 hazardous drinkers who met DSM-5 criterion A (trauma exposure) of a PTSD diagnosis | Script-driven imagery. Participants listened to a personalized neutral cue followed by either a neutral-social (n = 24) or a social conflict cue (n = 22). Each cue was 1 minute long followed by a 30 second visualization period. | State PTSD symptoms, subjective craving response, affect, and alcohol approach bias. | Cue-induced alcohol craving was measured using a VAS from 0 to 100. | Following the social conflict cue but not the neutral social cue, state PTSD symptoms increased. There were no differences in alcohol approach bias, affect, or craving between cues. |
| Trautmann et al. [54] | 95 healthy occasional drinkers who had experienced childhood trauma. | Standardized video. Participants watched either a 15-minute trauma film (n = 47) or a 15-minute neutral film (n = 48). | Subjective craving response, anxiety, and physiological reactivity (i.e., skin conductance, heart rate, and saliva cortisol levels) | Cue-induced alcohol craving was measured using the Alcohol Craving Questionnaire-Short Form [69]. | In females, the trauma film elicited greater craving responses compared to the neutral film. In males, the number of childhood traumas positively moderated the relationship between film condition and craving responses. In males, childhood trauma was associated with increases in skin conductance, heart rate, and cortisol levels; only skin conductance was related to craving responses. |

| First author (year) | Sample characteristics and context | Cue reactivity paradigm and method | Outcome(s) of interest | Craving measure | Relevant findings |
|---|---|---|---|---|---|
| Stauffer et al. [35]* | 47 males with comorbid PTSD-AUD and 37 healthy control males. | *In vivo* substance cues. Following either oxytocin or placebo administration, participants were presented with their preferred alcoholic beverage and a neutral water cue. | Effects of oxytocin as a treatment for comorbid PTSD-AUD, subjective craving responses, and heart rate variability. | Cue-induced alcohol craving was measured using a VAS from 0 to 100. | Craving responses and heart rate were higher following the alcohol cues compared to neutral cues. No effects of oxytocin compared to placebo on cue-induced craving or heart rate. |
| Ralevski et al. [38]* | 25 veterans with comorbid PTSD-AUD. | Script-driven imagery. All participants listened to personalized trauma, stress, and neutral audio cues. | Subjective craving responses, blood pressure, heart rate, negative affect, and salivary cortisol. | Cue-induced alcohol craving was measured using the Alcohol Craving Questionnaire-Short Form [69] and a VAS. | Craving responses, cardiovascular reactivity, and negative affect were highest following the trauma cue but were also high following the stress cue, both compared to the neutral cue. |
| Winokur [60] | 95 individuals with (n = 31) and without (n = 39) trauma histories who were heroin (n = 25) or nicotine (n = 70) dependent. | Standardized video. Participants watched standardized video cues related to either heroin or nicotine use, and a neutral video cue. | Subjective craving responses. | Cue-induced heroin or nicotine craving was measured using a Within Sessions Rating Scale (0–9). | Post substance cue-craving responses increased among both the opiate and nicotine-dependent groups, but were highest in the opiate-dependent group, and only among those with trauma histories. |
| Coffey et al. [39]* | 43 SUD inpatients with comorbid PTSD-AUD. 75% of participants who completed at least one clinical session were randomly assigned to receive six | Script-driven imagery and *in vivo* substance cues. Participants completed the following experimental cue reactivity trials: Trial 1: All participants listened to personalized | Subjective craving responses, affect, and emotional distress. | Cue-induced alcohol craving was measured using a VAS from 0 to 10. | Craving responses decreased from pre- to post-treatment among those in the imaginal exposure condition following the trauma-alcohol cue (trial 2) and |

| First author (year) | Sample characteristics and context | Cue reactivity paradigm and method | Outcome(s) of interest | Craving measure | Relevant findings |
|---|---|---|---|---|---|
| | sessions of either imaginal exposure therapy (n = 12) or relaxation (control) condition (n = 12). However, only 17 participants completed the study. | neutral and trauma cues. Trial 2: All participants listened to a personalized trauma cue followed by the presentation of either alcohol or water. | | | did not change in the relaxation condition. Craving responses also decreased in both groups following the trauma cue (trial 1). Negative affect was highest in trial 2. |
| Read et al. [13] | 232 undergraduate students with PTSD (n = 28), with trauma exposure but no PTSD (n = 113), or no trauma history (n = 91) taking part in a clinical trial. | Script-driven imagery. Participants listened to either a personalized trauma (n = 111) or neutral cue (n = 121). Participants wrote about the event while continuing to imagine the scene. | Subjective craving, affect, and performance on a Stroop attentional task with trauma and alcohol-specific stimuli. | Cue-induced alcohol craving was measured using a 10-point Likert scale rating urge to drink. | Participants with PTSD in the trauma cue condition showed a slowed response in the Stroop task. This effect was associated with an urge to drink only among those with PTSD in the trauma cue condition. |
| Kaag et al. [29] | 117 adults, half cocaine users (n = 59) and half healthy controls (n = 58) | Event-related cue-reactivity paradigm. All participants viewed substance-related photos, neutral photos, and photos of animals. They were instructed to press a button when photos of animals were presented. | Subjective craving and neural activation. | Cue-induced cocaine craving was measured using the Desire for Drug Questionnaire [21] at baseline and following the cue-reactivity paradigm. | Only among substance users, the presentation of cocaine cues led to neural activation in the frontal striatal circuit and the amygdala. Amygdala-striatal connectivity was associated with childhood trauma among substance users. |
| Coffey et al. [58] | 75 individuals receiving SUD treatment with PTSD who were cocaine (n = 30) or alcohol-dependent (n = 45) | Script-driven imagery and *in vivo* substance cues. All participants took part in four cue trials, which were counterbalanced. Participants listened to a | Subjective craving. | Cue-induced craving was measured using the Cocaine Craving Questionnaire-Now (CCQ-Now) [70] and Alcohol Craving Questionnaire- | Both alcohol-dependent and cocaine-dependent participants evidenced greater cravings following the trauma- and substance- |

| First author (year) | Sample characteristics and context | Cue reactivity paradigm and method | Outcome(s) of interest | Craving measure | Relevant findings |
|---|---|---|---|---|---|
| | | personalized cue (trauma or neutral). Immediately after, either a substance or neutral (i.e., alcohol or wood chips) *in vivo* cue was placed in front of them. | | Now (ACQ-Now) [71] | related cues compared to the neutral cues. |
| McHugh et al. [44] | 194 individuals with PTSD receiving treatment for a comorbid SUD. | Script-driven imagery. All participants listened to a personalized trauma and neutral cue, counterbalanced across two sessions, followed by a 1-minute visualization period. | Subjective craving and affect. | Cue-induced substance craving was measured on an 11-point scale. Ratings ranged from 0 (no cravings) to 11 (very strong cravings). | Craving and negative emotional reactivity were greater following the trauma cue compared to the neutral cue. Anxiety sensitivity was associated with greater emotional reactivity following the trauma cue, but there was no association between anxiety sensitivity and craving response. |
| McGuire et al. [36] | 29 veterans receiving treatment for comorbid PTSD-SUD. | Interview. All participants provided a detailed verbal description of their most traumatic lifetime event. | Subjective craving, resilience, and PTSD symptoms. | Cue-induced craving for alcohol and/or other substances was measured using the Alcohol Craving Questionnaire Short Form-Revised [71] | Posttreatment, participants evidenced a decrease in cue-induced craving and fewer PTSD symptoms, as well as increased resiliency, relative to pre-treatment baseline. |
| Saladin et al. [45] | 124 individuals with trauma histories receiving SUD treatment who were alcohol- (n = 70) or cocaine- | Script-driven imagery and *in vivo* substance cues. All participants took part in four cue trials, which were counterbalanced. | Subjective craving. | Cue-induced substance craving was measured using a 21-point VAS. | Craving was greater following the trauma- and substance-related cues in comparison to the neutral cues. |

| First author (year) | Sample characteristics and context | Cue reactivity paradigm and method | Outcome(s) of interest | Craving measure | Relevant findings |
|---|---|---|---|---|---|
| | dependent (n = 54). | Participants listened to a personalized cue (trauma or neutral). Immediately after, either a substance (e.g., Jack Daniels over ice) or neutral *in vivo* cue was placed in front of them. | | | PTSD symptom severity predicted greater craving responses, but only following the trauma + substance cue pairing. |
| Coffey et al. [18] | 40 individuals with comorbid PTSD-AUD receiving inpatient SUD treatment. | Script-driven imagery and *in vivo*. All participants listened to a personalized trauma or neutral imagery cue paired with an *in vivo* substance or neutral (water) cues. | Subjective and objective craving responses; emotional distress. | Cue-induced craving was measured using a VAS from 0 to 10 and salivary flow. | Subjective craving responses, distress, and salivary flow were greater following substance and trauma cues compared to the neutral cue. |
| Vujanovic et al. [43] | 58 low-income inner-city adults. | Script-driven imagery. All participants listened to personalized trauma, substance, and neutral audio cues. | Subjective craving responses. | Cue-induced craving was measured using a VAS from 0 to 100. | Lower distress tolerance was a significant predictor of higher craving responses following the trauma cue. |
| Rodriguez et al. [40] | 305 undergraduate students with no trauma (n = 127), trauma exposure (n = 106), and PTSD (n = 72). | Script-driven imagery. Participants were instructed to close their eyes and imagine their most traumatic event as if it was happening to them. Participants then wrote about the scene while continuing to imagine the scene. | Subjective craving responses and affect. | Cue-induced craving was measured using the Urge to Drink Questionnaire [22], on a scale from 1 to 10. | Emotional responses to the trauma cue mediated the relationship between trauma exposure and the urge to drink. |
| Bing-Canar et al. [41] | 184 young adults with trauma histories | Script-driven imagery and *in vivo* substance | Subjective and objective | Cue-induced craving was measured using | Depressive symptoms did not have any |

| First author (year) | Sample characteristics and context | Cue reactivity paradigm and method | Outcome(s) of interest | Craving measure | Relevant findings |
|---|---|---|---|---|---|
| | | cues. All participants listened to a personalized trauma or neutral imagery cue paired with an *in vivo* substance or neutral (water) cues | craving responses. | a three-item Alcohol Craving Scale [72] and salivation levels. | effect or interaction with the cue-reactivity paradigm to predict increased craving or salivation. |
| Zambrano-Vazquez et al. [61] | 85 individuals with comorbid PTSD-SUD and current alcohol dependence receiving SUD treatment. Only 66 participants who completed 8 or more prolonged exposure treatment sessions were included in the analyses. | Script-driven imagery and *in vivo* substance cues. Pre- and post-treatment, all participants listened to a personalized trauma or neutral imagery cue paired with an *in vivo* substance or neutral (water) cues. | Subjective and objective (salivation) craving, subjective distress, and domains of functioning. | Cue-induced craving was measured using the Alcohol Craving Questionnaire-Now [69] and salivation levels. | Severity in all domains of functional impairment (Negative Valence, Arousal, and Cognitive) decreased from pre to post-treatment, and this change was associated with a decrease from pre-treatment baseline in self-reported craving and salivation post-treatment following alcohol and trauma cue exposure. |
| Garland et al. [28]* | 36 opioid-treated chronic pain patients at risk for opioid use disorder, with adverse childhood experiences (ACEs). | Emotional Regulation Task. Participants were shown trauma-related images and were asked to both views or reappraise the images (dependent on the trial block) to regulate the emotions elicited by the image. | Subjective craving, heart rate variability, and negative affect. | Cue-induced opioid craving was measured using a 5-point scale, with 1 indicating no craving and 5 indicating very strong cravings. | Following the emotional regulation task, craving increased from the pre-task baseline. This change was related to the number of ACE exposures. ACEs and duration of opioid use also predicted a blunted heart rate variability when regulating negative emotions. |
| Zaso et al. [42] | 611 college students with | Script-driven imagery. | Subjective craving | Cue-induced craving was | Following the trauma cue, but |

| First author (year) | Sample characteristics and context | Cue reactivity paradigm and method | Outcome(s) of interest | Craving measure | Relevant findings |
|---|---|---|---|---|---|
| | PTSD (n = 50), with trauma exposure but no PTSD (n = 325), and no trauma (n = 236) who drink alcohol | Participants were randomized to listen to either a personalized trauma or neutral cue followed by a 2-minute writing period relating to the cues. | response and affect. | measured using a 10-point scale, with 1 indicating no urge to drink and 10 indicating a very strong urge to drink. | not the neutral cue, participants reported greater cravings and negative affect relative to baseline, which was associated with coping drinking motives. |
| Kwako et al. [32]* | 53 individuals with comorbid PTSD-AUD receiving inpatient SUD treatment. Participants received either aprepitant (n = 26) or a placebo (n = 27) prior to cue exposure. | Script-driven imagery, *in vivo* alcohol cues, standardized photos of alcohol, and neutral cues. Following the Trier Social Stress test, participants handled *in vivo* cues of their preferred substance. In another session, participants listened to either a personalized stress, alcohol, or neutral cue. In an fMRI session, participants viewed photos of substance-related and neutral stimuli. | Subjective craving, blood cortisol, and neural activation. | Cue-induced alcohol craving was measured using the Alcohol Urge Questionnaire [22] | Alcohol and stress cues induced more cravings compared to neutral cues. There was no significant neural activation following the substance-related relative to the neutral stimuli. |
| Nosen et al. [59] | 108 adults with comorbid PTSD-AUD who were receiving residential treatment for SUD. | Script-driven imagery and *in vivo* substance cues. All participants listened to a personalized trauma or neutral imagery cue paired with an *in vivo* substance or neutral (water) cues. (TN; TS; NS; NN). | Subjective and objective (salivation) craving and affect. | Cue-induced alcohol craving was measured using a three-item alcohol craving scale [72] and salivation levels. | Trauma and substance cue pairings elicited the greatest subjective craving responses, negative affect, and salivation vs. all other cue combinations. Ambivalent affective responses predicted the strongest craving. |

| First author (year) | Sample characteristics and context | Cue reactivity paradigm and method | Outcome(s) of interest | Craving measure | Relevant findings |
|---|---|---|---|---|---|
| Tull et al. [19] | 60 cocaine-dependent individuals with (n = 30) and without PTSD (n = 30) in treatment for a SUD | Script-driven imagery. Across two sessions, all participants listened to a personalized cue (trauma or neutral; 1 min) followed by a visualization period (1 min). | Subjective craving response and affect. | Cue-induced cocaine craving was measured using an 11-point scale, with 0 indicating no cravings and 10 indicating very strong cravings. | PTSD was associated with greater craving and negative affect following the trauma cue, but not the neutral cue. Among men, this relationship was mediated by self-conscious emotions. |
| Nosen et al. [53] | 120 individuals with comorbid PTSD-AUD in treatment for a SUD. Participants were assigned to receive exposure therapy (n = 52) or health and lifestyle treatment (n = 35); only those who completed treatment (n = 87) were included in analyses. | Script-driven imagery and *in vivo* substance cue exposure. All participants have presented with four counterbalanced cue combinations: They first listened to a personalized cue (trauma or neutral). Immediately after, either a substance or neutral *in vivo* cue was placed in front of them. | Subjective and objective (salivation) craving response, distress, and affect. | Cue-induced craving was measured using a three-item alcohol craving scale [72] and salivation levels. | Pre-treatment, the trauma + substance cue-elicited the strongest craving responses, negative affect, and distress. Post-treatment, trauma cues no longer elicited greater craving compared to substance cues alone. Both treatments led to a decrease in salivation and subjective craving following cue exposure. |
| Badour et al. [37]* | 54 veterans with comorbid PTSD-SUD taking part in a COPE RCT. | Participants were presented with personalized *in vivo* substance cues across nine sessions. | Subjective craving and distress. | Cue-induced craving for participants' preferred substance was measured using a VAS (0–100). | Between-session reduction of substance cue-induced craving and distress responses were associated with a decrease in PTSD symptom severity. |
| Tull et al. [52] | 133 individuals with trauma histories in treatment for a SUD. | Script-driven imagery. Participants listened to a personalized trauma cue (1 min) followed | Subjective craving, emotional regulation, negative affect, and salivary cortisol. | Cue-induced craving for participants' preferred substance was measured using an 11-point scale, with 0 | Following the trauma cue, craving increased relative to the pre-cue baseline. This change was |

| First author (year) | Sample characteristics and context | Cue reactivity paradigm and method | Outcome(s) of interest | Craving measure | Relevant findings |
|---|---|---|---|---|---|
| | | by a visualization period (1 min). | | indicating no cravings and 11 indicating very strong cravings. | associated with greater PTSD symptom severity. PTSD symptom severity was related to both adaptive and maladaptive emotional regulation strategies. |
| Beckham et al. [55] | 129 smokers with (n = 82) and without PTSD (n = 47) were randomly assigned to either a nicotine or a non-nicotine smoking condition. | Script-driven imagery. Participants listened to either a personalized trauma, neutral, or stress cue (30 sec) followed by a visualization period (30 sec) both before and after smoking a nicotine or denicotinized cigarette. | Subjective craving and affect. | Cue-induced craving to smoke was measured using the Questionnaire on Smoking Urges [73]. | Trauma-related cues produced greater cravings and negative affect compared to stress scripts and neutral scripts. This effect was most pronounced among those with PTSD. Smoking either the nicotine or non-nicotine cigarettes reduced craving, negative affect, and PTSD symptoms following the trauma and stress script relative to the neutral script. |
| Beckham et al. [30] | 25 veterans receiving PTSD treatment who smoke cigarettes. | Stroop task with combat/trauma-related words. Participants named the ink color of three blocks of trauma-related and three blocks of neutral words. | Subjective craving, affect somatic symptoms, and alertness. | Cue-induced craving to smoke was measured using a modified Smoking Withdrawal Questionnaire Short Form-Revised [71] | Craving, negative affect, somatic symptoms, and lack of alertness were all greater following the presentation of trauma-related words compared to neutral words. |

*randomized controlled trial.*

**Author details**

Sarah DeGrace[1], Pablo Romero-Sanchiz[2], Catherine Standage[1] and Sherry H. Stewart[1]*

1 Dalhousie University, Halifax, NS, Canada

2 University of Roehampton, London, UK

*Address all correspondence to: sstewart@dal.ca

## References

[1] American Psychiatric Association. Diagnostic and Statistical Manual of Mental Disorders. 5th ed. Arlington, VA: Author; 2013

[2] Smith NDL, Cottler LB. The epidemiology of post-traumatic stress disorder and alcohol use disorder. Alcohol Research: Current Reviews. 2018;**39**(2):113-120

[3] Bonn-Miller M, Harris A, Trafton J. Prevalence of cannabis use disorder diagnoses among veterans in 2002, 2008, and 2009. Psychological Services. 2012;**9**:404-416. DOI: 10.1037/a0027622

[4] Walsh K, Elliott JC, Aharonovich E, Strous R, Frisch A, Weizman A, et al. Trauma exposure, posttraumatic stress disorder, and risk for alcohol, nicotine, and marijuana dependence in Israel. Comprehensive Psychiatry. 2014;**55**(3):621-630. DOI: 10.1016/j.comppsych.2013.11.016

[5] Khoury L, Tang YL, Bradley B, Cubells JF, Ressler KJ. Substance use, childhood traumatic experience, and posttraumatic stress disorder in an urban civilian population. Depression and Anxiety. 2010;**27**(12):1077-1086. DOI: 10.1002/da.20751

[6] Berenz EC, Coffey SF. Treatment of co-occurring posttraumatic stress disorder and substance use disorders. Current Psychiatry Reports. 2012;**14**(5):469-477. DOI: 10.1007/s11920-012-0300-0

[7] McCauley JL, Killeen T, Gros DF, Brady KT, Back SE. Posttraumatic stress disorder and co-occurring substance use disorders: Advances in assessment and treatment. Clinical Psychology. 2012;**19**(3). DOI: 10.1111/cpsp.12006

[8] Jacobsen LK, Southwick SM, Kosten TR. Substance use disorders in patients with posttraumatic stress disorder: A review of the literature. American Journal of Psychiatry. 2001;**158**(8):1184-1190. DOI: 10.1176/appi.ajp.158.8.1184

[9] Mowrer OH. On the dual nature of learning: A re-interpretation of "conditioning" and "problem-solving". Harvard Educational Review. 1947;**17**:102-148

[10] Stasiewicz PR, Maisto SA. Two-factor avoidance theory: The role of negative affect in the maintenance of substance use and substance use disorder. Behavior Therapy. 1993;**24**(3):337-356. DOI: 10.1016/S0005-7894(05)80210-2

[11] Drobes DJ, Tiffany ST. Induction of smoking urge through imaginal and in vivo procedures: Physiological and self-report manifestations. Journal of Abnormal Psychology. 1997;**106**(1):15-25. DOI: 10.1037/0021-843X.106.1.15

[12] Blume AW. Negative reinforcement and substance abuse: Using a behavioral conceptualization to enhance treatment. The Behavior Analyst Today. 2001;**2**(2):86-91

[13] Read JP, Bachrach RL, Wardell JD, Coffey SF. Examining cognitive processes and drinking urge in PTSD. Behaviour Research and Therapy. 2017;**90**:159-168. DOI: 10.1016/j.brat.2016.12.014

[14] Reynolds EK, Monti PM. The cue-reactivity paradigm in addiction research. In: MacKillop J, de Wit H, editors. The Wiley-Blackwell Handbook of Addiction Psychopharmacology. Hoboken, NJ: Wiley Blackwell; 2013.

pp. 381-410. DOI: 10.1002/9781118384404.ch14

[15] Carter BL, Tiffany ST. Meta-analysis of cue-reactivity in addiction research. Addiction. 1999;**94**(3):327-340

[16] Drobes DJ. Cue-reactivity in alcohol and tobacco dependence. Alcoholism: Clinical and Experimental Research. 2002;**26**(12):1928-1929. DOI: 10.1097/00000374-200212000-00026

[17] Witteman J, Post H, Tarvainen M, de Bruijn A, Perna EDSF, Ramaekers JG, et al. Cue-reactivity and its relation to craving and relapse in alcohol dependence: A combined laboratory and field study. Psychopharmacology. 2015;**232**(20):3685-3696. DOI: 10.1007/s00213-015-4027-6

[18] Coffey SF, Schumacher JA, Stasiewicz PR, Henslee AM, Baillie LE, Landy N. Craving and physiological reactivity to trauma and alcohol cues in PTSD and alcohol dependence. Experimental and Clinical Psychopharmacology. 2010;**18**(4):340-349. DOI: 10.1037/a0019790

[19] Tull MT, Kiel EJ, McDermott MJ, Gratz KL. The effect of trauma cue exposure on cocaine cravings among cocaine dependent inpatients with and without posttraumatic stress disorder: Exploring the mediating role of negative affect and discrete negative emotional states. Journal of Experimental Psychopathology. 2013;**4**(5):485-501. DOI: 10.5127/jep.028812

[20] Romero-Sanchiz P, Mahu IT, Barrett SP, Salmon JP, Al-Hamdani M, Swansburg JE, et al. Craving and emotional responses to trauma and cannabis cues in trauma-exposed cannabis users: Influence of PTSD symptom severity. Addictive Behaviors. 2022;**125**:107126. DOI: 10.1016/j.addbeh.2021.107126

[21] Franken IHA, Hendriksa VM, van den Brink W. Initial validation of two opiate craving questionnaires the obsessive compulsive drug use scale and the desires for drug questionnaire. Addictive Behaviors. 2002;**27**(5):675-685. DOI: 10.1016/s0306-4603(01)00201-5

[22] Bohn MJ, Krahn DD, Staehler BA. Development and initial validation of a measure of drinking urges in abstinent alcoholics. Alcoholism: Clinical and Experimental Research. 1995;**19**(3):600-606. DOI: 10.1111/j.1530-0277.1995.tb01554.x

[23] Heishman SJ, Evans RJ, Singleton EG, Levin KH, Copersino ML, Gorelick DA. Reliability and validity of a short form of the Marijuana Craving Questionnaire. Drug and Alcohol Dependence. 2009;**102**(1–3):35-40. DOI: 10.1016/j.drugalcdep.2008.12.010

[24] Sayette MA, Shiffman S, Tiffany ST, Niaura RS, Martin CS, Shadel WG. The measurement of drug craving. Addiction. 2000;**95**(Suppl 2):S189-S210. DOI: 10.1080/09652140050111762

[25] Tricco A, Lillie E, Zarin W, O'Brien K, Colquhoun H, Levac D, et al. PRISMA extension for scoping reviews (PRISMA-ScR): Checklist and explanation. Annals of Internal Medicine. 2018;**169**:467-473. DOI: 10.7326/M18-0850

[26] McHugh ML. Interrater reliability: The kappa statistic. Biochemia Medica. 2012;**22**(3):276-282

[27] Peters MDJ, Godfrey CM, Khalil H, McInerney P, Parker D, Soares CB. Guidance for conducting systematic scoping reviews. International Journal of Evidence-Based Healthcare. 2015;**13**(3):141-146. DOI: 10.1097/XEB.0000000000000050

[28] Garland EL, Reese SE, Bedford CE, Baker AK. Adverse childhood experiences predict autonomic indices of emotion dysregulation and negative emotional cue-elicited craving among female opioid-treated chronic pain patients. Development and Psychopathology. 2019;**31**(3):1101-1110. DOI: 10.1017/S0954579419000622

[29] Kaag AM, Reneman L, Homberg J, van den Brink W, van Wingen GA. Enhanced amygdala-striatal functional connectivity during the processing of cocaine cues in male cocaine users with a history of childhood trauma. Frontiers in Psychiatry. 2018;**9**:article 70. DOI: 10.3389/fpsyt.2018.00070

[30] Beckham JC, Lytle BL, Vrana SR, Hertzberg MA, Feldman ME, Shipley RH. Smoking withdrawal symptoms in response to a trauma-related stressor among Vietnam combat veterans with posttraumatic stress disorder. Addictive Behaviors. 1996; **21**(1):93-101. DOI: 10.1016/0306-4603(95)00038-0

[31] Scarpina F, Tagini S. The stroop color and word test. Frontiers in Psychology. 2017;**8**:557. DOI: 10.3389/fpsyg.2017.00557

[32] Kwako LE, George DT, Schwandt ML, Spagnolo PA, Momenan R, Hommer DW, et al. The neurokinin-1 receptor antagonist aprepitant in co-morbid alcohol dependence and posttraumatic stress disorder: A human experimental study. Psychopharmacology. 2015;**232**(1): 295-304. DOI: 10.1007/s00213-014-3665-4

[33] Dutton C. An experimental test of the effects of social conflict on posttraumatic stress symptoms and alcohol craving. Graduate Theses and Dissertations. 2017. https://scholarworks.uark.edu/etd/2442

[34] Elton A, Smitherman S, Young J, Kilts CD. Effects of childhood maltreatment on the neural correlates of stress- and drug cue-induced cocaine craving. Addiction Biology. 2015;**20**(4): 820-831. DOI: 10.1111/adb.12162

[35] Stauffer CS, Meinzer NK, Morrison T, Wen J-H, Radanovich L, Leung D, et al. Effects of oxytocin administration on cue-induced craving in co-occurring alcohol use disorder and PTSD: A within-participant randomized clinical trial. Alcoholism: Clinical and Experimental Research. 2019;**43**(12): 2627-2636. DOI: 10.1111/acer.14217

[36] McGuire AP, Mota NP, Sippel LM, Connolly KM, Lyons JA. Increased resilience is associated with positive treatment outcomes for veterans with comorbid PTSD and substance use disorders. Journal of Dual Diagnosis. 2018;**14**(3):181-186. DOI: 10.1080/15504263.2018.1464237

[37] Badour CL, Flanagan JC, Gros DF, Killeen T, Pericot-Valverde I, Korte KJ, et al. Habituation of distress and craving during treatment as predictors of change in PTSD symptoms and substance use severity. Journal of Consulting and Clinical Psychology. 2017;**85**(3):274-281. DOI: 10.1037/ccp0000180

[38] Ralevski E, Southwick S, Jackson E, Jane JS, Russo M, Petrakis I. Trauma- and stress-induced response in veterans with alcohol dependence and comorbid post-traumatic stress disorder. Alcoholism: Clinical and Experimental Research. 2016;**40**(8):1752-1760. DOI: 10.1111/acer.13120

[39] Coffey SF, Stasiewicz PR, Hughes PM, Brimo ML. Trauma-focused imaginal exposure for individuals with comorbid posttraumatic stress disorder and alcohol dependence: Revealing mechanisms of alcohol craving in a cue-

reactivity paradigm. Psychology of Addictive Behaviors. 2006;**20**(4): 425-435. DOI: 10.1037/0893-164X.20.4.425

[40] Rodriguez L, Read JP. Momentary emotional responding and emotion regulation in PTSD-related drinking urge. Experimental and Clinical Psychopharmacology. 2020;**28**(1): 99-111. DOI: 10.1037/pha0000292

[41] Bing-Canar H, Demos A, Mermelstein RJ, Berenz EC. Evaluating the influences of major depression and posttraumatic stress disorder on trauma and alcohol cue-reactivity. Addictive Behaviors. 2021;**112**:106596. DOI: 10.1016/j.addbeh.2020.106596

[42] Zaso MJ, Read JP. Drinking motives as moderators of in-the-moment drinking risks in response to trauma-related distress. Alcoholism: Clinical and Experimental Research. 2020;**44**(12): 2561-2569. DOI: 10.1111/acer.14487

[43] Vujanovic AA, Wardle MC, Bakhshaie J, Smith LJ, Green CE, Lane SD, et al. Distress tolerance: Associations with trauma and substance cue-reactivity in low-income, inner-city adults with substance use disorders and posttraumatic stress. Psychology of Addictive Behaviors. 2018;**32**(3): 264-276. DOI: 10.1037/adb0000362

[44] McHugh RK, Gratz KL, Tull MT. The role of anxiety sensitivity in reactivity to trauma cues in treatment-seeking adults with substance use disorders. Comprehensive Psychiatry. 2017;**78**:107-114. DOI: 10.1016/j.comppsych.2017.07.011

[45] Saladin ME, Drobes DJ, Coffey SF, Dansky BS, Brady KT, Kilpatrick DG. PTSD symptom severity as a predictor of cue-elicited drug craving in victims of violent crime. Addictive Behaviors. 2003;**28**(9):1611-1629. DOI: 10.1016/j.addbeh.2003.08.037

[46] Sheehan DV, Lecrubier Y, Sheehan KH, Amorim P, Janavs J, Weiller E, et al. The Mini-International Neuropsychiatric Interview (M.I.N.I.): The development and validation of a structured diagnostic psychiatric interview for DSM-IV and ICD-10. Journal of Clinical Psychiatry. 1998;**59** (Suppl. 20):22-33

[47] First MB, Williams JBW, Karg RS, Spitzer RL. Structured Clinical Interview for DSM-5: Research Version (SCID-5 for DSM-5, Research Version; SCID-5-RV). Arlington, VA: American Psychiatric Association; 2015

[48] Blake DD, Weathers FW, Nagy LM, Kaloupek DG, Gusman FD, Charney DS, et al. The development of a Clinician-Administered PTSD Scale. Journal of Traumatic Stress. 1995;**8**(1):75-90. DOI: 10.1007/BF02105408

[49] Hooper LM, Stockton P, Krupnick JL, Green BL. Development, use, and psychometric properties of the Trauma History Questionnaire. Journal of Loss and Trauma. 2011;**16**(3):258-283. DOI: 10.1080/15325024.2011.572035

[50] Gray MJ, Litz BT, Hsu JL, Lombardo TW. Psychometric properties of the life events checklist. Assessment. 2004;**11**(4):330-341. DOI: 10.1177/1073191104269954

[51] Blevins CA, Weathers FW, Davis MT, Witte TK, Domino JL. The Posttraumatic Stress Disorder Checklist for *DSM-5* (PCL-5): Development and initial psychometric evaluation. Journal of Traumatic Stress. 2015;**28**:489-498. DOI: 10.1002/jts.22059

[52] Tull MT, Berghoff CR, Wheeless LE, Cohen RT, Gratz KL. PTSD symptom

severity and emotion regulation strategy use during trauma cue exposure among patients with substance use disorders: Associations with negative affect, craving, and cortisol reactivity. Behavior Therapy. 2018;**49**(1):57-70. DOI: 10.1016/j.beth.2017.05.005

[53] Nosen E, Littlefield AK, Schumacher JA, Stasiewicz PR, Coffey SF. Treatment of co-occurring PTSD-AUD: Effects of exposure-based and non-trauma focused psychotherapy on alcohol and trauma cue-reactivity. Behaviour Research and Therapy. 2014; **61**:35-42. DOI: 10.1016/j.brat.2014.07.003

[54] Trautmann S, Kräplin A, Dieterich R, Richter J, Muehlhan M. The role of childhood trauma and stress reactivity for increased alcohol craving after induced psychological trauma: An experimental analogue study. Psychopharmacology. 2018;**235**(10): 2883-2895. DOI: 10.1007/s00213-018-4979-4

[55] Beckham JC, Dennis MF, McClernon FJ, Mozley SL, Collie CF, Vrana SR. The effects of cigarette smoking on script-driven imagery in smokers with and without posttraumatic stress disorder. Addictive Behaviors. 2007;**32**(12):2900-2915. DOI: 10.1016/j.addbeh.2007.04.026

[56] Segal DL. Diagnostic interview schedule for DSM-IV (DIS-IV). In: The Corsini Encyclopedia of Psychology. Hoboken, NJ: John Wiley & Sons, Ltd; 2010. pp. 1-2. DOI: 10.1002/9780470479216.corpsy0273

[57] Saunders JB, Aasland OG, Babor TF, de la Fuente JR, Grant M. Development of the Alcohol Use Disorders Identification Test (AUDIT): WHO collaborative project on early detection of persons with harmful alcohol consumption: II. Addiction. 1993;**88**(6): 791-804. DOI: 10.1111/j.1360-0443.1993.tb02093.x

[58] Coffey SF, Saladin ME, Drobes DJ, Brady KT, Dansky BS, Kilpatrick DG. Trauma and substance cue-reactivity in individuals with comorbid posttraumatic stress disorder and cocaine or alcohol dependence. Drug and Alcohol Dependence. 2002;**65**(2): 115-127. DOI: 10.1016/s0376-8716(01)00157-0

[59] Nosen E, Nillni YI, Berenz EC, Schumacher JA, Stasiewicz PR, Coffey SF. Cue-elicited affect and craving: Advancement of the conceptualization of craving in co-occurring posttraumatic stress disorder and alcohol dependence. Behavior Modification. 2012;**36**(6):808-833. DOI: 10.1177/0145445512446741

[60] Winokur SB. The impact of gender and trauma on cue-induced drug craving [Psy.D., Widener University, Institute for Graduate Clinical Psychology]. 2011. http://search.proquest.com/docview/1370246150/abstract/8B644AE736944A95PQ/6

[61] Zambrano-Vazquez L, Levy HC, Belleau EL, Dworkin ER, Howard Sharp KM, Pittenger SL, et al. Using the research domain criteria framework to track domains of change in comorbid PTSD and SUD. Psychological Trauma: Theory, Research, Practice, and Policy. 2017;**9**(6):679-687. DOI: 10.1037/tra0000257

[62] Kirschbaum C, Pirke KM, Hellhammer DH. The'Trier Social Stress Test': A tool for investigating psychobiological stress responses in a laboratory setting. Neuropsychobiology. 1993;**28**(1–2):76-81. DOI: 10.1159/000119004

[63] Watson D, Clark LA, Tellegen A. Development and validation of brief measures of positive and negative affect: The PANAS scales. Journal of Personality and Social Psychology. 1988;**54**(6): 1063-1070

[64] Russell J, Weiss A, Mendelsohn G. Affect Grid: A single-item scale of pleasure and arousal. Journal of Personality and Social Psychology. 1989; **57**:493-502. DOI: 10.1037/0022-3514.57.3.493

[65] Betts JM, Dowd AN, Forney M, Hetelekides E, Tiffany ST. A meta-analysis of cue-reactivity in tobacco cigarette smokers. Nicotine & Tobacco Research. 2021;**23**(2):249-258. DOI: 10.1093/ntr/ntaa147

[66] Vujanovic AA, Lebeaut A, Zegel M, Smit T, Berenz EC. Post-traumatic stress and alcohol use disorders: Recent advances and future directions in cue-reactivity. Current Opinion in Psychology. 2019;**30**:109-116. DOI: 10.1016/j.copsyc.2019.04.003

[67] Drummond DC. What does cue-reactivity have to offer clinical research? Addiction. 2000;**95**(8s2):129-144. DOI: 10.1046/j.1360-0443.95.8s2.2.x

[68] Cheung MW-L, Chan W. Meta-analytic structural equation modeling: A two-stage approach. Psychological Methods. 2005;**10**(1):40-64. DOI: 10.1037/1082-989X.10.1.40

[69] Singleton EG, Tiffany ST, Henningfield JE. Development and validation of a new questionnaire to assess craving for alcohol. Proceedings of the 56th Annual Meeting, The College on Problems of Drug Dependence, Rockville, MD. 1994

[70] Tiffany S, Singleton E, Haertzen C, Henningfield J. The development of a Cocaine Craving Questionarie. Drug and Alcohol Dependence. 1993;**34**:19-28

[71] Singleton EG, Henningfield JE, Heishman TE, Douglas E, Tiffany ST. Multidimensional aspects of craving for alcohol. Proceedings of the 57th Annual Meeting of the College on Problems of Drug Dependence, Rockville, MD. 1995

[72] Kozlowski LT, Pillitteri JL, Sweeney CT, Whitfield KE, Graham JW. Asking questions about urges or cravings for cigarettes. Psychology of Addictive Behaviors. 1996;**10**(4):248

[73] Tiffany ST, Drobes DJ. The development and initial validation of a questionnaire on smoking urges. British Journal of Addiction. 1991;**86**(11): 1467-1476

Chapter 2

# Current Understanding of Biomarkers in Post Traumatic Stress Disorder and Mild Traumatic Brain Injury: A Systematic Review and Implications for Research and Treatment

*Jamie L. Scholl, Eric T. Graack, Michaela S. Ahrenholtz, Taylor J. Bosch and Lee A. Baugh*

## Abstract

For nearly 100 years, it was erroneously believed that the loss of consciousness and/or the altered mental status associated with a mild traumatic brain injury (mTBI) offered protection from the development of posttraumatic stress disorder (PTSD). However, it is now accepted that it is possible for PTSD to result from mTBI, and that the co-occurrence of these two conditions creates a more difficult condition to treat and worsens prognosis. In addition, it is known that the symptomology associated with PTSD and mTBI have a great deal of overlap, complicating diagnoses. The objective of this chapter is to review the current state of biomarkers aimed at diagnosing comorbid mTBI and PTSD that are useful on a single-patient basis and are not reliant on self-report or arduous interviews. Further, implications for future research and treatment are discussed.

**Keywords:** posttraumatic stress disorder, mild traumatic brain injury, biomarker, treatment

## 1. Introduction

Highlighted by recent world-conflicts, such as the wars in Afghanistan and Iraq, it has become evident that a better and more comprehensive understanding of the relationship between stress-related psychological disorders and traumatic brain injury is much-needed, in both military and civilian populations. For the purposes of this chapter, we will focus on posttraumatic stress disorder (PTSD) and mild traumatic brain injury (mTBI); however, this is not to underplay the crucial need to better understand the wide range of stress-related psychological conditions and brain injury. The prevalence rates of PTSD and mTBI in American military personnel returning from Operation Enduring Freedom (OEF) and Operation Iraqi Freedom (OIF) has been reportedly as high as approximately 14 and 20%, respectively [1]. Despite both PTSD and mTBI conditions being "invisible injuries" (injuries not outwardly observable), they are both capable of creating significant disruptions in normal living for individuals. Further, what little we know about the co-occurrence of these conditions suggests that, when combined, they are more difficult to treat and often result in poorer prognoses [2–4]. This understanding is a significant advancement, as it was once thought that the loss of consciousness or altered mental status that is often observed with brain injury offered protection from the development of stress disorders [5]. Although it is recent military engagements that have highlighted the need for a better understanding of concomitant PTSD and mTBI, these conditions are prevalent in both military and civilian contexts and are therefore issues of broad public health on a global scale.

Approximately 3.5–7.0% of adults within the United States develop PTSD every year. When examining military personnel, this number increases to anywhere between 33 and 65% [6]. On the global scale, approximately 25% of the world's population has been affected by PTSD, making it the most prevalent psychiatric disorder [7]. Traumatic brain injuries are also very commonplace, and well over one-million people within the U.S. seek care annually for brain injury [8], with the majority of these being classified as mild [9, 10]. Worldwide, up to 50-million people annually seek treatment [6]. However, this number is likely an underestimation as many individuals who suffer an mTBI do not seek medical care. Furthermore, those that do seek medical attention oftentimes are misdiagnosed or underdiagnosed, especially if symptoms are mild or transient and loss of consciousness is limited to a short period of time [11]. When examining PTSD comorbid with mTBI, it becomes clear that many of those that have been affected by trauma have also experienced mTBI. Within civilian populations, PTSD following accidents such as falls or automotive collisions in which an mTBI occurs, range from approximately 20–36% [12]. Within a military context, this number increases to roughly 34–44% [13, 14]. However, like the reporting of each condition in isolation, the potential for misdiagnosis or underdiagnosis is large.

The prevalence and impact of both mTBI and PTSD (whether it be together or in isolation) result in a high cost of treatment, increased suicide rates, and lost work, all of which place a substantial burden on healthcare systems. Although the true costs are difficult to quantify, estimates for the health services cost associated with an mTBI alone range from $10,000USD to $100,000+ per patient depending on severity, length of hospital stay, and costs of rehabilitation [15–19], with a mean cost of $96,000USD [20]. The numbers are equally startling for the treatment costs associated with PTSD, with annual costs in excess of 200 million USD in US military personnel alone [21], and civilian costs estimated at even greater levels [22–24]. This estimate does not include the loss of productivity associated with this condition, which easily exceeds billions of dollars at a national level [25]. Although both PTSD and mTBI have substantial costs of care in isolation, when combined, healthcare costs are certainly increased, largely due to the complexity of treating comorbid conditions.

Posttraumatic stress disorder and mild traumatic brain injury have overlapping symptomology yet require different therapeutic approaches. In classical diagnoses, detailed information is collected about the onset and progression of symptoms to arrive at a probable diagnosis, which is then further refined. When dealing with an individual that may meet diagnostic criteria for both conditions, this process becomes much more difficult. In theory, a pattern of symptom overlap and divergence could help differentiate etiologies when dealing with comorbid PTSD and mTBI, however, recent evidence suggests this is not the case. In a 2009 study, eight symptoms that are related to both PTSD and mTBI (fatigue, irritability, concentration problems, memory problems, depression, anxiety, insomnia, and dizziness) were examined and compared between patients who had experienced a recent mTBI or PTSD, revealing substantial overlap between both clinical groups. Although it was found that patients with PTSD had greater overall symptom severity, the degree of overlap prevented differential diagnoses based on the pattern of symptoms reported [26]. A meta-analysis conducted the same year [27] provided some evidence that there are symptoms unique to each when occurring in isolation (PTSD—shame, guilt, re-experiencing symptoms; mTBI—headache, sensitivity to light, dizziness, memory deficits), however, this information does not assist in the diagnosis of those that experience both mTBI and PTSD. Therefore, it remains unclear which aspects of these disorders play significant roles in disease onset following event exposure (whether it be set individual traits, epigenetic changes, alterations to specific brain area structure and function, or a combination of these and other factors), and ultimately which set of symptoms will manifest that are linked to the genuine presence of PTSD, mTBI, or both.

The objective of this chapter is to review our current understanding of comorbid mTBI and PTSD, with an emphasis on reviewing the current state of biomarkers used to diagnose comorbid mTBI and PTSD that offer promise on a single-patient basis. To best accomplish these goals, we will begin with providing definitions of what is meant by the terms PTSD and mTBI. Following, we will review the current understanding of the neurological underpinnings of each condition, with a focus on areas of overlap, and examine currently accepted methods of diagnosis and treatment options. Lastly, we will provide an account of the current researchers utilizing biomarkers for either diagnosis or prognosis of PTSD and mTBI, as well as discuss implications for future research and treatment.

## 2. Definitions

The lack of consistent definitions and assessments of mTBI and PTSD complicates the ability to capture accurate statistics for each condition. We focus on mild traumatic brain injury, as this is both the most common traumatic brain injury in civilian [28] and military populations [29], and is also the most likely to co-occur with PTSD [30]. Additionally, as mTBI is often the hardest to diagnose, the pursuit of biomarkers with clinical utility is of great importance. However, when it comes to describing what constitutes an mTBI, a large amount of ambiguity becomes apparent. What is clear is that for a diagnosis of mTBI, two things need to occur: (1) An external force must be exerted to the head; and (2) there must be a temporary change of mental status and/or other evidence of brain injury. Of course, for a traumatic brain injury to be classified as mild, there also needs to be an upper limit for the severity. This includes: (1) a loss of consciousness that does not exceed 30 minutes; and (2) posttraumatic amnesia that does not exceed 24 hrs. These criteria are largely accepted on a global scale [31–33] and will be used for this chapter as well.

Formal methods for the diagnosis of PTSD currently exist, making the definitions regarding the psychiatric condition somewhat consistent. In general, PTSD is characterized by four symptom clusters that develop in response to a traumatic event. The traumatic event must involve exposure to actual or perceived death, serious injury, or sexual violation. Furthermore, the event must be directly experienced or witnessed by the individual, or indirectly experienced by subsequently learning about the event after it happened to a close family member or friend. Specific clinical criteria include: (1) intrusive symptoms related to re-experiencing the trauma; (2) avoidance of the traumatic memory or cues; (3) negative mood and thoughts including emotional numbing and anhedonia; and (4) altered arousal including hypervigilance, irritability, aggression, and sleep disturbances [7, 34]. Additionally, symptoms result in significant social, personal, and vocational impairment [7]. PTSD is commonly comorbid with other anxiety or mood disorders, further complicating diagnosis, and is also associated with increased risk for numerous negative behavioral and health conditions, including substance use disorder, type II diabetes, and Alzheimer's disease [35–38], significantly expanding the costs of treatment. Although the criteria for diagnosing PTSD are rather straightforward, this does not mean that PTSD is a static phenomenon without gradation. It is known that PTSD symptoms appear on a continuum and can fluctuate in terms of their functional impact and presence across time. Furthermore, although the precipitating traumatic event is a critical component of PTSD, it is how an individual responds to that trauma that is essential in the diagnosis. An identical traumatic event for one individual may result in PTSD, whereas another person experiencing an identical event may not. Therefore, it is as much about the symptoms and functional impairment as it is about the event itself.

## 3. Neurobiological underpinnings

Research has shown that both mTBI and PTSD are correlated with both structural and functional changes in the brain, as evidenced by advanced neuroimaging. As can

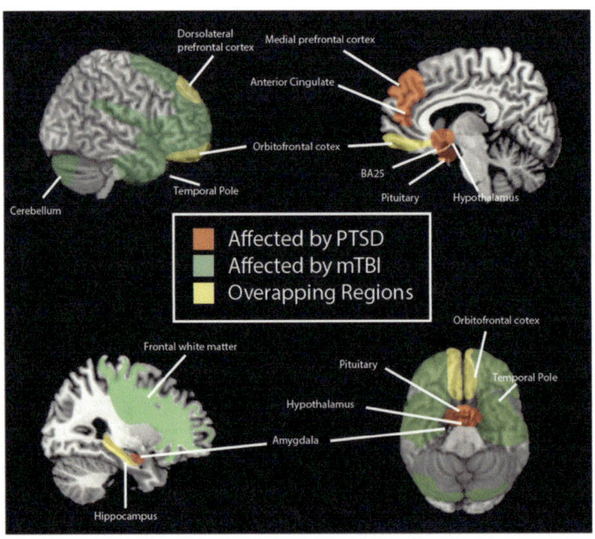


**Figure 1.**
*Multiple brain regions have been suggested as vulnerable to mTBI (green), including the dorsolateral prefrontal cortex, the temporal pole, cerebellum, and frontal white matter tracts connecting the amygdala and medial prefrontal cortex. PTSD has been correlated with numerous brain regions as well (red) including the amygdala, hippocampus, dorsolateral and dorsomedial prefrontal cortex, and orbitofrontal cortex. Areas in common to both PTSD and mTBI are displayed in yellow.*

be seen in **Figure 1**, there are many regions of the brain that are known to be particularly susceptible to both mTBI and PTSD.

Within PTSD, structural and functional imaging studies have shown a wide range of brain regions that are affected. These regions include the amygdala, hippocampus, dorsolateral and dorsomedial prefrontal cortex, and the orbitofrontal cortex. As should be apparent, many of these regions have functional implications for the onset and maintenance of PTSD symptomology [39, 40]. When examining brain structure, many studies (including two large meta-analyses) have shown reduced volume in the hippocampus, a brain area that is known to mediate declarative memories [41, 42]. Similarly, reduced volume within the anterior cingulate cortex and insula have also been shown to be related to PTSD onset [43]. When examining the functional neuroimaging data related to PTSD, exposure to stimuli related to an individual's trauma is associated with increased PTSD symptoms in concert with decreased activity within the medial prefrontal cortex and anterior cingulate [44–46]. Additional areas of decreased function during exposure to trauma-related stimuli include the inferior frontal gyrus, parietal cortex, visual association cortex, and hippocampus [44, 47, 48]. In contrast, areas of increased activity relative to controls include the amygdala [49, 50], parahippocampal gyrus [44, 51], and posterior cingulate [44, 45, 51]. Taken together, the existing literature provides strong evidence of dysfunction within a network of brain regions that are highly related to PTSD symptoms including the hippocampus and amygdala, cingulate cortex, and medial prefrontal cortex [52].

When examining the neurological correlates of mTBI, brain regions are most often damaged if the shearing forces that the brain undergoes during an mTBI are of sufficient magnitude to deform neural cells beyond normal tolerance levels [53]. If this deformation is of sufficient force to cause axonal tearing, the effects of the mTBI are likely to consist of longer-lasting neurological sequelae resulting from alterations to functional connectivity or difficulty with neuronal processing of information [54]. In comparison, if such forces are of a lesser magnitude, the neurological, cognitive, and behavioral symptoms are more likely to be short lived. In general, these forces particularly affect the longer white-matter tracts of the brain including the hypothalamic-pituitary–adrenal (HPA) axis, frontal, temporal, and limbic areas [55]. Specifically, these include the dorsolateral prefrontal cortex, the temporal pole, cerebellum, and frontal white matter tracts connecting the amygdala and medial prefrontal cortex [39, 40, 55–67]—all aforementioned areas that are also implicated in PTSD.

Although the role each of these regions play in the formation of cognition is beyond the scope of this chapter, it is apparent that many of these regions are involved in both emotional regulation and executive function, especially those that are affected in both PTSD and mTBI, including the prefrontal cortex and hippocampus [58, 68]. Perhaps not surprisingly, with the large amount of overlap in the neural substrates that are affected by both PTSD and mTBI, there is a fair degree of overlapping symptomology that has a significant impact on optimal methods for both diagnosing and treating PTSD concurrent with mTBI.

## 4. Current methods of diagnosis and treatment options

As stated previously, due to the overlap of symptoms in both PTSD and mTBI (**Table 1**), it is more difficult to both diagnose and treat PTSD when comorbid with mTBI. For example, in a recent study of 630,000+ veterans diagnosed with PTSD,

| | PTSD | mTBI | PTSD/mTBI |
|---|---|---|---|
| Behavioral symptoms | Aggression<br>Agitation<br>Avoidance of cues<br>Hostility<br>Hypervigilance<br>Irritability<br>Self-Destructive Behavior | Aggression<br>Impulsivity<br>Irritability | Aggression<br>Impulsivity/Self Destructive Behaviors<br>Irritability |
| Physical/cognitive symptoms | Inability to concentrate or focus on tasks Insomnia<br>Nightmares<br>Sensitivity to sound | Coordination problems/loss of balance Amnesia<br>Disorientation<br>Dizziness<br>Fatigue<br>Headache<br>Inability to concentrate or focus on tasks<br>Insomnia<br>Sensitivity to sound | Inability to concentrate or focus on tasks<br>Insomnia<br>Sensitivity to sound |
| Psychological Symptoms | Anhedonia/loss of interest Anxiety<br>Depression<br>Intrusive thoughts/ Unwanted thoughts<br>Reexperiencing the event/ Flashbacks<br>Shame/Guilt<br>Social Isolation/Loneliness | Anxiety<br>Apathy<br>Depression | Anhedonia/Apathy<br>Anxiety<br>Depression |

**Table 1.**
*Symptomologies of PTSD and mTBI.*

only 30% had PTSD alone, with most suffering from concurrent psychiatric conditions, of which mTBI was a prominent co-condition [69].

Diagnosis of PTSD usually consists of a combination of self-report measures and structured and/or semi-structured interview procedures. These procedures are often based on soliciting the information required to determine whether DSM-5 criteria [34] (or alternatives such as the ICD-10 [70]) have been met and include components of the trauma, symptoms/symptom clusters, and subtypes of the disorder. Common structured interviews, such as the Clinician-Administered PTSD Scale (CAPS), are considered both reliable and valid, however, they are time intensive [71]. Furthermore, due to upwards of 93% of PTSD cases co-reporting another psychiatric disorder, it can become difficult to differentiate between disorders with overlapping symptoms [6].

Unlike the diagnosis of TBI, where CT and MRI structural images readily demonstrate contusions or bleeds verifying their presence, there is a lack of interdisciplinary consensus as to what constitutes an mTBI. Although some criteria have been generally accepted (such as those described within the introduction of this chapter), there are diagnostic criteria available from the American Congress of Rehabilitation Medicine (ACRM), the US Centers for Disease Control and Prevention (CDC), and the World

Health Organization (WHO) [72]. Therefore, the utility of a consistent and universally accepted measure of mTBI presence would be of great benefit when diagnosing a mTBI in isolation, and especially when attempting to diagnose in the presence of the overlapping symptoms commonly reported in PTSD.

As should be apparent from this cursory examination, the current process of diagnosing both PTSD and mTBI is largely reliant on often erroneous self-report techniques and arduous clinical interviews that have an inherent lack of consensus, necessitating improvements in both speed of diagnosis and consistency to best offer care and interventions to patients with PTSD and mTBI. One such avenue of providing this information may be found through the discovery of diagnostic biomarkers, which will be the primary focus of discussion for the remainder of this chapter. Before such a discussion takes place, it is important to further highlight the need for improved methods of diagnosing comorbid mTBI and PTSD by examining the implications such discoveries may have on treatment of each condition.

Although there are recognized "gold-standard" treatments for PTSD, there is still much room for improvement. For PTSD, Cognitive Behavioral Therapy (CBT) [73] and psychopharmacological treatment with selective serotonin reuptake inhibitors (SSRIs) and/or serotonin noradrenaline reuptake inhibitors (SNRIs) are often used for treatment. Similarly, both psychological and pharmacological treatments are recommended for the treatment of mTBI, such as CBT [74] in conjunction with pharmacological treatment of the sequalae associated with mTBI [75]. However, in a recent study of the evaluations of 41 guidelines related to the treatment of mTBI, only three were founded in what was determined to be an evidenced-based fashion [76], highlighting the need for more rigorous and evidence-based treatment regimens. There is even less evidence-based guidance when it comes to the treatment of comorbid mTBI and PTSD, making research on how to best identify multimorbidity in PTSD patients critical to developing effective treatment strategies.

## 5. Current biomarker research

As should be evident from the previous sections from this chapter, both the ability to diagnose PTSD comorbid with mTBI and the ability to effectively monitor treatment of the concurrent conditions would benefit from the identification of biomarkers. For this discussion we adapt the definition of a biomarker using a conceptual framework that is useful for clinical research and treatment purposes. This may include any information that can be used as an objective indication of a relevant medical state observed from outside the patient. Importantly, these signs must be able to be measured accurately and have high levels of replicability. This is captured in the WHO's definition of a biomarker as "any substance, structure, or process that can be measured in the body or its products and influence or predict the incidence of outcome or disease" [77] and can be expanded to "… almost any measurement reflecting an interaction between a biological system and a potential hazard…[and] may be functional and physiological, biochemical at the cellular level, or a molecular interaction" [78]. In alignment with these requirements, our discussion will focus on the relevance and validity of the suggested biomarkers, allowing for it to be used as a surrogate endpoint [79]. There are a wide range of biomarkers and targets currently being researched for roles in both mTBI and PTSD. A summary of biomarkers currently undergoing research that meet the criteria previously discussed can be seen in **Table 2**, with in-depth discussion of each following.

| | | | |
|---|---|---|---|
| HPA axis dysregulation | Cortisol | Adrenal glucocorticoid hormone that modulates the HPA axis | PTSD |
| Monoamine Dysfunction | Norepinephrine (NE) | Endogenous neurotransmitter and stress hormone | PTSD |
| | Serotonin (5-HT) | Monoamine neurotransmitter | PTSD |
| Inflammatory and immune function | Interleukin-1ß (IL-1ß)<br>Interleukin-2 (IL-2)<br>Interleukin-6 (IL-6)<br>Interleukin-8 (IL-8)<br>Interleukin-10 (IL-10) | Cytokine protein involved in inflammation<br>Cytokine protein involved in immune function regulation<br>Cytokine protein with pro- and antiinflammatory actions<br>Cytokine protein involved in inflammation<br>Cytokine protein with anti-inflammatory actions | PTSD<br>PTSD<br>PTSD<br>and mTBI<br>mTBI<br>mTBI |
| | C-reactive protein (CRP) | Circulating protein released in response to inflammation | PTSD |
| | Tumor Necrosis Factor alpha subunit (TNF-α) | Cytokine protein with pro-inflammatory actions | PTSD |
| | Interferon gamma (IFN-γ) | Cytokine protein involved in immune function regulation | PTSD |
| | Marinobufagenin (MBG) | Endogenous steroid related to myocardial infarction, heart failure, and kidney failure | mTBI |
| Genetic variation | FKBP Prolyl Isomerase 5 (FKBP5)<br>Serotonin transporter gene linked polymorphic region (5-HTTLPR) | Protein coding gene regulating neuroendocrine stress<br>Gene promotor region on the serotonin<br>transporter gene linked to neuropsychiatric disorders | PTSD<br>PTSD |
| | Nuclear receptor subfamily 3 group C, member 1 (NR3C-1) | Promotor region of the glucocorticoid receptor gene related to metabolism and immune response | PTSD |
| | Apolipoprotein E (APOE) | Protein coding gene that regulates fat metabolism | mTBI |
| | brain-derived neurotrophic factor (BDNF) | Protein coding gene that promotes neuronal survival | PTSD and mTBI |
| Functional and structural neuroimaging | Amygdala<br>Medial Prefrontal Cortex<br>Rostral Anterior Cingulate Cortex<br>Hippocampus | Involved in emotional processing, and conditioned fear<br>Involved in inhibition and goal-directed behaviors<br>Cortical structure involved in mediating emotion and cognitive function<br>Involved in memory and cognition | PTSD<br>PTSD<br>PTSD<br>PTSD |
| | Diffusion weighted imaging (DWI) | Noninvasive technique using a specific form of Magnetic Resonance Imaging (MRI) to view water diffusion in images | mTBI |
| | Magnetic resonance spectroscopy (MRS) | Noninvasive technique to analyze metabolic changes in tissue | mTBI |

| | | | |
|---|---|---|---|
| Neuronal and axonal injury | Tau Protein<br>Ubiquitin C-terminal hydrolase isozyme L1 (UCHL1)<br>Neuron-specific enolase (NSE) | Protein expressed primarily in neurons, involved in stabilizing microtubules<br>Enzyme involved in axonal transport and integrity<br>Enzyme involved in glycolytic metabolism in the brain | mTBI<br>mTBI<br>mTBI |
| | Neutrophil gelatinaseassociated lipocalin (NGAL) | Polypeptide released in response to systemic inflammation | mTBI |
| Blood Brain Barrier Disturbances | CSF/serum albumin ratio<br>Astrocyte-specific SNS protein S100B | Measure of cerebrospinal fluid components in the periphery following injury<br>Binding protein produced by astrocytes involved in intracellular functions | mTBI<br>mTBI |
| | PrPc-cellular prion protein | Glycoprotein typically anchored to plasma membranes, proposed to be involved in neurodegenerative prion disease | mTBI |
| Cerebral Blood Flow Changes | Vasoreactivity | MRI measurable changes that could impair smooth muscle and affect cognition | mTBI |

**Table 2.**
*Summary of current biomarker research.*

## 5.1 PTSD

Most of the promising biomarkers for the presence of PTSD are related to either dysfunction of the HPA axis, monoamine systems, heightened inflammation, genetic and epigenetic changes thought to be a result of methylation brought about through exposure to prolonged stress, or functional and structural neuroimaging. There has also been growing interest and research in the examination of psychophysical biomarkers of PTSD, such as indicators of hyperarousal (heart rate, blood pressure, skin conductance, etc.). However, examination of these forms of hyperactivity through psychological testing is beyond the scope of this chapter.

*HPA Axis Dysregulation.* Cortisol, a circulating adrenal glucocorticoid hormone that modulates the HPA axis is known to be involved in anxiety responses and sleep regulation [80]. Research has shown that within a PTSD population, lower salivary cortisol levels were found when compared to control participants, especially when measurements were taken in the morning [80]. Typically, there is a diurnal cycle of salivary cortisol with peak concentration observed shortly after waking, and then drops across the waking hours. In addition to a lower morning level of cortisol, PTSD patients have also demonstrated a blunted cortisol response throughout the day [81]. This blunted cortisol reactivity in response to exposure to acute stress may offer more promise as it removes confounds associated with the measurement of baseline cortisol, such as sex differences and time of day effects. Therefore, although not specific to the presence of PTSD, measurements of circulating cortisol levels may form part of a panel of assays designed to detect the presence of PTSD in a clinical population due to its non-invasive status when measured from a saliva sample.

*Monoamine Dysfunction.* As PTSD includes increased sympathetic nervous system tone, it is not surprising that levels of norepinephrine (NE) are also heightened [82]. In a prospective study of motor vehicle accident survivors, urinary levels of NE were positively correlated with the likelihood of development of PTSD in the month following trauma, but only in males [83]. Changes in the serotonergic (5-HT) system have also been observed in PTSD. Specifically, 5-HT transporter binding within the amygdala is reduced in PTSD and correlated with both anxiety and depression within PTSD patients [84].

*Inflammatory and Immune Function.* Stemming from the high comorbidity between PTSD and general physical illnesses [85], there has been extensive examination of the potential role of markers of inflammation as a proxy for PTSD and PTSD symptomology. In all instances examined, there is a positive correlation between inflammatory markers and PTSD symptomology. This includes interleukin (IL) -6 [86], IL-2 [87], IL-1β [88]. Additionally, increased C-reactive protein (CRP) levels are shown to be elevated in individuals with PTSD [89–91], but also has been shown to be predictive of post-deployment PTSD when examined in a prospective study [92]. Continuing this trend, PTSD is also positively correlated with higher levels of TNF-α and IFN-γ when compared to healthy controls, likely as a result of the persistent stress experienced [93]. In general, data concerning the relationship between inflammatory responses and PTSD confirm that PTSD is likely associated with chronic inflammation. Although this may lead to inflammation as a viable therapeutic target to alleviate at least some of the symptoms associated with PTSD, they do not serve well as a general biomarker of PTSD presence or prognosis due to its status as a hallmark finding in many other diseased states, including those that are often comorbid with PTSD [85, 94–97].

*Genetic Variation.* Most genetic and epigenetic findings have clustered around modulators of HPA axis function either before or following trauma. Perhaps the most cited modulator is FKBP5, a protein encoding gene involved in immunoregulation [98]. Polymorphisms on FKBP5, specifically Val66Met, have been associated PTSD [99]. Met-allele carriers are also reported to have greater severity in PTSD symptoms amongst veterans compared to Val/Val genotypes [100]. However, FKBP5 is also associated with depression [101], a condition known to often co-occur with PTSD therefore making its use as a solitary differential marker of PTSD unlikely. The serotonin transporter gene linked polymorphic region (5-HTTLPR short and long) has also been linked to trauma exposure and depression. Individuals with the LL genotype exhibit lower intrusion and avoidance symptoms compared to those with the S-allele, though no differences were found in other PTSD symptoms [102]. Increased methylation levels at 4 promotor sites on BDNF were found in PTSD patients that experienced high combat exposure compared to those without PTSD [103]. Reduced glucocorticoid receptor NR3C1-1F promotor methylation was found in combat veterans that developed PTSD when compared to those that did not [104]. Hypermethylation at NR3C1 gene promoters were associated with lower risk of PTSD in male genocide survivors, but not female [105].

As has become apparent, many (if not all) of these genetic regions have been associated with other psychiatric conditions and may therefore be a better marker of stress-induced psychopathology in general rather than PTSD specifically, and there has yet to be a single genetic or epigenetic factor that reliably predicts the presence or severity of PTSD in isolation of other psychiatric conditions.

*Functional and Structural Neuroimaging.* One of the most consistent findings regarding neuroimaging of PTSD is the presence of increased amygdala activation when compared to controls when patients have been exposed to fear inducing stimuli [106]. For example, there have now been a number of studies that demonstrate hyperactivity of the amygdala when PTSD participants have been exposed to trauma-relevant words when compared to amygdala activity of control participants [107–110]. Further studies have shown that this increased activity may be a result of weakened inhibitory control of the amygdala by the medial prefrontal cortex [106, 108, 110]. Furthering these findings, a recent meta-analysis of imaging studies during emotional tasks for individuals with PTSD, anxiety, and phobia revealed that only the PTSD patients demonstrated decreased activity within the rostral anterior cingulate cortex, offering a potential mechanism to distinguish between aberrant functional activity observed in PTSD and not in other anxiety disorders [111].

In addition to functional studies, a number of structural examinations of PTSD have taken place using neuroimaging techniques. Early studies examining structural differences between PTSD and non-PTSD patients demonstrated that smaller hippocampal volume may be associated with an increased risk of developing PTSD [112], though this finding has more recently been questioned with hippocampal volume reductions being acquired with trauma exposure [113]. When examining specific regions of the hippocampus using structural MRI, it appears as though reductions in specific subregions can be associated with PTSD symptoms. Specifically, reductions within the cornu ammonis 3 (CA3) layer of the hippocampus and the dentate gyrus are related to PTSD symptomology [114].

### 5.2 mTBI

Currently, mTBI is typically diagnosed based solely on clinical presentation, in comparison to TBI which has prominent and objective neuroimaging findings. This has several implications as to the utility of biomarkers of mTBI. Perhaps of primary concern is the fact that any biomarker that would offer clinical benefits must be correlated with clinical symptom presentation. For example, a marker that elevates with impacts to the head without observable changes in clinical presentation in the patient would be of little clinical use. Potential biomarkers for mTBI are most often related to, or spawned, by the axonal injury that occurs following the much smaller forces related to a mTBI. These can be broadly categorized as those that are related to neuronal and axonal injury, blood brain barrier disturbances, neuroinflammation, cerebral blood flow changes, and genetic variation.

*Neuronal and Axonal Injury*. Disturbances of the cellular environment often occur following the shearing forces that often accompany mTBI [115], and while this usually is not to the extend to the point of axonal disconnection, it can indirectly affect membrane homeostasis which ultimately results in cell damage [53, 116]. There are several potential biomarkers associated with neuronal damage. Tau protein is known to be changed in response to injury [117] including mTBI, at least in animal models [118]. In one of the larger human studies (196 patients), the ratio of phosphorylated-tau to total tau had both a good diagnostic and prognostic marker for acute TBI, including those with a mild severity [119]. Other biomarkers of neuronal and axonal injury that have been explored as potentials include ubiquitin carboxyl-terminal hydrolase isozyme L1 (UCHL1), [120–122], neuron-specific enolase (NSE) [123–125], and neutrophil gelatinase-associated lipocalin (NGAL) [126]. However, current research into their utility has not demonstrated sufficient levels of specificity and/or replicability to be discussed in detail, but likely warrant further examination.

*Blood Brain Barrier Disturbances.* Although it has been well demonstrated that blood brain barrier (BBB) disruptions are associated with TBI [127], there is growing evidence that there are BBB disruptions following mTBI during both the chronic and the acute phase [128]. There are a number of non-invasive indirect measures of BBB dysfunction that rely on the detection of cerebrospinal fluid (CSF) components within peripheral serum, however, there has been little convincing evidence that suggests it will be a suitable biomarker of mTBI if used in isolation. The CSF/serum albumin ratio is the standard biomarker for BBB integrity [129] but is not sensitive enough to detect the presence of BBB disruption as a result of mTBI [130]. Perhaps the most studied is the astrocyte-specific SNS protein S100B. Research has shown that the detection of this marker approaches the same levels of sensitivity as the CSF/serum albumin ratio [127], and has been used to rule out mTBI in emergency medicine already, where S100B levels have a high (99 + %) predictive value [131]. However, there is relative non-specificity of elevated S100B (as there are extracerebral sources of S100B in peripheral blood), and it has also shown to be elevated in clinical cases without head trauma [132]. Further dampening enthusiasm, there is still conflicting evidence as to whether S100B levels are positively correlated with mTBI [133]. A less explored, though perhaps more promising marker is the glycoprotein PrPc—cellular prion protein. Since this plasma-soluble prion protein is located within the plasma membrane, is has been suggested that it may be released following an mTBI as a result of BBB dysfunction [134], with animal models showing increased serum levels following blast exposure induced mTBI [135, 136]. Within humans, a small (N = 6) study amongst athletes demonstrated PrPc levels increased and remained elevated following mTBI [134]. More recently, a slightly larger study conducted within a hospital setting (N = 20) confirmed this effect with elevated PrPc levels following TBI, with 8 of the 20 being classified as mild injuries. However, PrPc did levels did not correlate with severity of trauma [137]. A third study confirmed the ability for PrPc levels to differentiate TBI with cognitive symptoms versus TBI in which no cognitive symptoms were present [138]. Although additional study is required, these specific features of PrPc make it a particularly attractive candidate biomarker for mTBI. Specifically, its relative specificity with regard to cognitive dysfunction, and ability to be detected years following trauma, are likely of great utility.

*Neuroinflammation.* Following TBI, including mTBI, there is a cascade of events that ultimately results in the presence of inflammation [139–142], offering an opportunity to examine markers of the neuroinflammatory response as a marker of brain injury. Two promising classes of markers of neuroinflammation are the inflammatory interleukin proteins and the cardiotonic steroid marinobufagenin. There have been many studies demonstrating elevated levels of interleukins including IL-6, IL-8 and IL-10 following brain injury [143–148], as well as studies showing these levels are related to clinical outcome in mTBI [149, 150]. In a small (N = 6) study, marinobufagenin (MBG) levels were initially increased following mTBI, along with symptomology [151]. As MBG levels decreased, symptom scores also decreased, suggesting there may be a relationship between symptoms and MBG. A larger study (N = 110) found MBG levels were elevated following mTBI, and were also correlated with reported symptoms [151] adding further evidence for the potential utility of MBG.

A further drawback to most biofluid based biomarkers of mTBI is the timescale at which they can be detected, necessitating their examination within the acute stage of the injury as they return to baseline levels rather quickly (though PrPc is an exception to this). As an alternative, potentially longer-lasting biomarker, advanced neuroimaging techniques such as diffusion weighted imagery (DWI) and magnetic resonance spectroscopy (MRS) for diagnosing the presence of an mTBI at a timescale that extends beyond the acute stage. Genetic information may offer additional information not available through the other methods discussed, such as the susceptibility to mTBI following head trauma, reflected in the likelihood of developing symptoms based on genetic variation.

*Cerebral Blood Flow Changes.* Recent research has shown that following mTBI, there are changes in vasoreactivity that impair smooth muscle response [152], ultimately affecting cerebral blood flow that animal models have shown can persist up to a year after initial damage [153]. Due to the extended period of blood flow changes, this may be an ideal candidate for evaluating whether long-term changes in cognition are a result of a previously acquired mTBI [154]. These changes in blood flow can be detected using modern magnetic resonance imaging techniques as hypoperfusion in many of the anatomical regions previously described as particularly susceptible to mTBI injury including the prefrontal, frontal, and temporal regions of the brain [118].

*Genetic Variation.* The two leading genetic candidates are the genetic mutations in the genes encoding for apolipoprotein E (APOE) and brain-derived neurotrophic factor (BDNF). It is important to note that both of these genes are already being explored as they pertain to the risk of generating various types of neurodegeneration disorders, such as Alzheimer's disease [155]. This finding is not all that unexpected considering the building link between mTBI and subsequent neurodegenerative conditions [156–159]. The APOE ε4 allele has been shown to be a significant risk factor for the development of Alzheimer's disease, but systematic review [160] has shown it is unrelated to mTBI diagnosis. Interestingly, this same allele confers increased risk to some of the cognitive impairment associated with the longer-term symptoms of mTBI [161]. When it comes to studies examining the role of BDNF, a small sample (at least on the scale of genetic studies; N = 110) showed a link between carriers of the minor allele of rs115769 and the memory impairments often associated with mTBI [162], as well as the BDNF Val66Met allele being linked to a higher risk of experiencing an mTBI [163], and increased experience of emotional symptoms following the occurrence of an mTBI [164]. Further, it was been shown that mutations of BDNF rs6265 Val66Met polymorphisms affect neurocognitive performance in patients following mTBI, offering the potential for predicting which patients will go on to develop neurocognitive symptoms following mTBI [165].

## 6. Summary and conclusions

*Biomarkers for PTSD.* At this time, there are a number of biomarkers that are associated with PTSD risk, symptoms, and symptom progression. Despite this association, due to the common comorbidity with both other psychiatric conditions and general health status, there is currently little chance of using any single marker as a diagnostic characterization. Future studies must do a more thorough examination of biological and psychological states within PTSD to be able to characterize a combination of biomarkers that may cluster around symptoms and symptom progression in a meaningful way. One way that this may be accomplished is through the use of biomarkers to identify features associated with PTSD, rather than with markers that are consistent with the DSM criteria [166]. For example, it may be that reduced hippocampal volume is associated both with PTSD and comorbid depressive state and can serve as a biomarker of the cluster of symptoms associated with both. This approach would necessitate a panel of biomarkers to increase the specificity, sensitivity, and replicability of any proposed tool. In fact, such an approach utilizing signals from multiple biological domains totaling in excess of one million unique markers was used to define 343 candidate biomarkers via a combination of data-driven and hypothesis driven approaches. These features were further reduced to 28 based on performance and ability to track phenotype, resulting in a final panel which obtained impressive levels of accuracy, sensitivity, and specificity (81, 85, and 77%, respectively) [167].

*Biomarkers for mTBI.* Currently, there is insufficient evidence to support a relationship between biomarkers of mTBI and clinical outcomes, though many offer promise of acting in this capacity. For this relationship to be drawn, it is imperative that future research includes clinical outcome measures and that a standardized study design is utilized. From the non-exhaustive work cited here, it is clear that differences in methodology, especially related to the timing of sample collection, the length of follow-up, the clinical measurements performed, and the clinical population studied all could be leading to the sometimes-conflicting results reported and the relatively small, unconvincing effect sizes. Further, it is also apparent that although many of the reported biomarkers are sensitive to the presence of head impact, unless the candidate biomarker scales with symptoms reported, it will be of little clinical utility. In fact, there is often little disagreement as to whether an impact to the head has occurred, but rather, the intent of the biomarker is to assess whether that impact is going to result (or is the cause) of symptoms being reported.

## 7. Summary of differential features

Differential features of biomarkers specific to PTSD

- HPA Axis Dysregulation (cortisol)
- Monoamine Dysfunction (norepinephrine and serotonin)
- Inflammatory and Immune Function (interleukins 2 and 1ß, C-reactive protein)
- Genetic Variation (polymorphisms and methylation on genes FKBP5, 5-HTTLPR, and NR3C1)
- Functional and Structural Neuroimaging (differential activation in amygdala, prefrontal cortex, hippocampus and rostral anterior cingulate cortex)

Differential features of biomarkers specific to mTBI

- Neuronal and Axonal Injury (Tau protein, ubiquitin carboxyl-terminal hydrolase, neuron-specific enolase, neutrophil gelatinase-associated lipocalin)
- Blood Brain Barrier Disturbances (CSF/serum albumin ratio, S100B, PrPC levels)
- Neuroinflammation (interleukins 8 and 10, marinobufagenin)
- Cerebral Blood Flow Changes (magnetic resonance imaging techniques to detect hypoperfusion)

*Biomarkers for PTSD comorbid with mTBI.* It should be apparent from the lack of conclusive biomarkers for PTSD and mTBI when occurring in isolation that there is currently little prospect for a single biomarker that will be able to diagnose PTSD concurrent with mTBI versus detecting the presence of each condition in isolation. Part of this difficulty directly stems from the current method of diagnoses for each of these conditions. As previously discussed, although mTBI is most certainly a neurological event, it is diagnosed in a manner consistent with a psychiatric condition—based on the collection of symptoms reported. With the overlap of symptoms between both mTBI and PTSD, many of the identified biomarker candidates would be expected to be present in both PTSD and mTBI, ultimately hindering a differential diagnosis. In essence, the same conditions that necessitate the identification of a biomarker of these conditions also prevents its discovery. In addition to the necessity for larger and better designed studies, it is clear that examining the potential of any biomarker in isolation is ultimately a futile event. What may be possible in the near future is the union of several different biomarkers that are selected based on their specificity and replicability in differentially identifying PTSD and mTBI. This will require larger scale studies that collect a wide range of neuropsychological and biological samples, as well as neuroimaging, and combine them to truly accomplish these goals. In recent years there has been some progress in this regard [168, 169], at least signifying that within the field there is a recognized need and attempt to combine biomarkers not only from separate conditions, but indeed separate disciplines to discover ways to diagnose PTSD concurrent with mTBI in a more rigorous and efficient manner. This use of a collective intelligence approach, common in other fields such as finance [170], would allow for domain area expertise to identify successful candidates from what is a current, and continually growing, set of candidate biomarkers.

In summary, posttraumatic stress disorder and mTBI are both significant problems that lead to reduced quality of life for a wide range of people. Due to the nature of symptoms, diagnosis and treatment is inefficient and often delayed, resulting in additional complications in patient outcomes. Determining consistent and accurate biomarkers to improve diagnostic measures of both PTSD and mTBI as well as to differentiate between the two would improve outcomes for both disorders. In the near future, the combination of a selection of the individual biomarkers discussed could be used to design a comprehensive screening tool for individuals following a traumatic event. Additionally, identification of biomarkers involved in the transition post-injury to long-term post-concussive symptoms could allow for early intervention and prevent development of PTSD following trauma. Further, the monitoring and classification of individual responses to screening arrays could dictate the best treatment options, and inform recommendations of medication, therapies, neuromodulation techniques and various combinations from those currently available. Ultimately, this could allow patients and physicians to better direct treatment and response measures based on the individual's biological makeup.

## Author details

Jamie L. Scholl[1,2], Eric T. Graack[1,2], Michaela S. Ahrenholtz[1,3], Taylor J. Bosch[1,2] and Lee A. Baugh[1,2]*

1 Center for Brain and Behavioral Research, Vermillion, SD, USA

2 Basic Biomedical Sciences, Sanford School of Medicine, University of South Dakota, Vermillion, SD, USA

3 Department of Psychology, University of South Dakota, Vermillion, SD, USA

*Address all correspondence to: lee.baugh@usd.edu

## References

[1] Tanielian T et al. Invisible Wounds: Mental Health and Cognitive Care Needs of America's Returning Veterans. Santa Monica, CA: Rand Corporation; 2008

[2] Tanev KS et al. PTSD and TBI co-morbidity: Scope, clinical presentation and treatment options. Brain Injury. 2014;**28**(3):261-270

[3] Otis JD et al. Complicating factors associated with mild traumatic brain injury: Impact on pain and posttraumatic stress disorder treatment. Journal of Clinical Psychology in Medical Settings. 2011;**18**(2):145-154

[4] McAllister TW. Psychopharmacological Issues in the Treatment of TBI and PTSD. The Clinical Neuropsychologist. 2009;**23**(8):1338-1367

[5] Adler A. Neuropsychiatric complications in victims of Boston's cocoanut grove disaster. Journal of the American Medical Association. 1943;**123**(17):1098-1101

[6] Van Praag DLG et al. Post-traumatic stress disorder after civilian traumatic brain injury: A systematic review and meta-analysis of prevalence rates. Journal of Neurotrauma. 2019;**36**(23):3220-3232

[7] Jorge RE. Posttraumatic stress disorder. Continuum: Lifelong Learning in Neurology. 2015;**21**(3):789-805

[8] Faul M. et al. Traumatic Brain Injury in the United States; Emergency Department Visits, Hospitalizations, and Deaths, 2002-2006. Atlanta (GA): Centers for Disease Control and Prevention, National Center for Injury Prevention and Control; 2010

[9] Vos PE et al. EFNS guideline on mild traumatic brain injury: Report of an EFNS task force. European Journal of Neurology. 2002;**9**(3):207-219

[10] Corrigan JD, Selassie AW, Orman JAL. The epidemiology of traumatic brain injury. The Journal of Head Trauma Rehabilitation. 2010;**25**(2):72-80

[11] Carroll LJ et al. Systematic review of the prognosis after mild traumatic brain injury in adults: Cognitive, psychiatric, and mortality outcomes: Results of the international collaboration on mild traumatic brain injury prognosis. Archives of Physical Medicine and Rehabilitation. 2014;**95**(3):S152-S173

[12] Craig A et al. Psychological impact of injuries sustained in motor vehicle crashes: Systematic review and meta-analysis. BMJ Open. 2016;**6**(9):e011993-e011993

[13] Hoge CW et al. Mild traumatic brain injury in US soldiers returning from Iraq. New England Journal of Medicine. 2008;**358**(5):453-463

[14] Lew HL et al. Prevalence of chronic pain, posttraumatic stress disorder, and persistent postconcussive symptoms in OIF/OEF veterans: Polytrauma clinical triad. Journal of Rehabilitation Research & Development. 2009;**46**(6):697-702

[15] Borg J et al. Non-surgical intervention and cost for mild traumatic brain injury: Results of the WHO collaborating centre task force on mild traumatic brain injury. Journal of Rehabilitation Medicine. 2004;**36**(0):76-83

[16] Hu J et al. Trend and geographic analysis for traumatic brain injury

mortality and cost based on MarketScan database. Journal of Neurotrauma. 2013;**30**(20):1755-1761

[17] Davis KL et al. The direct economic burden of blunt and penetrating trauma in a managed care population. Journal of Trauma and Acute Care Surgery. 2007;**62**(3):622-630

[18] McGarry LJ et al. Outcomes and costs of acute treatment of traumatic brain injury. Journal of Trauma and Acute Care Surgery. 2002;**53**(6):1152-1159

[19] Kreutzer JS et al. Charges and lengths of stay for acute and inpatient rehabilitation treatment of traumatic brain injury 1990-1996. Brain Injury. 2001;**15**(9):763-774

[20] Thompson K, Antony A, Holtzman A. The costs of traumatic brain injury. North Carolina Medical Journal. 2001;**62**(6):376-379

[21] Harrison JP, Satterwhite LF, Ruday W. The financial impact of post traumatic stress disorder on returning US military personnel. Journal of Health Care Finance. 2010;**36**(4):65-74

[22] Ferry FR et al. The economic burden of PTSD in Northern Ireland. Journal of Traumatic Stress. 2015;**28**(3):191-197

[23] Konnopka A, König H. Economic burden of anxiety disorders: A systematic review and meta-analysis. PharmacoEconomics. 2020;**38**(1):25-37

[24] Greenberg PE et al. The economic burden of anxiety disorders in the 1990s. Journal of Clinical Psychiatry. 1999;**60**(7):427-435

[25] Wilson S, Guliani H, Boichev G. On the economics of post-traumatic stress disorder among first responders in Canada. Journal of Community Safety and Well-Being. 2016;**1**(2):26-31

[26] Vanderploeg RD, Belanger HG, Curtiss G. Mild traumatic brain injury and posttraumatic stress disorder and their associations with health symptoms. Archives of Physical Medicine and Rehabilitation. 2009;**90**(7):1084-1093

[27] Stein MB, McAllister TW. Exploring the convergence of posttraumatic stress disorder and mild traumatic brain injury. American Journal of Psychiatry. 2009;**166**(7):768-776

[28] Silverberg ND, Duhaime A-C, Iaccarino MA. Mild traumatic brain injury in 2019-2020. JAMA. 2020;**323**(2):177-178

[29] Cameron KL et al. Trends in the incidence of physician-diagnosed mild traumatic brain injury among active duty US military personnel between 1997 and 2007. Journal of Neurotrauma. 2012;**29**(7):1313-1321

[30] Zatzick DF et al. Multisite investigation of traumatic brain injuries, posttraumatic stress disorder, and self-reported health and cognitive impairments. Archives of General Psychiatry. 2010;**67**(12):1291-1300

[31] Menon DK et al. Position statement: Definition of traumatic brain injury. Archives of Physical Medicine and Rehabilitation. 2010;**91**(11):1637-1640

[32] Prevention, N.C.f.I. and Control, Report to Congress on mild traumatic brain injury in the United States: Steps to prevent a serious public health problem. 2003: Centers for Disease Control and Prevention

[33] Ruff RM et al. Recommendations for diagnosing a mild traumatic brain injury: A National Academy of Neuropsychology

education paper. Archives of Clinical Neuropsychology. 2009;**24**(1):3-10

[34] American Psychiatric Association. Diagnostic and Statistical Manual of Mental Disorders: DSM-5. Arlington, VA: American Psychiatric Association; 2013

[35] Gaher RM et al. An experience sampling study of PTSD and alcohol-related problems. Psychology of Addictive Behaviors. 2014;**28**(4):1013

[36] Sareen J. Posttraumatic stress disorder in adults: Impact, comorbidity, risk factors, and treatment. The Canadian Journal of Psychiatry. 2014;**59**(9):460-467

[37] Weiner MW et al. Effects of traumatic brain injury and posttraumatic stress disorder on Alzheimer's disease in veterans, using the Alzheimer's disease neuroimaging initiative. Alzheimer's & Dementia. 2014;**10**:S226-S235

[38] Roberts AL et al. Posttraumatic stress disorder and incidence of type 2 diabetes mellitus in a sample of women: A 22-year longitudinal study. JAMA Psychiatry. 2015;**72**(3):203-210

[39] Jovanovic T, Ressler KJ. How the neurocircuitry and genetics of fear inhibition may inform our understanding of PTSD. American Journal of Psychiatry. 2010;**167**(6):648-662

[40] Lanius RA et al. Emotion modulation in PTSD: Clinical and neurobiological evidence for a dissociative subtype. American Journal of Psychiatry. 2010;**167**(6):640-647

[41] Kitayama N et al. Magnetic resonance imaging (MRI) measurement of hippocampal volume in posttraumatic stress disorder: A meta-analysis. Journal of Affective Disorders. 2005;**88**(1):79-86

[42] Smith ME. Bilateral hippocampal volume reduction in adults with post-traumatic stress disorder: A meta-analysis of structural MRI studies. Hippocampus. 2005;**15**(6):798-807

[43] Kasai K et al. Evidence for acquired pregenual anterior cingulate gray matter loss from a twin study of combat-related posttraumatic stress disorder. Biological Psychiatry. 2008;**63**(6):550-556

[44] Bremner JD et al. Neural correlates of memories of childhood sexual abuse in women with and without posttraumatic stress disorder. American Journal of Psychiatry. 1999;**156**(11):1787-1795

[45] Lanius RA et al. Recall of emotional states in posttraumatic stress disorder: An fMRI investigation. Biological Psychiatry. 2003;**53**(3):204-210

[46] Lanius RA et al. Neural correlates of traumatic memories in posttraumatic stress disorder: A functional MRI investigation. American Journal of Psychiatry. 2001;**158**(11):1920-1922

[47] Shin LM et al. Regional cerebral blood flow during script-driven imagery in childhood sexual abuse-related PTSD: A PET investigation. American Journal of Psychiatry. 1999;**156**(4):575-584

[48] Shin LM et al. Visual imagery and perception in posttraumatic stress disorder: A positron emission tomographic investigation. Archives of General Psychiatry. 1997;**54**(3):233-241

[49] Rauch SL et al. A symptom provocation study of posttraumatic stress disorder using positron emission tomography and script-driven imagery. Archives of General Psychiatry. 1996;**53**(5):380-387

[50] Shin LM et al. Regional cerebral blood flow in the amygdala and medial

prefrontalcortex during traumatic imagery in male and female vietnam veterans with ptsd. Archives of General Psychiatry. 2004;**61**(2):168-176

[51] Bremner JD et al. Neural correlates of exposure to traumatic pictures and sound in Vietnam combat veterans with and without posttraumatic stress disorder: A positron emission tomography study. Biological Psychiatry. 1999;**45**(7):806-816

[52] Bremner JD. Neuroimaging studies in post-traumatic stress disorder. Current Psychiatry Reports. 2002;**4**(4):254-263

[53] Büki A, Povlishock J. All roads lead to disconnection?–Traumatic axonal injury revisited. Acta Neurochirurgica. 2006;**148**(2):181-194

[54] Biasca N, Maxwell WL. Minor traumatic brain injury in sports: A review in order to prevent neurological sequelae. Progress in Brain Research. 2007;**161**:263-291

[55] Hamberger A et al. Concussion in professional football: Morphology of brain injuries in the NFL concussion model—part 16. Neurosurgery. 2009;**64**(6):1174-1182

[56] Yehuda R. Post-traumatic stress disorder. New England Journal of Medicine. 2002;**346**(2):108-114

[57] McAllister TW, Stein MB. Effects of psychological and biomechanical trauma on brain and behavior. Annals of the New York Academy of Sciences. 2010;**1208**(1):46-57

[58] Thurmond VA et al. Advancing integrated research in psychological health and traumatic brain injury: Common data elements. Archives of Physical Medicine and Rehabilitation. 2010;**91**(11):1633-1636

[59] Daniels JK et al. Switching between executive and default mode networks in posttraumatic stress disorder: Alterations in functional connectivity. Journal of Psychiatry & Neuroscience: JPN. 2010;**35**(4):258

[60] Panenka WJ et al. Neuropsychological outcome and diffusion tensor imaging in complicated versus uncomplicated mild traumatic brain injury. PLoS One. 2015;**10**(4):e0122746

[61] Meier TB et al. Longitudinal assessment of white matter abnormalities following sports-related concussion. Human Brain Mapping. 2016;**37**(2):833-845

[62] Orrison WW Jr et al. Traumatic brain injury: A review and high-field MRI findings in 100 unarmed combatants using a literature-based checklist approach. Journal of Neurotrauma. 2009;**26**(5):689-701

[63] Dretsch MN. Enhancing operational readiness through neuroimaging: Mapping the pathophysiology of mild traumatic brain injury in warfighters. In: The 71F Advantage: Applying army research psychology for health and performance gains. Washington D.C.: National Defense University Press; 2010. pp. 261-282

[64] Huisman TA et al. Diffusion tensor imaging as potential biomarker of white matter injury in diffuse axonal injury. American Journal of Neuroradiology. 2004;**25**(3):370-376

[65] Kennis M et al. Treatment outcome-related white matter differences in veterans with posttraumatic stress disorder. Neuropsychopharmacology. 2015;**40**(10):2434

[66] Bierer LM et al. White matter abnormalities in Gulf War veterans

with posttraumatic stress disorder: A pilot study. Psychoneuroendocrinology. 2015;**51**:567-576

[67] Sanjuan PM et al. Reduced white matter integrity in the cingulum and anterior corona radiata in posttraumatic stress disorder in male combat veterans: A diffusion tensor imaging study. Psychiatry Research: Neuroimaging. 2013;**214**(3):260-268

[68] Rosenfeld JV, Ford NL. Bomb blast, mild traumatic brain injury and psychiatric morbidity: A review. Injury. 2010;**41**(5):437-443

[69] Hefner K, Rosenheck R. Multimorbidity among veterans diagnosed with PTSD in the veterans health administration nationally. Psychiatric Quarterly. 2019;**90**(2):275-291

[70] World Health Organization. The ICD-10 Classification of Mental and Behavioural Disorders: Clinical Descriptions and Diagnostic Guidelines. Geneva: World Health Organization; 1992

[71] Blake DD et al. The development of a clinician-administered PTSD scale. Journal of Traumatic Stress. 1995;**8**(1):75-90

[72] Prince C, Bruhns ME. Evaluation and treatment of mild traumatic brain injury: The role of neuropsychology. Brain Sciences. 2017;**7**(8):105

[73] Kar N. Cognitive behavioral therapy for the treatment of post-traumatic stress disorder: A review. Neuropsychiatric Disease and Treatment. 2011;**7**:167

[74] Cicerone KD et al. Evidence-based cognitive rehabilitation: Updated review of the literature from 2003 through 2008. Archives of Physical Medicine and Rehabilitation. 2011;**92**(4):519-530

[75] Warden DL et al. Guidelines for the pharmacologic treatment of neurobehavioral sequelae of traumatic brain injury. Journal of Neurotrauma. 2006;**23**(10):1468-1501

[76] Borg J, Carroll L. Critical evaluation of the existing guidelines on mild traumatic brain injury. Journal of Rehabilitation Medicine. 2004;**43**:106-112

[77] World Health Organization. International Programme on Chemical Safety. Biomarkers in Risk Assessment: Validity and Validation. Geneva: WHO; 2001. p. 2016

[78] World Health Organization. Biomarkers and Risk Assessment: Concepts and Principles-Environmental Health Criteria 155. Geneva: WHO; 1993

[79] Strimbu K, Tavel JA. What are biomarkers? Current Opinion in HIV and AIDS. 2010;**5**(6):463-466

[80] Pan X et al. Salivary cortisol in post-traumatic stress disorder: A systematic review and meta-analysis. BMC Psychiatry. 2018;**18**(1):324-324

[81] Speer KE et al. HPA axis function and diurnal cortisol in post-traumatic stress disorder: A systematic review. Neurobiology of Stress. 2019;**11**: 100180-100180

[82] Geracioti TD et al. CSF norepinephrine concentrations in posttraumatic stress disorder. American Journal of Psychiatry. 2001;**158**(8):1227-1230

[83] Hawk LW et al. Urinary catecholamines and cortisol in recent-onset posttraumatic stress disorder after motor vehicle accidents. Psychosomatic Medicine. 2000;**62**(3):423-434

[84] Murrough JW et al. Reduced amygdala serotonin transporter binding in posttraumatic stress disorder. Biological Psychiatry. 2011;**70**(11):1033-1038

[85] Boscarino JA. Posttraumatic stress disorder and physical illness: Results from clinical and epidemiologic studies. Annals of the New York Academy of Sciences. 2004;**1032**(1):141-153

[86] Maes M et al. Elevated serum interleukin-6 (IL-6) and IL-6 receptor concentrations in posttraumatic stress disorder following accidental man-made traumatic events. Biological Psychiatry. 1999;**45**(7):833-839

[87] Smith AK et al. Differential immune system DNA methylation and cytokine regulation in post-traumatic stress disorder. American journal of medical genetics. Part B: Neuropsychiatric Genetics : The Official Publication of the International Society of Psychiatric Genetics. 2011;**156B**(6):700-708

[88] Spivak B et al. Elevated levels of serum interleukin-1β in combat-related posttraumatic stress disorder. Biological Psychiatry. 1997;**42**(5):345-348

[89] Michopoulos V et al. Association of CRP genetic variation and CRP level with elevated PTSD symptoms and physiological responses in a civilian population with high levels of trauma. The American Journal of Psychiatry. 2015;**172**(4):353-362

[90] Miller RJ et al. C-reactive protein and interleukin6 receptor in post-traumatic stress disorder: A pilot study. Cytokine. 2001;**13**(4):253-255

[91] Plantinga L et al. Association between posttraumatic stress disorder and inflammation: A twin study. Brain, Behavior, and Immunity. 2013;**30**:125-132

[92] Eraly SA et al. Assessment of plasma C-reactive protein as a biomarker of posttraumatic stress disorder risk. JAMA Psychiatry. 2014;**71**(4):423-431

[93] Passos IC et al. Inflammatory markers in post-traumatic stress disorder: A systematic review, meta-analysis, and meta-regression. The Lancet Psychiatry. 2015;**2**(11):1002-1012

[94] Boscarino JA. Diseases among men 20 years after exposure to severe stress. Psychosomatic Medicine. 1997;**59**(6):605-614

[95] Boscarino JA, Chang J. Electrocardiogram abnormalities among men with stress-related psychiatric disorders: Implications for coronary heart disease and clinical research. Annals of Behavioral Medicine. 1999;**21**(3):227-234

[96] Raison CL, Capuron L, Miller AH. Cytokines sing the blues: Inflammation and the pathogenesis of depression. Trends in Immunology. 2006;**27**(1):24-31

[97] Weiss T et al. Posttraumatic stress disorder is a risk factor for metabolic syndrome in an impoverished urban population. General Hospital Psychiatry. 2011;**33**(2):135-142

[98] Wang Q, Shelton RC, Dwivedi Y. Interaction between early-life stress and FKBP5 gene variants in major depressive disorder and post-traumatic stress disorder: A systematic review and meta-analysis. Journal of Affective Disorders. 2018;**225**:422-428

[99] Zhang L et al. PTSD risk is associated with BDNF Val66Met and BDNF overexpression. Molecular Psychiatry. 2013;**19**(1):8-10

[100] Pitts BL et al. BDNF Val66Met polymorphism and posttraumatic

stress symptoms in U.S. military veterans: Protective effect of physical exercise. Psychoneuroendocrinology. 2019;**100**:198-202

[101] Hosang GM et al. Interaction between stress and the BDNF Val66Met polymorphism in depression: A systematic review and meta-analysis. BMC Medicine. 2014;**12**:7-7

[102] Liu L et al. Serotonin transporter 5-HTTLPR genotype is associated with intrusion and avoidance symptoms of DSM-5 posttraumatic stress disorder (PTSD) in Chinese earthquake survivors. Anxiety, Stress, & Coping. 2017;**31**(3):318-327

[103] Kim TY et al. Epigenetic alterations of theBDNFgene in combat-related post-traumatic stress disorder. Acta Psychiatrica Scandinavica. 2016;**135**(2):170-179

[104] Yehuda R et al. Lower methylation of glucocorticoid receptor gene promoter 1F in peripheral blood of veterans with posttraumatic stress disorder. Biological Psychiatry. 2015;**77**(4):356-364

[105] Vukojevic V et al. Epigenetic modification of the glucocorticoid receptor gene is linked to traumatic memory and post-traumatic stress disorder risk in genocide survivors. The Journal of Neuroscience: The Official Journal of the Society for Neuroscience. 2014;**34**(31):10274-10284

[106] Hughes KC, Shin LM. Functional neuroimaging studies of post-traumatic stress disorder. Expert Review of Neurotherapeutics. 2011;**11**(2):275-285

[107] Protopopescu X et al. Differential time courses and specificity of amygdala activity in posttraumatic stress disorder subjects and normal control subjects. Biological Psychiatry. 2005;**57**(5):464-473

[108] Rauch SL et al. Exaggerated amygdala response to masked facial stimuli in posttraumatic stress disorder: A functional MRI study. Biological Psychiatry. 2000;**47**(9):769-776

[109] Shin LM et al. A functional magnetic resonance imaging study of amygdala and medial prefrontal cortex responses to overtly presented fearful faces in posttraumatic stress disorder. Archives of General Psychiatry. 2005;**62**(3):273

[110] Stevens JS et al. Disrupted amygdala-prefrontal functional connectivity in civilian women with posttraumatic stress disorder. Journal of Psychiatric Research. 2013;**47**(10):1469-1478

[111] Etkin A, Wager TD. Functional neuroimaging of anxiety: A meta-analysis of emotional processing in PTSD, social anxiety disorder, and specific phobia. The American Journal of Psychiatry. 2007;**164**(10):1476-1488

[112] Gilbertson MW et al. Smaller hippocampal volume predicts pathologic vulnerability to psychological trauma. Nature Neuroscience. 2002;**5**(11):1242-1247

[113] Admon R, Milad MR, Hendler T. A causal model of post-traumatic stress disorder: Disentangling predisposed from acquired neural abnormalities. Trends in Cognitive Sciences. 2013;**17**(7):337-347

[114] Neylan TC et al. Insomnia severity is associated with a decreased volume of the CA3/dentate gyrus hippocampal subfield. Biological Psychiatry. 2010;**68**(5):494-496

[115] Smith DH, Hicks R, Povlishock JT. Therapy development for diffuse axonal injury. Journal of Neurotrauma. 2013; **30**(5):307-323

[116] Smith DH et al. High tolerance and delayed elastic response of cultured axons to dynamic stretch injury. Journal of Neuroscience. 1999;**19**(11):4263-4269

[117] Wang Y, Mandelkow E. Tau in physiology and pathology. Nature Reviews Neuroscience. 2016;**17**(1):22-35

[118] Choe MC. The pathophysiology of concussion. Current Pain and Headache Reports. 2016;**20**(6):42

[119] Rubenstein R et al. Comparing plasma phospho tau, total tau, and phospho tau–total tau ratio as acute and chronic traumatic brain injury biomarkers. JAMA Neurology. 2017;**74**(9):1063-1072

[120] Kou Z et al. Combining biochemical and imaging markers to improve diagnosis and characterization of mild traumatic brain injury in the acute setting: Results from a pilot study. PLoS One. 2013;**8**(11):e80296

[121] Papa L et al. Serum levels of Ubiquitin C-terminal Hydrolase (UCH-L1) distinguish mild traumatic brain injury (TBI) from trauma controls and are elevated in mild and moderate TBI patients with intracranial lesions and neurosurgical intervention. The Journal of Trauma and Acute Care Surgery. 2012;**72**(5):1335

[122] Puvenna V et al. Significance of ubiquitin carboxy-terminal hydrolase L1 elevations in athletes after sub-concussive head hits. PLoS One. 2014;**9**(5):e96296

[123] Böhmer AE et al. Neuron-specific enolase, S100B, and glial fibrillary acidic protein levels as outcome predictors in patients with severe traumatic brain injury. Neurosurgery. 2011;**68**(6):1624-1631

[124] Chiaretti A et al. NGF, DCX, and NSE upregulation correlates with severity and outcome of head trauma in children. Neurology. 2009;**72**(7):609-616

[125] Ross S et al. Neuron-specific enolase as an aid to outcome prediction in head injury. British Journal of Neurosurgery. 1996;**10**(5):471-476

[126] Zhao J et al. Early expression of serum neutrophil gelatinase-associated lipocalin (NGAL) is associated with neurological severity immediately after traumatic brain injury. Journal of the Neurological Sciences. 2016;**368**:392-398

[127] Marchi N et al. Consequences of repeated blood-brain barrier disruption in football players. PLoS One. 2013;**8**(3):e56805

[128] Shlosberg D et al. Blood–brain barrier breakdown as a therapeutic target in traumatic brain injury. Nature Reviews Neurology. 2010;**6**(7):393-403

[129] Tibbling G, Link H, Öhman S. Principles of albumin and IgG analyses in neurological disorders. I. Establishment of reference values. Scandinavian Journal of Clinical and Laboratory Investigation. 1977;**37**(5):385-390

[130] Zetterberg H, Blennow K. Fluid biomarkers for mild traumatic brain injury and related conditions. Nature Reviews Neurology. 2016;**12**(10):563-574

[131] Zongo D et al. S100-B protein as a screening tool for the early assessment of minor head injury. Annals of Emergency Medicine. 2012;**59**(3):209-218

[132] Neher MD et al. Serum biomarkers for traumatic brain injury. Southern Medical Journal. 2014;**107**(4):248-255

[133] Metting Z et al. GFAP and S100B in the acute phase of mild traumatic brain injury. Neurology. 2012;**78**(18):1428-1433

[134] Pham N et al. Plasma soluble prion protein, a potential biomarker for sport-related concussions: A pilot study. PLoS One. 2015;**10**(2):e0117286

[135] Kochanek PM et al. Screening of biochemical and molecular mechanisms of secondary injury and repair in the brain after experimental blast-induced traumatic brain injury in rats. Journal of Neurotrauma. 2013;**30**(11):920-937

[136] Pham N et al. Primary blast-induced traumatic brain injury in rats leads to increased prion protein in plasma: A potential biomarker for blast-induced traumatic brain injury. Journal of Neurotrauma. 2015;**32**(1):58-65

[137] Persad A et al. Plasma PrPC and ADAM-10 as novel biomarkers for traumatic brain injury and concussion: A pilot study. Brain Injury. 2021:1-8

[138] Goetzl EJ et al. Neuron-derived plasma exosome proteins after remote traumatic brain injury. Journal of Neurotrauma. 2020;**37**(2):382-388

[139] Loane DJ, Byrnes KR. Role of microglia in neurotrauma. Neurotherapeutics : The Journal of the American Society for Experimental NeuroTherapeutics. 2010;**7**(4):366-377

[140] Habgood MD et al. Changes in blood-brain barrier permeability to large and small molecules following traumatic brain injury in mice. European Journal of Neuroscience. 2007;**25**(1):231-238

[141] Shitaka Y et al. Repetitive closed-skull traumatic brain injury in mice causes persistent multifocal axonal injury and microglial reactivity. Journal of Neuropathology and Experimental Neurology. 2011;**70**(7):551-567

[142] Khuman J et al. Tumor necrosis factor alpha and Fas receptor contribute to cognitive deficits independent of cell death after concussive traumatic brain injury in mice. Journal of Cerebral Blood Flow and Metabolism : Official Journal of the International Society of Cerebral Blood Flow and Metabolism. 2011;**31**(2):778-789

[143] Csuka E et al. IL-10 levels in cerebrospinal fluid and serum of patients with severe traumatic brain injury: Relationship to IL-6, TNF-α, TGF-β1 and blood–brain barrier function. Journal of Neuroimmunology. 1999;**101**(2):211-221

[144] Kossmann T et al. Intrathecal and serum interleukin-6 and the acute-phase response in patients with severe traumatic brain injuries. Shock. 1995;**4**(5):311-317

[145] Semple BD et al. Role of CCL2 (MCP-1) in traumatic brain injury (TBI): Evidence from severe TBI patients and CCL2−/− mice. Journal of Cerebral Blood Flow and Metabolism : Official Journal of the International Society of Cerebral Blood Flow and Metabolism. 2010;**30**(4):769-782

[146] Goodman JC et al. Pro-inflammatory and pro-apoptotic elements of the neuroinflammatory response are activated in traumatic brain injury. In: Acta Neurochirurgica Supplements. Vienna: Springer; 2008. pp. 437-439

[147] Buttram SDW et al. Multiplex assessment of cytokine and chemokine levels in cerebrospinal fluid following severe pediatric traumatic brain injury: Effects of moderate hypothermia. Journal of Neurotrauma. 2007;**24**(11):1707-1718

[148] Phillips DJ et al. Activin a release into cerebrospinal fluid in a subset of patients with severe traumatic brain injury. Journal of Neurotrauma. 2006;**23**(9):1283-1294

[149] Kumar RG et al. Acute CSF interleukin-6 trajectories after TBI: Associations with neuroinflammation, polytrauma, and outcome. Brain, Behavior, and Immunity. 2015;**45**:253-262

[150] Csajbok LZ et al. In-hospital C-reactive protein predicts outcome after aneurysmal subarachnoid haemorrhage treated by endovascular coiling. Acta Anaesthesiologica Scandinavica. 2015;**59**(2):255-264

[151] Oliver J et al. Comparison of neurocognitive testing and the measurement of marinobufagenin in mild traumatic brain injury: A preliminary report. Journal of Experimental Neuroscience. 2015;**9**:S27921

[152] DeWitt DS, Prough DS. Traumatic cerebral vascular injury: The effects of concussive brain injury on the cerebral vasculature. Journal of Neurotrauma. 2003;**20**(9):795-825

[153] Jünger EC et al. Cerebral autoregulation following minor head injury. Journal of Neurosurgery. 1997;**86**(3):425-432

[154] Xiong Y, Mahmood A, Chopp M. Animal models of traumatic brain injury. Nature Reviews. Neuroscience. 2013;**14**(2):128-142

[155] Liu C-C et al. Apolipoprotein E and Alzheimer disease: Risk, mechanisms and therapy. Nature Reviews. Neurology. 2013;**9**(2):106-118

[156] Brett BL et al. Traumatic brain injury and risk of neurodegenerative disorder. Biological Psychiatry. 2021;91(5):498-507

[157] Gardner RC, Yaffe K. Epidemiology of mild traumatic brain injury and neurodegenerative disease. Molecular and Cellular Neuroscience. 2015;**66**:75-80

[158] Graham NS, Sharp DJ. Understanding neurodegeneration after traumatic brain injury: From mechanisms to clinical trials in dementia. Journal of Neurology, Neurosurgery & Psychiatry. 2019;**90**(11):1221-1233

[159] Johnson VE et al. Traumatic brain injury as a trigger of neurodegeneration. Neurodegenerative Diseases. 2017:383-400

[160] Lawrence DW et al. The role of apolipoprotein E episilon (ε)-4 allele on outcome following traumatic brain injury: A systematic review. Brain Injury. 2015;**29**(9):1018-1031

[161] Yang S-T et al. Accumulation of amyloid in cognitive impairment after mild traumatic brain injury. Journal of the Neurological Sciences. 2015;**349**(1-2):99-104

[162] Hayes JP et al. BDNF genotype is associated with hippocampal volume in mild traumatic brain injury. Genes, Brain, and Behavior. 2018;**17**(2):107-117

[163] Dretsch MN et al. Brain-derived neurotropic factor polymorphisms, traumatic stress, mild traumatic brain injury, and combat exposure contribute to postdeployment traumatic stress. Brain and Behavior. 2015;**6**(1):e00392-e00392

[164] Wang Y-J et al. The association between BDNF Val66Met polymorphism and emotional symptoms after mild traumatic brain injury. BMC Medical Genetics. 2018;**19**(1):1-7

[165] Narayanan V et al. Missense mutation of brain derived neurotrophic factor (BDNF) alters neurocognitive performance in patients with mild traumatic brain injury: A longitudinal study. PLoS One. 2016;**11**(7):e0158838

[166] Michopoulos V, Norrholm SD, Jovanovic T. Diagnostic biomarkers for

posttraumatic stress disorder: Promising horizons from translational neuroscience research. Biological Psychiatry. 2015;**78**(5):344-353

[167] Dean KR et al. Multi-omic biomarker identification and validation for diagnosing warzone-related post-traumatic stress disorder. Molecular Psychiatry. 2020;**25**(12):3337-3349

[168] Huang M, Risling M, Baker DG. The role of biomarkers and MEG-based imaging markers in the diagnosis of post-traumatic stress disorder and blast-induced mild traumatic brain injury. Psychoneuroendocrinology. 2016;**63**:398-409

[169] Rangaprakash D et al. Compromised hippocampus-striatum pathway as a potential imaging biomarker of mild-traumatic brain injury and posttraumatic stress disorder. Human Brain Mapping. 2017;**38**(6):2843-2864

[170] Ray R. Prediction markets and the financial "Wisdom of Crowds". The Journal of Behavioral Finance. 2006;**7**(1):2-4

Section 2

# New Advances in Aetiology

Chapter 3

# Stress, Microglial Activation, and Mental Disorders

*Shingo Enomoto and Takahiro A. Kato*


## Abstract

Microglia play a major role in immune response in the brain. Recent progress in studies for microglia suggests that stress causes morphological alterations in microglia and affects microglial humoral release and phagocytosis. In this review, we present a molecular mechanism by which stress impacts microglia. Then, we describe current findings for the involvement of microglia in stress-related mental disorders including posttraumatic stress disorder (PTSD), depression, and pain enhancement. We focus on preclinical and clinical studies. Preclinical PTSD studies using animal models with fear memory dysregulation show neuroinflammation by microglia and altered microglial phagocytosis, two imaging studies and a postmortem study assessing neuroinflammation in PTSD patients show contradictory results. Imaging studies suggest neuroinflammation in depressed patients, postmortem studies show no microglial inflammatory changes in non-suicidal depressed patients. Although it has been established that microglia in the spinal cord play a pivotal role in chronic neuropathic pain, several preclinical studies suggest microglia also participate in stress-induced pain. A clinical study with induced microglia-like (iMG) cells and an imaging study indicate neuroinflammation by microglia in fibromyalgia patients. We believe that progress in interactive research between humans and animals elucidates the role of microglia in the pathophysiology of stress-related mental disorders.


**Keywords:** microglia, neuroinflammation, cytokine, neurotrophic factors, phagocytosis, PTSD, depression, pain, animal studies, PET, postmortem studies

## 1. Introduction

Microglia is a glial cell that is widely distributed in the central nervous system occupying 10–15% of cells in the brain. Microglia are derived from the mesoderm as well as blood cells and peripheral immune cells. As other cells in the brain are derived from the ectoderm, microglia are similar in nature to peripheral immune cells and play an important role in immune response in the brain. In the steady-state, microglial protrusions are extended in a tree-shape to monitor the intracerebral environment, but when faced with infection, ischemia, exposure to harmful substances, trauma, etc., they are activated and changes morphologically. Activated microglia have enlarged cell bodies, thickened and shortened protrusions, and become amoebic. Microglia move to the target site and release humoral factors such as cytokines and neurotrophic factors [1]. In addition, microglia have a phagocytic ability similar to peripheral macrophages and have the function of digesting waste products in the brain.

Since 2006, rodent studies that report that stress causes microglial morphological changes in various areas of the brain have been accumulated [2, 3]. It has also been investigated how stress affects the release of cytokines and neurotrophic factors from microglia and the phagocytosis of synapses by microglia. Along with this, imaging studies focusing on microglia have been conducted in humans with stress-related mental disorders. Inflammatory changes in microglia in the human brain can be partially evaluated by positron emission tomography (PET) techniques targeting translocator proteins (TSPO). Depression and posttraumatic stress disorder (PTSD) are representative stress-related psychiatric disorders and are closely associated with suicide. Fibromyalgia is also closely related to stress in its onset and chronicity. Currently, the findings of PET studies targeting TSPO in patients with depression are accumulating, and PET studies targeting patients with PTSD and fibromyalgia have been reported since 2019. A few postmortem studies investigating the association between stress-related mental disorders and microglia have also been conducted.

In this chapter, we first describe the effects of stress on the release of cytokines and neurotrophic factors from microglia and the phagocytosis of synapses by microglia, and their molecular mechanisms. Second, we outline animal and human studies investigating the involvement of microglia in the pathologies of PTSD, depression, suicide, and stress-induced pain.

## 2. Microglia and stress

Some studies have reported that stress promoted the production and release of cytokines by microglia, while others have reported that it suppressed them. It seems to depend on the type and intensity of stress and the brain region where microglia are present. Water immersion restraint stress is a stress paradigm in which mice are confined to a conical tube and then immersed in water to the chest level. Ohgidani et al. reported that a single water immersion restraint stress for 2 h increased the production of tumor necrosis α (TNF-α), an inflammatory mediator, from microglia in the mouse hippocampus [4]. Chronic unpredictable stress (CUS) is a stress paradigm in which multiple stressors are applied daily, including cage rotation, radio noise, food or water deprivation, light on or off all day, single breeding, overcrowding, no bedding, and wet bedding. Wholeb et al. reported that 14-day chronic unpredictable stress reduced the production of TNF-α and interleukin-1β (IL-1β) in microglia in the mouse prefrontal cortex [5].

Increased production of damage-associated molecular patterns (DAMPs) in the brain such as high-mobility group box 1 (HMGB1), heat-shock protein 72 (HSP72), and ATP is a pivotal molecular mechanism by which stress promotes cytokine release from microglia. These DAMPs bind to toll-like receptors (TLRs) on microglial cell membranes to induce nuclear factor-κB (NF-κB) and increase the production of pro-IL-1β, IL-6, and TNF-α. In addition, DAMPs activate nucleotide-binding oligomerization domain, leucine-rich repeat, and pyrin domain protein 3 (NLRP3) inflammasomes in microglia that act on pro-IL-1β processing to increase IL-1β production [6]. Stress activates the hypothalamus-pituitary-adrenal (HPA) axis and sympathetic nerves, then glucocorticoid and noradrenaline increase in the brain. It is proposed that both glucocorticoid and noradrenaline regulate cytokine release from microglia, but their effects on microglia are complex. Glucocorticoid is considered to suppress cytokine release from microglia through suppression of NF-κB. On the other hand, a few studies have shown that administration of glucocorticoid to the hippocampus after inducing inflammation by kainic acid increased inflammatory cytokines and the number of microglia in the hippocampus [7, 8]. CXCR1 and CD200R are receptors that are expressed in microglia and act in a direction that suppresses microglial inflammatory changes. Glucocorticoid promotes inflammatory responses in microglia to future stress by reducing CXCR1 and CD200R expression and increasing HMGB1 release, which is referred microglial priming [6]. Noradrenaline acts on the β-receptor of microglia to promote their activation and stimulate cAMP/protein kinase leading to the release of IL-1β. On the other hand, when noradrenaline acts on the α-receptor of microglia, it works in the direction of suppressing their activation [9].

Brain-derived neurotrophic factor (BDNF), which is released from neurons and microglia, is involved in neurogenesis and neurite branching. It has been reported

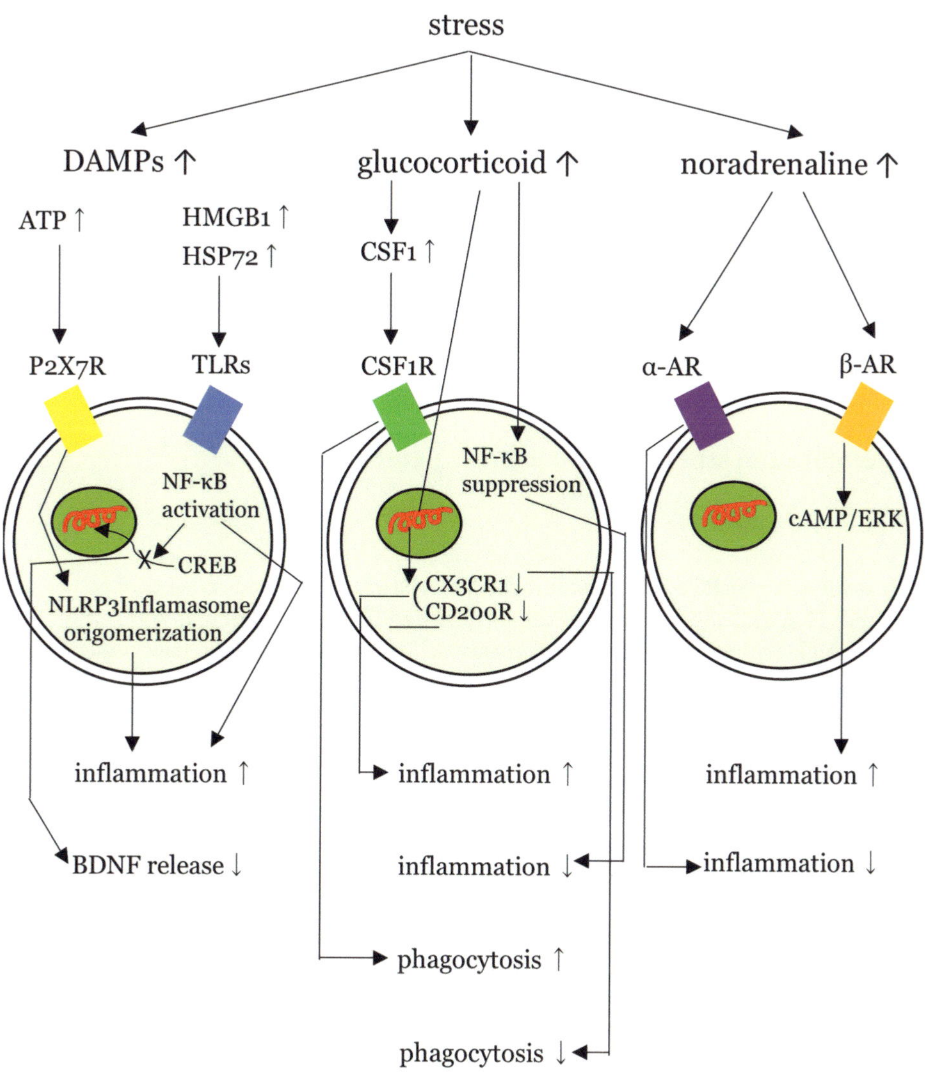


**Figure 1.**
*Schematic of the proposed molecular mechanism by which stress influences microglia.*

that various stress paradigms such as repeated restraint stress and CUS reduce BDNF expression in the hippocampus and prefrontal cortex of rodents [10, 11]. A recent study reported that when CUS was loaded into a rat model of stroke, CUS reduced BDNF release from microglia in the amygdala [12]. One of the possible mechanisms of this microglial-derived BDNF decrease is the decrease in binding of the cAMP response element-binding protein to the promoter region of the BDNF gene due to overactivation of NF-κB [13].

It has recently been suggested that the phagocytic capacity of microglia is also affected by stress. Several studies have reported that 14-day CUS increased the uptake of neuronal structures, including synapses, by microglia in the hippocampus and medial prefrontal cortex [5, 14, 15]. A recent study in which male mice were loaded with CUS extended to 28 days observed no increase of uptake of neuronal structures by microglia at 28-day loading despite an increase at 14-day loading [16]. This result indicates that repeated stress exposure changes microglial function dynamically. In addition to CUS, the effects of restraint stress exposure on microglial phagocytosis have been investigated. Piirainen et al. found that 10-day restraint stress enhanced the phagocytosis of pre-glutamatergic synapses by CD206-positive microglia in the hippocampus and reduced microglial-synaptic contact in the amygdala [17]. In another study with 7-day restraint, stress loading showed increased rat microglial process branching and contacts between microglial processes and synapses, using two-photon microscopy [18]. As a molecular mechanism behind stress-enhanced microglial synaptic phagocytosis, a pathway in which an increase in glucocorticoid enhances phagocytosis via a colony-stimulating factor 1 (CSF1) signal has been reported [15]. Given that CX3CR1 knockout mice were shown to inhibit stress-enhanced microglial phagocytosis [14], CX3CL1/CX3CR1 signaling may also be one of the candidates of the mechanism. We summarize the molecular mechanisms above mentioned in **Figure 1**.

## 3. Microglia and stress-related mental disorders

### 3.1 Microglia and PTSD

Fear memory of PTSD has several characteristics. First, fear extinction is impaired. Fear extinction refers to the diminished fear of a particular traumatic stimulus by learning that it is safe to be exposed to that stimulus. In case measuring the degree of fear extinction in animal experiments, after loading the foot electric shock stimulus in a chamber, researchers repeatedly expose the animal to the chamber or the sound that was heard when the stimulus was applied, without the stimulus, and observe whether the freezing behavior weakens or if it can be maintained once weakened. Lai et al. loaded single prolonged stress (restraint, forced swim, and ether anesthesia) to rats. Then, the authors gave a foot shock stimulus to rats in a specific chamber 7 days later to measure the degree of fear extinction to the chamber at a later date and examined changes in the inflammatory response and microglial cell number. SPS impaired fear extinction and increased the microglial cell number and the expression of HMGB1 and TLR4 in the amygdala. Intra-BLA administration of HMGB1 inhibitor or TLR4 antagonist normalized these behavioral and molecular changes [19]. A separate SPS study reported that the degree of fear extinction was inversely correlated with the number of IL-10 genes, which is anti-inflammatory, expressed by microglia in the prefrontal cortex [20]. Another recent study showed that microglial synaptic phagocytosis in the hippocampal dentate gyrus was enhanced by foot electric shock stimulation, which impaired fear extinction [21].

The second characteristic of PTSD fear memory is an excessive fear generalization. Fear generalization refers to showing fear response to stimuli that are similar to those that remind us of past traumatic experiences. Excessive fear generalization leads to perceiving an inherently neutral stimulus as dangerous and causes unnecessary anxiety and fear. In case measuring the degree of fear generalization in animal experiments, after loading the foot electric shock stimulus in a chamber, researchers put animals in a chamber that is different in color, shape, and odor from those used for electric shock stimulation, and measure the freezing behavior. Nguyen et al. focused on the interaction of neurons and microglia in the hippocampus via the IL-33 signal and investigated the effect of inhibition of that signal on fear generalization. The authors showed that when IL-33 released from neurons acted on the IL-33 receptor (IL1RL1) in microglia, it promoted extracellular matrix phagocytosis by microglia and increased synaptogenesis in the hippocampus, and that fear generalization was enhanced in IL-33 or IL1RL1 conditional knockout mice [22].

If the fear of a particular stimulus diminishes without going through the process of fear extinction, it is defined as forgetting of fear memory. Being not to be able to forget is the third feature of PTSD fear memory [23]. Memories are considered to be stored in engrams, a specific neuronal population. Wang et al. generated mice that express CD55 only in hippocampal engram cells.CD55 is supposed to suppress microglial phagocytosis by inhibiting complement pathways. In these mice, microglial phagocytosis for components of engram cells was reduced and fear forgetting was impaired [24].

The fourth feature of PTSD fear memory is that while the sensory information of the trauma is clearly preserved, the contextual information of when/where/why/how it happened is not well integrated. A protocol of animal experiments was proposed to investigate such characteristics. In the protocol, in an environment where the sound of a specific frequency is regularly generated, an electric foot shock stimulus is given to an animal in a chamber, and after a certain period of time, freezing time is measured for the chamber and the sound, respectively under a condition without a shock stimulus [25]. If the freezing response to sound is enhanced while the response to the chamber is not enhanced, it is considered to capture the fourth feature described above. Although the association between this feature and microglia has not been directly investigated, it was reported that glucocorticoid variability in the hippocampus and norepinephrine variability in the amygdala were associated with this behavioral change. Changes in microglial cytokine release by these stress hormones may be associated with the fourth feature of PTSD fear memory.

Since 2020, imaging studies and postmortem brain studies in PTSD patients have been reported. Bhatt et al. showed that expression of TSPO in the insula and ventromedial prefrontal cortex was reduced in patients with PTSD and suggested that less microglia that release neurotrophic factors might be behind it. In addition, they have genetically analyzed postmortem brain samples from female PTSD patients and found reduced expression of the microglial-related genes TNFRSF14 and TSPOAP1 in addition to TSPO in the prefrontal cortex [26]. Conversely, Deri et al. reported in a similar PET study that the severity of PTSD symptoms was positively correlated with TSPO expression in the hippocampus and prefrontal cortex [27]. We summarize animal, PET, and postmortem studies in **Table 1**.

| **Animal studies** | | | | |
|---|---|---|---|---|
| Stress/manipulation | Behavioral change | Brain region | Cellular and molecular changes | References |
| SPS | Fear extinction ↓ | AMY | Iba1 ↑, TLR 4 ↑, HMGB1 ↑ | |
| /HMGB1 inhibitor or TLR4 antagonist (intra BLA administration) | /Recovery | | /Suppression | [19] |
| SPS | Fear extinction ↓ | PFC | IL10 mRNA in microglia ↓ | [20] |
| Foot shock | Fear extinction ↓ | DG in HIP | Synaptic phagocytosis by microglia ↑ | |
| /CSF1R inhibitor | /Recovery | | /Suppression | [21] |
| Foot shock /IL33 cKO IL1RL 1 cKO | /Fear generalization ↑ | DG in HIP | /Phagocytosis of ECM by microglia ↓ | [22] |
| Foot shock /CD55 expression in only engram cells | /Forgetting of fear ↓ | HIP | /Phagocytosis by microglia for parts of engram cells | [24] |
| **PET with TSPO** | | | | |
| Subjects | Paper type | Brain region | TSPO availability | References |
| PTSD patients | Original article | Insula, VMPFC | Down | [26] |
| PTSD patients | Original article | HIP, PFC | Up | [27] |
| **Postmortem study** | | | | |
| Subjects | Brain region | | Molecular changes | Reference |
| Female PTSD patients | PFC | | TNFRSF14 ↓ TSPOAP1 ↓ TSPO ↓ | [26] |

*AMY, amygdala; PFC, prefrontal cortex; DG, dentate gyrus; HIP, hippocampus; cKO, conditional knockout; ECM, extracellular matrix; VMPFC, ventromedial prefrontal cortex.*

**Table 1.**
*List of papers of microglia and PTSD including animal studies, PET with TSPO, and a post mortem study.*

## 3.2 Microglia, depression, and suicide

CUS, social defeat stress, repeated restraint stress, and social isolation stress are known as stress-induced animal models of depression. In these models, immobility time during forced swimming or when hung upside down is evaluated as an index of depressive symptoms [28]. While many studies report that microglia cause neuroinflammation in these model rodents [29–32], a few studies report reduced production of inflammatory mediators in microglia [5, 21]. However, depressive mood and suicidal ideation, which are important in the clinical setting of depression, are inherently subjective symptoms, and it is difficult to evaluate them from the behavior of model animals. In addition, it is not clear whether the phenomenon of suicide exists in animals other than humans, thus research on humans is indispensable for understanding the pathophysiology of depression and suicide.

Several PET studies using TSPO as a ligand have been conducted in depressed patients, and two systematic reviews have ever been reported. Gritti et al. examined nine original articles and reported that most studies suggested increased TSPO expression in the anterior cingulate gyrus, prefrontal cortex, hippocampal formation, and insula of depressed patients. In addition, the authors suggested treatment with antidepressants and cognitive-behavioral therapy might reduce TSPO expression [33]. Enache et al. performed a meta-analysis on six of the nine original articles above mentioned. The authors concluded that TSPO expression was increased in depressed patients in the anterior cingulate gyrus, prefrontal cortex, temporal lobe, insula, and hippocampus [34].

The results of postmortem brain studies in depressed patients examining microglial changes are mixed. One study showed an increase in the number of Iba-1 positive amoeboid-like microglia in the ventrolateral prefrontal cortex of depressed patients [35], while another study showed that the number of HLA-positive microglia in the amygdala did not change [36]. In the tryptophan-serotonin alternative pathway, the tryptophan-kynurenine pathway, microglia synthesize neurotoxic quinolinic acid. It has ever been reported that quinolinic acid expression is reduced in the hippocampus and ventrolateral prefrontal cortex of depressed patients [35, 37]. Several studies observed microglial changes in the brains of suicide victims. Steiner et al. found increases in HLA-DR-positive microglia in the dorsolateral prefrontal cortex, anterior cingulate gyrus, and mediodorsal thalamus, of suicide victims [38]. On the other hand, Brisch et al. found a decrease in HLA-DR-positive microglia in the dorsal raphe nuclei of non-suicidal depressed patients [39]. Schneider et al. observed an increase in CD68 highly positive microglia in the ventral prefrontal white matter of suicide victims [40]. In another study, the number of IBA-1-positive microglia did not change in the dorsal anterior cingulate gyrus of depressed suicide victims, but microglia in suicide victims had wider cell bodies than control groups [41]. In a recent study, Snijders et al. isolated and extracted microglia from the medial frontal gyrus, superior temporal gyrus, thalamus, and subventricular zone in the postmortem brain of depressed patients, and investigated gene and protein expression changes extensively. No inflammatory changes in microglia were detected in these regions, the expression levels of CX3CR1 and TMEM119 increased, and the expression levels of CD14 and CD163 decreased [42]. The authors hypothesize that these results reflect changes in microglial homeostatic function other than inflammation in depressed patients.

We are conducting reverse translational research to elucidate the dynamics of microglia in depression at the molecular level using the peripheral blood of patients. We performed a blood metabolome/lipidome analysis in patients with first-time depressive episodes who are not receiving medication and found that multiple metabolites in the tryptophan-kynurenine pathway, which are closely associated with microglial activation, correlate with the severity of depressive symptoms and the intensity of suicidal ideation [43]. In a separate study of peripheral blood samples from depressed patients, we evaluated nerve-derived exosomes in blood by the sandwich ELISA (enzyme-linked immune sorbent assay) method and found that IL-34 was increased in the patient group and that synaptophysin and TNF-α correlated with the severity of depression [44]. IL-34 is a cytokine essential for maintaining the function of microglia. We envision a process in which activated microglia damage synapses and lead to the formation of depressive symptoms. Additionally, we are developing our own technology to generate induced microglia-like (iMG) cells from human peripheral blood monocytes and obtained a US patent in 2018. Human iMG cells can be produced in 2 weeks by separating monocytes from the collected human peripheral blood and adding two types of cytokines, granulocyte colony-stimulating factor and IL-34. We analyzed gene profiling patterns of iMG cells from three patients

| **PET with TSPO** | | | | |
|---|---|---|---|---|
| Subject | Paper type | Brain region | TSPO availability | References |
| Depressed patients | Systematic review | ACC, PFC Hippocampal formation, insula | Up | [33] |
| Depressed patients | Systematic review meta-analysis | ACC, PFC, HIP temporal lobe, insula | Up | [34] |
| **Postmortem study** | | | | |
| Subject | | Brain region | Molecular changes | References |
| Depressed patients | | AMY | No change in the number of HLA positive microglia | [36] |
| Suicide victims | | DLPFC, ACC, mediodorsal thalamus | HLA-DR positive microglia ↑ | [38] |
| Depressed suicides | | dACC white matter | Microglia having a wider cell body ↑ | [41] |
| Suicide victims | | Ventral prefrontal white matter | CD68 highly positive microglia ↑ | [40] |
| Depressed patients | | HIP | Quinolinic acid ↓ | [37] |
| Non suicidal depressed patients | | DRN | HLA-DR positive microglia ↓ | [39] |
| Depressed patients | | VLPFC | Iba-1 positive microglia ↑ quinolinic acid ↓ | [35] |
| Subject | | Brain region | Molecular changes | References |
| Depressed patients | | Medial frontal gyrus, superior temporal gyrus, thalamus, subventricular zone | CX3CR1 ↑, TMEM119 ↑ CD163 ↓, CD14 ↓ no change in HLA-DRA, IL6, IL1β | |
| | | | *These are expressions in isolated microglia | [42] |
| **iMG study** | | | | |
| Subject | | | Molecular changes | Reference |
| Depressed state (bipolar patients) | | | CD206 ↑ (compared to manic state) | [45] |

*ACC, anterior cingulate cortex; dACC, dorsal anterior cingulate cortex; PFC, prefrontal cortex; HIP, hippocampus; AMY, amygdala; DLPFC, dorsolateral prefrontal cortex; DRN, dorsal raphe nuclei, VLPFC, ventrolateral prefrontal cortex.*

**Table 2.**
*List of papers of microglia in depression and suicide including PET with TSPO, postmortem studies.*

with rapid cycling bipolar disorder during both manic and depressive states, respectively. We revealed that CD206 gene expression was upregulated in the depressive state compared to the manic state among all three patients [45]. We summarize PET, postmortem, and iMG studies in **Table 2**.

## 3.3 Microglia and stress-induced pain

It has been established that microglia in the dorsal horn of the spinal cord play major roles in the mechanism of chronic neuropathic pain. Activated microglia highly express $P_2X_4$ and $P_2X_7$ receptors, which enhance ATP/$P_2$ receptors signaling and increase IL-1β, TNFα, BDNF release, leading to increased glutamatergic receptor function and decreased GABA receptor function in dorsal horn neurons of the spinal cord. This is the mechanism of chronic neuropathic pain by microglial activation [46].

As a mechanism by which pain is enhanced by stress, changes at the respective levels of the spinal cord and the central nervous system can be considered. Several animal studies have investigated the relationship between stress-induced pain and changes in microglia. Sawacki loaded social defeat stress for 6 days to mice and evaluated pain behavior, gene expressions of inflammatory mediators in the spinal cord. Social defeat stress enhanced mechanical allodynia and increased the number of microglia and expressions of IL-1, TNF, TLR4, CC chemokine ligand2. Selective removal of microglia by CSF-1 inhibitor attenuated these changes [47]. Another series of studies using SPS reported that SPS also enhances mechanical allodynia, increases the number of microglia and expressions of inflammatory mediators in the spinal cord, and induces microglial priming there. Administration of respectively, angiotensin II type 1 receptor antagonist, alpha-7 nicotinic acetylcholine receptor agonist,

| **Animal studies** | | | | |
|---|---|---|---|---|
| Stress/manipulation | Behavioral change | Region | Cellular and molecular change | References |
| Social defeat stress | Allodynia ↑ | Spinal cord | IL-1β ↑, TNF-α ↑, CCL2 ↑ TLR4 ↑ | |
| /CSF1 inhibitor | /Suppression | | /Suppression | [47] |
| SPS | Allodynia ↑ | Spinal cord | Iba1 positive cells ↑ TNF-α ↑, IL-1β ↑, NFκB in microglia ↑, microglial priming ↑ | |
| /α7 nAChR agonist (intrathecal injection) | /Suppression | | /Suppression | [49] |
| /AT1R antagonist (intrathecal injection) | /Suppression | | /Suppression | [48] |
| /GR antagonist | /Suppression | | /Suppression | [50] |
| SPS | Allodynia ↑ | HIP | Iba1 positive cells ↑ TNF-α ↑, IL-1β ↑ | |
| /minocycline (intrahippocampal injection) | /Suppression | | /Suppression | [51] |
| **PET with TSPO** | | | | |
| Subjects | Brain region | | TSPO availability | Reference |
| Fibromyalgia | Anterior and posterior middle cingulate cortices | | Up | [54] |
| **iMG study** | | | | |
| Subject | | | Molecular change | Reference |
| Fibromyalgia patients | | | TNFα release ↑ | [55] |

*HIP, hippocampus.*

**Table 3.**
*List of papers regarding microglia in stress induced pain, which include animal studies, PET with TSPO, and an study with iMG cells.*

and glucocorticoid receptor antagonist were shown to attenuate rat pain sensitivity and inflammatory changes in the spinal cord [48–50]. Thus, these receptors may be involved in the mechanism of stress-induced pain.

Activation of microglia in the central nervous system as well as in the spinal cord may also be involved in stress-induced pain. Intrahippocampal injection of minocycline was shown to normalize SPS-induced hippocampal microglial inflammatory changes and mechanical allodynia [51]. The rostral ventromedial medulla (RVM) is considered to be one of the brain regions that directly project to the dorsal horn of the spinal cord to regulate pain. In pathological pain, serotonin neurons in the RVM are excited to increase serotonin release in the spinal cord. Wei et al. induced postoperative chronic pain in rats by skin/muscle incision and retraction. It caused inflammatory changes in microglia and elevated serotonin levels in the RVM. Inhibiting microglial inflammatory changes in the RVM reduced rat pain sensitivity and serotonin levels in the spinal cord [52]. Given that it has been reported that chronic restraint stress increases serotonin levels in the RVM and increases pain [53], inflammatory changes in microglia in the RVM may be relevant to the stress-induced pain.

Fibromyalgia is characterized by a wide range of pain for a long period of 3 months or more, strong stiffness, and various symptoms such as severe fatigue, insomnia, headache, and depressed mood. Psychosocial stress is related to its onset and chronicity. A PET study targeting TSPO in patients with fibromyalgia was reported in 2019. The expression level of TSPO in the anterior and posterior middle cingulate cortex increased in the patient group and was also correlated with clinical symptoms [54].

In our laboratory, we generated iMG cells from patients with fibromyalgia and investigated the details of their activation at the cellular level. We found that patient-derived iMG cells have an increased ability to release TNF-α and it correlates with the degree of pain [55]. We summarize animal, PET, and iMG studies indicating microglial involvement in stress-induced pain and fibromyalgia in **Table 3**.

## 4. Conclusion

Given that microglia play major roles in brain inflammation and express many receptors for neurotransmitters in addition to stress hormones, we speculate that microglia are deeply involved in the pathophysiology of stress-related psychiatric disorders. In this chapter, we described findings regarding microglia ever obtained from animal and human studies of stress-related psychiatric disorders. The animal study is an indispensable research method for stress-related psychiatric disorders because it can control the type and intensity of stress to be applied and the molecular mechanism related to the pathological condition and therapeutic mechanism can be investigated in detail. There is a limit to extrapolating human higher brain dysfunction from animal behaviors. On the other hand, the greatest advantage of a human-samples study is the ability to capture detailed psychopathological symptoms. There are also drawbacks in human imaging studies, postmortem brain studies, and studies using peripheral blood. Current PET imaging with TSPO ligands can measure only a small portion of microglial changes and has an inadequate resolution. Postmortem brain study is not easy to carry out due to various technical and ethical constraints. It is not clear how far we can infer events in the central nervous system from the results of studies using peripheral blood. It has been shown that human iMG cells made from monocytes in our laboratory share many features with microglia [56, 57]. We expect that iMG cells play a role as a biomarker for psychiatric disorders, and have the potential to reproduce in vitro the dynamics of microglia actually occurring in the brain. We are planning to generate iMG cells in patients with stress-related psychiatric disorders and perform morphological and molecular analysis, and further analyze the correlation with clinical findings such as diagnosis, various test scores, severity. We hope that progress in bidirectional research between animals and humans by making the best use of the strengths of each research method and improving the weaknesses elucidates the role of microglia in stress-related psychiatric disorders and develops treatment targeting them.

## Acknowledgements

Our studies shown in this chapter were partially supported by Grant-in-Aid for Scientific Research on (1) Innovative Areas "Will-Dynamics" of The Ministry of Education, Culture, Sports, Science, and Technology, Japan (JP16H06403 to T.A.K.), (2) The Japan Agency for Medical Research and Development (AMED) (JP19dk0307047 & JP19dk0307075, JP19dm0107095, and JP21wm0425010 to T.A.K.), (3) KAKENHI - the Japan Society for the Promotion of Science ("Wakate A" JP26713039 and "Kiban A" JP18H04042 to T.A.K.) and (4) SENSHIN Medical Research Foundation (to T.A.K.). The funders had no role in study design, data collection and analysis, decision to publish, or preparation of the manuscript.

## Conflict of interest

The authors declare no conflict of interest.

## Author details

Shingo Enomoto[1,2] and Takahiro A. Kato[2*]

1 Self Defense Force, Fukuoka Hospital, Fukuoka, Japan

2 Department of Neuropsychiatry, Graduate School of Medical Sciences, Kyushu University, Fukuoka, Japan

*Address all correspondence to: kato.takahiro.015@m.kyushu-u.ac.jp

## References

[1] Prinz M, Jung S, Priller J. Microglia biology: One century of evolving concepts. Cell. 2019;**179**(2):292-311. DOI: 10.1016/j.cell.2019.08.053

[2] Sugama S, Fujita M, Hashimoto M, Conti B. Stress induced morphological microglial activation in the rodent brain: Involvement of interleukin-18. Neuroscience. 2007;**146**(3):1388-1399. DOI: 10.1016/j.neuroscience.2007.02.043

[3] Tynan RJ, Naicker S, Hinwood M, Nalivaiko E, Buller KM, Pow DV, et al. Chronic stress alters the density and morphology of microglia in a subset of stress-responsive brain regions. Brain, Behavior, and Immunity. 2010;**24**(7):1058-1068. DOI: 10.1016/j.bbi.2010.02.001

[4] Ohgidani M, Kato TA, Sagata N, Hayakawa K, Shimokawa N, Sato-Kasai M, et al. TNF-alpha from hippocampal microglia induces working memory deficits by acute stress in mice. Brain, Behavior, and Immunity. 2016;**55**:17-24. DOI: 10.1016/j.bbi.2015.08.022

[5] Wohleb ES, Terwilliger R, Duman CH, Duman RS. Stress-induced neuronal colony stimulating factor 1 provokes microglia-mediated neuronal remodeling and depressive-like behavior. Biological Psychiatry. 2018;**83**(1):38-49. DOI: 10.1016/j.biopsych.2017.05.026

[6] Johnson JD, Barnard DF, Kulp AC, Mehta DM. Neuroendocrine regulation of brain cytokines after psychological stress. Journal of the Endocrine Society (JES). 2019;**3**(7):1302-1320. DOI: 10.1210/js.2019-00053

[7] MacPherson A, Dinkel K, Sapolsky R. Glucocorticoids worsen excitotoxin-induced expression of pro-inflammatory cytokines in hippocampal cultures. Experimental Neurology. 2005;**194**(2):376-383. DOI: 10.1016/j.expneurol.2005.02.021

[8] Dinkel K, MacPherson A, Sapolsky RM. Novel glucocorticoid effects on acute inflammation in the CNS. Journal of Neurochemistry. 2003;**84**(4):705-716. DOI: 10.1046/j.1471-4159.2003.01604.x

[9] Sugama S, Kakinuma Y. Noradrenaline as a key neurotransmitter in modulating microglial activation in stress response. Neurochemistry International. 2021;**143**:104943. DOI: 10.1016/j.neuint.2020.104943

[10] Bath KG, Schilit A, Lee FS. Stress effects on BDNF expression: Effects of age, sex, and form of stress. Neuroscience. 2013;**239**:149-156. DOI: 10.1016/j.neuroscience.2013.01.074

[11] Fanous S, Hammer RP Jr, Nikulina EM. Short- and long-term effects of intermittent social defeat stress on brain-derived neurotrophic factor expression in mesocorticolimbic brain regions. Neuroscience. 2010;**167**(3):598-607. DOI: 10.1016/j.neuroscience.2010.02.064

[12] Zhu HX, Cheng LJ, Ou Yang RW, Li YY, Liu J, Dai D, et al. Reduced amygdala microglial expression of brain-derived neurotrophic factor and tyrosine kinase receptor B (TrkB) in a rat model of poststroke depression. Medical Science Monitor. 2020;**26**:e926323. DOI: 10.12659/MSM.926323

[13] Zou J, Crews F. CREB and NF-kappaB transcription factors regulate sensitivity to excitotoxic and oxidative

stress induced neuronal cell death. Cellular and Molecular Neurobiology. 2006;**26**(4-6):385-405. DOI: 10.1007/s10571-006-9045-9

[14] Milior G, Lecours C, Samson L, Bisht K, Poggini S, Pagani F, et al. Fractalkine receptor deficiency impairs microglial and neuronal responsiveness to chronic stress. Brain, Behavior, and Immunity. 2016;**55**:114-125. DOI: 10.1016/j.bbi.2015.07.024

[15] Horchar MJ, Wohleb ES. Glucocorticoid receptor antagonism prevents microglia-mediated neuronal remodeling and behavioral despair following chronic unpredictable stress. Brain, Behavior, and Immunity. 2019;**81**:329-340. DOI: 10.1016/j.bbi.2019.06.030

[16] Woodburn SC, Bollinger JL, Wohleb ES. Synaptic and behavioral effects of chronic stress are linked to dynamic and sex-specific changes in microglia function and astrocyte dystrophy. Neurobiology of Stress. 2021;**14**:100312. DOI: 10.1016/j.ynstr.2021.100312

[17] Piirainen S, Chithanathan K, Bisht K, Piirsalu M, Savage JC, Tremblay ME, et al. Microglia contribute to social behavioral adaptation to chronic stress. Glia. 2021;**69**(10):2459-2473. DOI: 10.1002/glia.24053

[18] Liu T, Lu J, Lukasiewicz K, Pan B, Zuo Y. Stress induces microglia-associated synaptic circuit alterations in the dorsomedial prefrontal cortex. Neurobiology of Stress. 2021;**15**:100342. DOI: 10.1016/j.ynstr.2021.100342

[19] Lai S, Wu G, Jiang Z. Glycyrrhizin treatment facilitates extinction of conditioned fear responses after a single prolonged stress exposure in rats. Cellular Physiology and Biochemistry. 2018;**45**(6):2529-2539. DOI: 10.1159/000488271

[20] Cotrone TS, Hocog CB, Ramsey JT, Sanchez MA, Sullivan HM, Scrimgeour AG. Phenotypic characterization of frontal cortex microglia in a rat model of post-traumatic stress disorder. Brain and Behavior: A Cognitive Neuroscience Perspective. 2021;**11**(3):e02011. DOI: 10.1159/000488271

[21] Cui X, Zhou S, Xia G, Chen J, Jiang L, Huang J, et al. A multispecies probiotic accelerates fear extinction and inhibits relapse in mice: Role of microglia. Neuropharmacology. 2021;**193**:108613

[22] Nguyen PT, Dorman LC, Pan S, Vainchtein ID, Han RT, Nakao-Inoue H, et al. Microglial remodeling of the extracellular matrix promotes synapse plasticity. Cell. 2020;**182**(2):388-403. DOI: 10.1016/j.cell.2020.05.050

[23] Brewin CR. The nature and significance of memory disturbance in posttraumatic stress disorder. Annual Review of Clinical Psychology. 2011;**7**:203-227. DOI: 10.1146/annurev-clinpsy-032210-104544

[24] Wang C, Yue H, Hu Z, Shen Y, Ma J, Li J, et al. Microglia mediate forgetting via complement-dependent synaptic elimination. Science. 2020;**367**(6478):688-694. DOI: 10.1126/science.aaz2288

[25] Al Abed AS, Sellami A, Ducourneau EG, Bouarab C, Marighetto A, Desmedt A. Protocols to induce, prevent, and treat post-traumatic stress disorder-like memory in mice: Optogenetics and behavioral approaches. Bio-protocol. 2021;**11**(19):e4174. DOI: 10.21769/BioProtoc.4174

[26] Bhatt S, Hillmer AT, Girgenti MJ, Rusowicz A, Kapinos M, Nabulsi N, et al.

PTSD is associated with neuroimmune suppression: Evidence from PET imaging and postmortem transcriptomic studies. Nature Communications. 2020;**11**(1):2360. DOI: 10.1038/s41467-020-15930-5

[27] Deri Y, Clouston SAP, DeLorenzo C, Gardus JD 3rd, Bartlett EA, Santiago-Michels S, et al. Neuroinflammation in world trade center responders at midlife: A pilot study using [18 F]-FEPPA PET imaging. Brain, Behavior, and Immunity - Health (BBI - Health). 2021;**16**:100287. DOI: 10.1016/j.bbih.2021.100287

[28] Becker M, Pinhasov A, Ornoy A. Animal models of depression: What can they teach us about the human disease? Diagnostics (Basel). 2021;**11**(1):123. DOI: 10.3390/diagnostics11010123

[29] Nozaki K, Ito H, Ohgidani M, Yamawaki Y, Sahin EH, Kitajima T, et al. Antidepressant effect of the translocator protein antagonist ONO-2952 on mouse behaviors under chronic social defeat stress. Neuropharmacology. 2020;**162**:107835. DOI: 10.1016/j.neuropharm.2019.107835

[30] Liu HY, Yue J, Hu LN, Cheng LF, Wang XS, Wang XJ, et al. Chronic minocycline treatment reduces the anxiety-like behaviors induced by repeated restraint stress through modulating neuroinflammation. Brain Research Bulletin. 2018;**143**:19-26. DOI: 10.1016/j.brainresbull.2018.08.015

[31] Niu L, Luo SS, Xu Y, Wang Z, Luo D, Yang H, et al. The critical role of the hippocampal NLRP3 inflammasome in social isolation-induced cognitive impairment in male mice. Neurobiology of Learning and Memory. 2020;**175**:107301. DOI: 10.1016/j.nlm.2020.107301

[32] Duan CM, Zhang JR, Wan TF, Wang Y, Chen HS, Liu L. SRT2104 attenuates chronic unpredictable mild stress-induced depressive-like behaviors and imbalance between microglial M1 and M2 phenotypes in the mice. Behavioural Brain Research. 2020;**378**:112296. DOI: 10.1016/j.bbr.2019.112296

[33] Gritti D, Delvecchio G, Ferro A, Bressi C, Brambilla P. Neuroinflammation in major depressive disorder: A review of PET imaging studies examining the 18-kDa translocator protein. Journal of Affective Disorders. 2021;**292**:642-651. DOI: 10.1016/j.jad.2021.06.001

[34] Enache D, Pariante CM, Mondelli V. Markers of central inflammation in major depressive disorder: A systematic review and meta-analysis of studies examining cerebrospinal fluid, positron emission tomography and post-mortem brain tissue. Brain, Behavior, and Immunity. 2019;**81**:24-40. DOI: 10.1016/j.bbi.2019.06.015

[35] Clark SM, Pocivavsek A, Nicholson JD, Notarangelo FM, Langenberg P, McMahon RP, et al. Reduced kynurenine pathway metabolism and cytokine expression in the prefrontal cortex of depressed individuals. Journal of Psychiatry & Neuroscience. 2016;**41**(6):386-394. DOI: 10.1503/jpn.150226

[36] Hamidi M, Drevets WC, Price JL. Glial reduction in amygdala in major depressive disorder is due to oligodendrocytes. Biological Psychiatry. 2004;**55**(6):563-569. DOI: 10.1016/j.biopsych.2003.11.006

[37] Busse M, Busse S, Myint AM, Gos T, Dobrowolny H, Muller UJ, et al. Decreased quinolinic acid in the hippocampus of depressive patients: Evidence for local anti-inflammatory and

neuroprotective responses? European Archives of Psychiatry and Clinical Neuroscience. 2015;**265**(4):321-329. DOI: 10.1007/s00406-014-0562-0

[38] Steiner J, Bielau H, Brisch R, Danos P, Ullrich O, Mawrin C, et al. Immunological aspects in the neurobiology of suicide: Elevated microglial density in schizophrenia and depression is associated with suicide. Journal of Psychiatric Research. 2008;**42**(2):151-157. DOI: 10.1016/j.jpsychires.2006.10.013

[39] Brisch R, Steiner J, Mawrin C, Krzyzanowska M, Jankowski Z, Gos T. Microglia in the dorsal raphe nucleus plays a potential role in both suicide facilitation and prevention in affective disorders. European Archives of Psychiatry and Clinical Neuroscience. 2017;**267**(5):403-415. DOI: 10.1007/s00406-017-0774-1

[40] Schnieder TP, Trencevska I, Rosoklija G, Stankov A, Mann JJ, Smiley J, et al. Microglia of prefrontal white matter in suicide. Journal of Neuropathology and Experimental Neurology. 2014;**73**(9):880-890. DOI: 10.1097/NEN.0000000000000107

[41] Torres-Platas SG, Cruceanu C, Chen GG, Turecki G, Mechawar N. Evidence for increased microglial priming and macrophage recruitment in the dorsal anterior cingulate white matter of depressed suicides. Brain, Behavior, and Immunity. 2014;**42**:50-59. DOI: 10.1016/j.bbi.2014.05.007

[42] Snijders G, Sneeboer MAM, Fernandez-Andreu A, Udine E, et al. Distinct non-inflammatory signature of microglia in post-mortem brain tissue of patients with major depressive disorder. Molecular Psychiatry. 2021;**26**(7):3336-3349. DOI: 10.1038/s41380-020-00896-z

[43] Setoyama D, Kato TA, Hashimoto R, Kunugi H, Hattori K, Hayakawa K, et al. Plasma metabolites predict severity of depression and suicidal ideation in psychiatric patients-a multicenter pilot analysis. PLoS One. 2016;**11**(12):e0165267. DOI: 10.1371/journal.pone.0165267

[44] Kuwano N, Kato TA, Mitsuhashi M, Sato-Kasai M, Shimokawa N, Hayakawa K, et al. Neuron-related blood inflammatory markers as an objective evaluation tool for major depressive disorder: An exploratory pilot case-control study. Journal of Affective Disorders. 2018;**240**:88-98. DOI: 10.1016/j.jad.2018.07.040

[45] Ohgidani M, Kato TA, Haraguchi Y, Matsushima T, Mizoguchi Y, Murakawa-Hirachi T, et al. Microglial CD206 gene has potential as a state marker of bipolar disorder. Frontiers in Immunology. 2017;7:676. DOI: 10.3389/fimmu.2016.00676

[46] Inoue K, Tsuda M. Microglia in neuropathic pain: Cellular and molecular mechanisms and therapeutic potential nature reviews. Neuroscience. 2018;**19**(3):138-152

[47] Sawicki CM, Kim JK, Weber MD, Faw TD, McKim DB, Madalena KM, et al. Microglia promote increased pain behavior through enhanced inflammation in the spinal cord during repeated social defeat stress. The Journal of Neuroscience. 2019;**39**(7):1139-1149. DOI: 10.1523/JNEUROSCI.2785-18.2018

[48] Hong Y, Wu W, Wang S, Hao Q, Zheng H, Li S, et al. Angiotensin II type 1 receptor blockade attenuates posttraumatic stress disorder-related chronic pain by inhibiting glial activation in the spinal cord. Neuropharmacology. 2021;**196**:108704. DOI: 10.1016/j.neuropharm.2021.108704

[49] Sun R, Liu Y, Hou B, Lei Y, Bo J, Zhang W, et al. Perioperative activation of spinal alpha7 nAChR promotes recovery from preoperative stress-induced prolongation of postsurgical pain. Brain, Behavior, and Immunity. 2019;**79**:294-308. DOI: 10.1016/j.bbi.2019.02.017

[50] Sun R, Zhao Z, Feng J, Bo J, Rong H, Lei Y, et al. Glucocorticoid-potentiated spinal microglia activation contributes to preoperative anxiety-induced postoperative hyperalgesia. Molecular Neurobiology. 2017;**54**(6):4316-4328. DOI: 10.1007/s12035-016-9976-1

[51] Sun R, Zhang Z, Lei Y, Liu Y, Lu C, Rong H, et al. Hippocampal activation of microglia may underlie the shared neurobiology of comorbid posttraumatic stress disorder and chronic pain. Molecular Pain. 2016;**12**:1744806916679166. DOI: 10.1177/1744806916679166

[52] Wang W, Zhong X, Li Y, Guo R, Du S, Wen L, et al. Rostral ventromedial medulla-mediated descending facilitation following P2X7 receptor activation is involved in the development of chronic post-operative pain. Journal of Neurochemistry. 2019;**149**(6):760-780. DOI: 10.1111/jnc.14650

[53] Imbe H, Murakami S, Okamoto K, Iwai-Liao Y, Senba E. The effects of acute and chronic restraint stress on activation of ERK in the rostral ventromedial medulla and locus coeruleus. Pain. 2004;**112**(3):361-371. DOI: 10.1016/j.pain.2004.09.015

[54] Albrecht DS, Forsberg A, Sandstrom A, Bergan C, Kadetoff D, Protsenko E, et al. Brain glial activation in fibromyalgia - a multi-site positron emission tomography investigation. Brain, Behavior, and Immunity. 2019;**75**:72-83. DOI: 10.1016/j.bbi.2018.09.018

[55] Ohgidani M, Kato TA, Hosoi M, Tsuda M, Hayakawa K, Hayaki C, et al. Fibromyalgia and microglial TNF-alpha: Translational research using human blood induced microglia-like cells. Scientific Reports. 2017;7(1):11882. DOI: 10.1038/s41598-017-11506-4

[56] Banerjee A, Lu Y, Do K, Mize T, Wu X, Chen X, et al. Validation of induced microglia-like cells (iMG cells) for future studies of brain diseases. Frontiers in Cellular Neuroscience. 2021;**15**:629279. DOI: 10.3389/fncel.2021.629279

[57] Tanaka S, Ohgidani M, Hata N, Inamine S, Sagata N, Shirouzu N, et al. CD206 expression in induced microglia-like cells from peripheral blood as a surrogate biomarker for the specific immune microenvironment of neurosurgical diseases including glioma. Frontiers in Immunology. 2021;**12**:670131. DOI: 10.3389/fimmu.2021.670131

Chapter 4

# Stress-induced Anger and Hypertension: An Evaluation of the Effects of Homeopathic Treatment

*Leena S. Bagadia and Arun More*


## Abstract

Excessive pressure or demand on an individual resulting in adverse reaction affecting mentally and physically is termed "stress." Chronic stress has been assumed as a risk factor for hypertension which constitutes an important public health issue. According to the latest data, it affects 30% of the world population. Hypertension (HTN) rates are not decreasing despite improved detection and treatments. People experiencing increased anger, anxiety, depression brought on by globalization, and stress leading to high-risk behaviors are increasing many folds. There is the possibility that blood pressure (BP) may positively correlate with anger variables leading to essential hypertension (EHT). Homeopathy considers the human being having an integrated mind and body. It works holistically, helping the patient cope with environmental and psychosocial changes. The following research is one such example. It was conducted on 172 patients (108 males and 64 females) randomized and divided into intervention and control groups. The intervention group was administered individualized homeopathic treatment. We found that most EHT patients, especially those with a family history of HTN, suppress their anger and hostile impulses. Most appropriate homoeopathic medicine lessens anger and thereby has a reduction in elevated BP. Also, it relieves associated ailments.


**Keywords:** essential hypertension, anger-state, trait, STAXI-2

## 1. Introduction

Despite the common acceptance that psychological stress causes disease, the biomedical populace remains skeptical of this outcome. Stress contributes to many disease processes. Exposures to chronic stress are considered the most deleterious as it leads to everlasting distortion in the emotional, physiological, and behavioral reverberation that accelerates susceptibility to and course of disease like essential hypertension. It is now well established that the total variability in the aetiology of HTN cannot be solely explained by physiological, genetic, and lifestyle factors. Several physiological and behavioural mechanisms are suggested to explain the link between psychological stress, hypertension, and cardiovascular diseases (CVD). The hypothalamus–pituitary–adrenal axis and the sympathetic nervous system are activated by psychological stress, due to which hemodynamic and hormonal responses are generated [1]. Mimicking chronic stress by experimentally elevating glucocorticoids within the brain produces enhanced adrenocorticotropic hormone (ACTH) responses [2]. It increases both baseline arterial blood pressure [3] and blood pressure and heart responses to an acute novel stressor [4], as seen in many animal studies. There is a vast body of documentation to support the role of psychosocial factors as the primary risk for HTN [5–7]. As a result, national HTN guidelines recommend psychosocial intervention as a means to prevent or delay the onset of HTN [8–10].

Hypertension (HTN) is a rapidly pervasive condition observed in different parts of the world. It brings about a variety of chronic conditions in the human body [11] without apparently noticeable symptoms and hence is often called a silent killer [12]. It affects the overall body functioning and human life in various ways. Untreated patients with HTN have an average life expectancy between 50 and 60 years, compared with 71 years for the population at large.

What causes essential hypertension is still unknown. The intensity and duration of exposure to chronic stressors are presumed to be important determinants of risk. Effects of acute stressors on blood pressure (BP) have been demonstrated, but ongoing exposure to stress may be more plausibly linked to sustained BP elevations and hypertension incidence [5]. The effects of chronic stress in several domains are being investigated, including work-related stress, relationship stress, low socioeconomic status (SES). The adrenal gland is a major site that coordinates the stress response via the hypothalamic-pituitary–adrenal axis and the sympathetic-adrenal system. There is a fight or flight response to the stress stimulus. Due to which catecholamines are released from the adrenal medulla, they function in the neurohormonal regulation of blood pressure and have a well-established link to hypertension.

The psychological status of an individual greatly affects his physical condition. Hypertension is among the seven psychosomatic diseases for which mental aetiologies were proposed in the 1950s [13]. Studies conducted during the last decade have reported significant relationships between HT and psychological factors such as anger, anxiety, and depression. Usually, as individuals experience stress, they activate the sympathetic nervous system and the hypothalamic-pituitary–adrenal–cortical axis system. As a result of this activation, catecholamines (e.g., epinephrine and norepinephrine) and glucocorticoids (e.g., cortisol) are released, contributing to increases in blood pressure and heart rate [14]. Although the exact mechanism that explains the relationship between cardiovascular reactivity (CVR) and high blood pressure (and the subsequent development of coronary artery disease) is still under debate, research has focused on releasing catecholamines and glucocorticoids [15]. Early research in this field investigated trait anger and whether it was related to overall increased physiological reactivity [14]. These researchers assumed physiological reactivity was a person-based trait associated with a constellation of emotional, cognitive, and behavioural anger reactions. Anger could contribute to the elevation of BP directly through the psychophysiological activation and indirectly by facilitating the emergence of a coping style that contributes to the maintenance of elevated BP [16–18].

Also, anger and hostility are associated with adverse lifestyle behaviour, such as excess alcohol consumption and smoking, higher BMI values, and increased total energy intake [19], which are recognized as critical behavioural risk factors for HT and cardiovascular diseases.

## 2. Risk factors for hypertension

### 2.1 Non-modifiable

#### *2.1.1 Age*

The prevalence of hypertension is reported to increase with age linearly [20–22].

#### *2.1.2 Genetic*

Positive family history is commonly found in hypertensive patients, with the heritability varying between 35% and 50% in most studies [17, 23]. Family history of hypertension doubles the risk of developing hypertension [24] independent of other risk factors, such as weight, age, and smoking status.

#### *2.1.3 Gender*

Gender is also a critical social determinant of Health to which global forums have increasingly drawn attention. Gender encompasses various practices, beliefs, roles, opportunities, and constraints, shaping men's and women's Health differently. In both men and women, the subjective experience of psychophysiological wellbeing significantly correlates with cardiovascular risk factors [25]. It seems that men must defend their status more often than women. The effects of job strain on BP tend to be stronger among men than women [26].

### 2.2 Modifiable

#### *2.2.1 Behavioural*

Excess alcohol consumption and smoking, higher BMI values, and increased total energy intake [19] are recognized as critical behavioural risk factors for HT.

#### *2.2.2 Deprivation and socioeconomic status*

Epidemiologic studies consistently demonstrate graded associations between SES and risk of hypertension, cardiovascular disease, and mortality [27–29]. Low SES is associated with hypertension-related BP patterns, including reduced nocturnal BP dipping [24] and delayed BP recovery following laboratory stress [30].

#### *2.2.3 Type of job*

Employed men are healthier than their unemployed counterparts even after adjusting for low income and low educational attainment [31]. The same holds for women [32], although employment does not affect all women in the same way [33].

#### *2.2.4 Job strain*

Psychosocial stress was defined under four domains: social, work, financial, and environment. Women and young adults reported higher psychological stress levels,

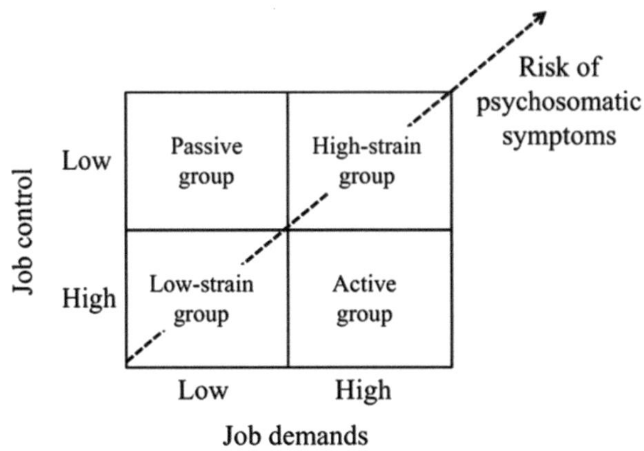


**Figure 1.**
*Karasek job strain model.*

particularly at work, which raised age-and sex-related job strain issues with high demand and low control (**Figure 1**) [34, 35].

Modifying effect of suppressed anger on the relationship between job stress and hypertension were studied by Cottington et al. [36], and they found that high blood pressure was markedly associated with self-reporting of ambiguous job future, disappointment with colleagues, and advancements in ranks among employees who suppress their anger. These findings advocate that anger expression, a coping mechanism, maybe an important factor that can modify the relation between occupational stress and essential hypertension.

## 3. Anger

Anger is the most basic emotion varying from mild irritation to intense fury in response to feeling threatened or hurt.

It has three components:

- Physical – fight or flight response.
- Cognitive – angry thoughts.
- Behavioural – anger expressed verbally, physically, or just withdrawal.

Unfortunately, anger is also poorly understood in current diagnostic practices. For example, in DSM V, there are no Axis I disorders that directly address the emotion of anger, unlike anxiety and mood disorders.

Anger as such is a natural emotion, but if it increases, it can cause devastating effects upon the body and most conspicuously upon the heart [37]. It is observed that healthy persons may also occasionally have a conspicuous boost in their blood pressure occasionally when they are angry [38, 39] explain that anger is an arousing state with feelings varying from slight irritation to intense fury or rage. It is reported that anger-arousing situations also become an important contributing factor for increased blood pressure [17]. Historically, its roots back to 1939, when Alexander

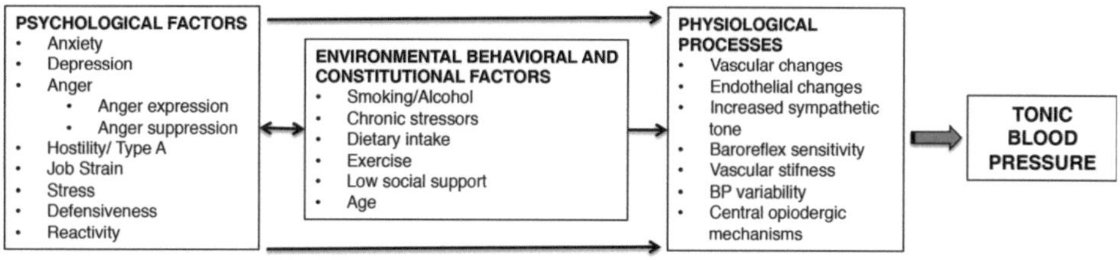


**Figure 2.**
*Proposed biological and behavioral pathways linking psychological factors to an increased risk of incident essential hypertension [41].*

identified the suppression of anger as a major cause of HTN and further investigated its lethal outcomes in the human body. The reactivity hypothesis describes that individuals prone to HTN react to environmental stress with intense anger [23]. In an earlier study on people with HTN [24] reports that blood pressure rises remarkably during anger states. The association of anger with HTN has been confirmed by many researchers [40, 41], and is a well-established risk factor for CHD [40, 42] further augmenting the association between HTN and cardiovascular diseases.

Anger is an important variable in essential hypertension. Cardiovascular reactivity to stress in which a recurrent pattern of exaggerated sympathetic nervous system activity is proposed to up-regulate basal blood pressure levels over time.

The neurohormonal model shows that psychological characteristics may predispose to CVR and hypertension development by altering the central nervous system control of baroreceptor function, opioid activity, and neurotransmitter levels. Unresolvable anger causes prolonged sympathetic nervous system over-activity. Anxiety and guilt of consequences of expressing anger results in suppression of anger. In vulnerable individuals, neural mediation of repetitive high BP episodes causes structural adjustments in arterioles culminating in sustained hypertension. Anger could be contributing to the elevation of BP directly through psychophysiological activation via the HPA axis and indirectly by facilitating the emergence of a coping style that contributes to the maintenance of elevated BP (**Figure 2**).

According to Addotta [43] anger comes from the reptilian part of our body, known as the amygdala, an almond-shaped structure located just above the hypothalamus, one on each side. They consist of several nerves connected to various parts of the brain, such as the neocortex and the visual cortex. Amygdala is an excellent indicator of threats. Its primary purpose is emotional and social processing. One can react to a threat before the prefrontal cortex, responsible for the brain's thoughts and judgments, can assess the rationality of the reaction. The amygdala is responsible for the brain to react to a threat or fear before the prefrontal cortex can consider the consequences. Resilient people can make rapid recoveries from stress, with their prefrontal cortex working to calm the amygdala. However, the brain cannot release itself out of an emotional rut; and, the body is flooded with the cascade of cortisol or stress hormones ("Effects of Anger,", para. 18).

Before one feels anger, a primary emotion is felt. It can be a feeling of fear, offense, disrespect, force, entrapment, or pressure. When the primary emotions become too intense, the secondary emotion of anger is experienced.

In some cases, minor irritation can trigger full-blown anger within a shorter period. According to Dr. Sietse d Boer of the University of Groningen, "serotonin deficiency appears to be related to pathological, violent forms of aggressiveness, but not to the normal aggressive behaviour that animals and humans use to adapt to everyday survival" (as cited in Society for Neuroscience, 2007, para. 19).

Anger can assemble psychological resources for corrective action. Uncontrolled anger can negatively affect personal and social wellbeing. Many philosophers and writers have cautioned against the spontaneous, wild fits of rage, but they disagree on anger's intrinsic value. Coping with anger has been addressed in the writings of the earliest philosophers up to modern times. Most notable being Bhagvad Geeta in its Chapter 2, Verse 63, says:

क्रोधाद्भवति सम्मोहः सम्मोहात्स्मृतिविभ्रमः |स्मृतिभ्रंशाद् बुद्धिनाशो बुद्धिनाशात्\ ्रणश्यति|| Meaning: Anger distorts thought & perception leading to errors in reasoning which results in damage & destruction [44].

Modern psychologists and psychiatrists have also pointed out the harmful effects of suppressing anger.

Anger is a predominant feeling expressed behaviorally, cognitively, and physiologically when a person consciously chooses to stop the threatening behaviour of another outside force immediately [45].

## 3.1 Concept and assessment of anger

Anger is a universal emotion. It has long been recognized as a significant constituent of human life since long. Individuals face many problems in their daily lives and solve them [46]. While solving these problems, they exhibit different emotional and behavioral reactions, and anger is one of them. Anger is one of the basic emotions felt by almost everyone at times. Simultaneously, it can be suggested that it is one of the most interesting and least understood feelings [47].

Kassinove and Tafrate [48] asserted that anger is often a learned emotion. They believe that anger is partly an inborn quality but mostly modeled from family and the surrounding environment. However, people learn from the social environment about what and when they will get angry and the kind of behaviors they will exhibit [49–52].

Anger is a multidimensional construct that consists of physiological (general sympathetic arousal, hormone/neurotransmitter function), cognitive (irrational beliefs, automatic thoughts, inflammatory imagery), phenomenological (subjective awareness and labeling of angry feelings), and behavioral (facial expressions, verbal/behavioral anger expression strategies) variables [53–55]

## 3.2 Anger expression/anger subcategories

Spielberger et al. [56] stated that the expression of anger must be distinguished conceptually and empirically from the experience of anger as an emotional state (S-anger) and individual differences in anger as a personality trait (T-anger).

- Anger-In (AX-In): mean anger held in or suppression of angry feelings.
- Anger-Out (AX-O): this is defined as the frequency at which angry feelings are expressed in verbally or physically aggressive behavior.
- Anger Control (AX-Con): this refers to attempts to control and suppress or mitigate anger expression.

## 4. Mode of action of homoeopathic medicine

Homeopathy is an over 226-year-old system of complementary and alternative medicine (CAM) developed by the German physician Samuel Hahnemann, MD. This mode of healing is based on distinct principles, comprehensive case history-based clinical findings], noteworthy patient contentment, and an expanding contemporary research database. It deals with the patient holistically and looks at the patient's ailment as a multicausative phenomenon. Dynamic forces that derail need dynamic intervention, and homeopathy provides a solution. It focuses on the patient with hypertension rather than on hypertension itself.

### 4.1 Essential principles of classical homeopathy

1. Potentially therapeutic substances must be tested carefully in healthy subjects in order to document their 'pure', direct effects on physical as well as mental sphere; this is the basis of the medical matter.

2. The remedy capable of causing a similar state in a healthy subject causes a counter-reaction in a patient that is stronger than the pathological stimulus of the disease itself.

3. The disease must be studied as a whole (and not only in terms of its main symptom or pathology but also the state of mind it causes in an individual) in order to ensure that it and the drug interact in a global manner; the choice of the remedy must be based on the complex of individual symptoms rather than on the name of the disease and the organ or system affected.

4. The dose must be the minimal effective dose and therefore adjusted on the basis of individual sensitivity.

The original method of preparing homeopathic medicines comprises trituration in lactose and/or serial dilution in ethanol–water solutions and succession (vigorous replicated cycles of pounding by hand or standardized mechanical arm pounding on a hard surface) in glass vials containing ethanol–water solutions [37]. This generates "top–down" nanoparticles of the source material. Nanoparticles range in size from 1 nanometer (nm) on a side up to 1000 nm or more. Thus, insoluble substances were converted into effective remedial agents for the first time in the history of western medicine. He also observed that as these potentization methods ascend the scale, the capacity of the drug to produce mental symptoms increased. By potentization, the drug energy is released in a form best suited to restoring the lost harmony through the use of a similar force. The physico-chemical effects of the remedy cease, and it acts at the dynamic level where it follows the rules applicable to the field of dynamics.

The action of homoeopathic remedy on a living organism (**Figure 3**) [57]

Fundamental research in basic science indicates that authentically-prepared homeopathic medicines:

A. contain calculable source nanoparticles (NPs) and/or silica nanoparticles with adsorbed original materials [57–60], which are compositely dispersed in colloidal solution;

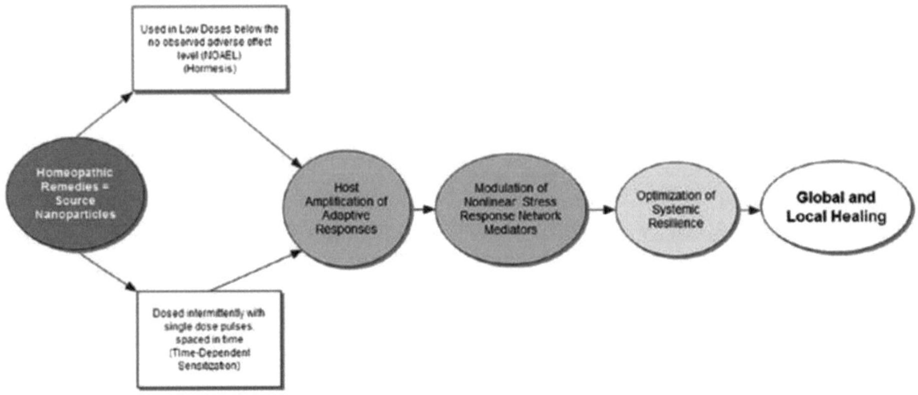


**Figure 3.**
*Nanoparticle model for homeopathic remedy action: hormesis, allostatic cross-adaptation, and time-dependent sensitization of the nonlinear stress response mediator network. Global and local healing occur across the person as a self-organized complex adaptive system in response to the individualized remedy serving as personalized hermetic stressor, i.e., holistic nanomedicine: an exogenous nanoparticle stimulating self-amplified, bidirectional adaptive change (see text).*

B. act by regulating the biological function of the allostatic stress response network [61, 62], including cytokines, oxidative stress, and heat shock proteins [63, 64], as well as immune, endocrine, metabolic, autonomic, and central nervous system functions [65, 66];

C. evoke biphasic actions on the adaptive plasticity of living systems [67–71] via organism-dependent, endogenously amplified, rather than agent-dependent pharmacological effects [72]. The effects of homeopathic remedy nanoparticles involve state- and time-dependent adaptive changes [63, 64, 73–76] within the complex adaptive organism [75–78]. The main clinical outcome is

D. improvement in intrinsic resilience to future environmental stressors and recovery back to normal healthy homeostatic operating [79]. The disease resolves as an indirect result of changing the system dynamics that had supported its initial development [78, 80], rather than as a downright consequence of suppressing end-organ symptoms.

The action of homoeopathic medicines can be explained with the help of the biopsychosocial model. The biopsychosocial model reflects the development of illness through the complex interaction of biological factors (genetic, infections, trauma, nutrition, etc.), psychological factors (mood, personality, emotional turmoil, negative thinking, etc.), and social factors (cultural, socioeconomic, technological, etc.) [81]. According to the biopsychosocial model, individuals as per their present state and personal history, respond differently to one and the same substance. Homeopathy is the pioneer of personalized medicine where the patient's complete data of health issues is considered for a precisely aimed therapy. The homoeopath considers the case a disease phenomenon that is a modification in the whole individual from his original state of health. It is the totality of alterations that comprises all the patient's mental, physical, and psychological changes.

The prescription of a homoeopath is based on the totality of the symptoms, which includes patient's life span, counting past illnesses, family history, constitution and

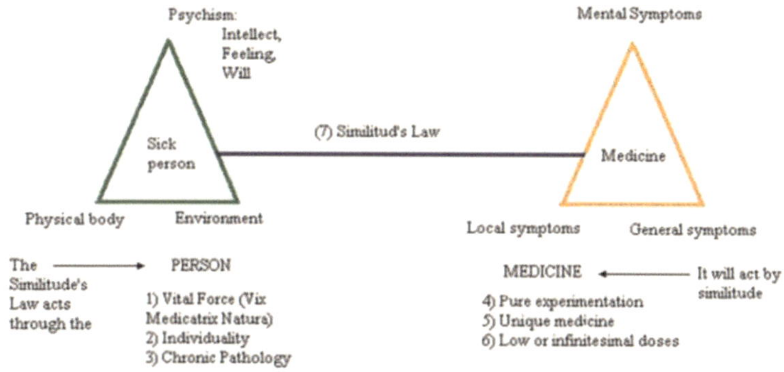


**Figure 4.**
*Application of the law of similia in homeopathy.*

temperament, and peculiar symptoms of the present illnesses. A patient's portrait is created on this base, and this disease partite is correlated with a remedy picture. When these two portraits match, a homeopathic response is established, and the body shall make efforts to cure the illness. It is called the similia principle. The fundamental law of homoeopathy is based on nature's law of "Like cures like," also known as the "Law of similars." According to this law, the prescribed homeopathic medicine faces very little resistance as the patient exhibits an enhanced susceptibility to it (**Figure 4**).

Modern anti-hypertensive drugs are not always well-tolerated due to their many harmful side effects [82]. They have the inconvenience of drug treatment despite its unchallenged efficacy [83, 84]; side effects [85] and difficulties with drug compliance occur in up to 70% of the patients [86]. They have no impact on depression, general psychopathology, and quality of life scores compared to those who use only a dietary program [87]. Such drugs do not have any effect on reducing the anger of hypertensive patients. Homeopathic medicines do not have unwanted side effects [88].

This research studies the relationship between essential hypertension (EHT), higher levels of negative emotion such as high trait anger and perceived stress, and their homeopathic treatment. This anger research has mainly explored the experience and expression of anger. The purpose of this study is to ascertain the efficacy of a homeopathic similimum in treating anger and thereby controlling EHT. Homeopathic treatment is much more cost-effective, has no adverse effects, and improves the quality of life, making it more readily accepted.

## 5. Materials and methods

This trial was randomized, placebo-controlled, comparative, and open-label conducted at an urban and a rural charitable homoeopathic hospital and a plastic factory. About 1187 adults were screened for hypertension. They were asked about the history of hypertension as well. We found 303 patients with either history of hypertension or were detected with hypertension during screening on BP measurements. The screening was carried out at a rural and an urban charitable hospital and a plastic factory. Secondary hypertension was ruled out among these 303 hypertensive patients by checking routine blood biochemistry, Ultrasonography (USG), electrocardiogram (ECG), and x-ray chest. However, eight patients were found to have secondary causes like renal artery stenosis, Conn's syndrome, coarctation of the aorta; these patients were excluded from moving into the study. One-hundred and seventy-two patients (108 males and 64 females) between 18 and 65 years who gave their informed, voluntary consent were enrolled in the study as per the approval from the ethics committee of Dr. M.L. Dhawale Memorial Homoeopathic Institute's approval. By simple randomization, they were allocated their respective groups, i.e., placebo and intervention groups. More than 50% of patients in both groups were on Antihypertensives prescribed by the physician at the beginning of the study.

All the patients were given necessary lifestyle management advice, also suggested a dietary approach to stop hypertension (DASH diet) [89] and regular exercises. Thorough homeopathic case-taking was done, and the STAXI-2 scale was applied at the beginning and after a 6-months study period to measure the change in anger for all the patients. Every 2 weeks, these patients were followed up for subjective criteria like anger, anger episodes, fights, and moods. Also, objective criteria were assessed like BP, pulse rate, physical complaints. Regular follow-up was done every 2 weeks to check all the patients' subjective and objective parameters.

Data were entered in MS Excel and then transferred to SPSS SW V. 21 for analysis. The quantitative data were represented as mean ± SD & compared using Student's *t*-test. In addition, a Pearson correlation test was performed to find correlations between variables.

## 5.1 STAXI-2

Spielberger's State-Trait Anger Expression Inventory-2 (STAXI-2) is a measure of anger experience and expression used to assess aggression and violence, given the close association between anger dysregulation and aggressive and violent behavior. The STAXI-2 is one of the most widely used measures in clinical and research settings (**Table 1**) [56].

| | STAXI-2 scale/subscale | Description of scale/subscale |
|---|---|---|
| 1 | **State anger (*S-Ang*)** | Measures the intensity of angry feelings and the extent to which a person feels like expressing anger at a particular time |
| A | Feeling angry (*S-Ang/F*) | Measures the intensity of the angry feelings the person is currently experiencing |
| B | Feel like expressing anger verbally (*S-Ang/V*) | Measures the intensity of current feelings related to the verbal expression of anger |
| C | Feel like expressing anger physically (*S-Ang/P*) | Measures the intensity of current feelings related to the physical expression of anger |
| 2 | **Trait anger (*T-Ang*)** | Measures how often angry feelings are experienced over time |
| A | Angry temperament (*T-Ang/T*) | Measures the disposition to experience anger without specific provocation |
| B | Angry reaction (*T-Ang/R*) | Measures the frequency that angry feelings are experienced in situations that involve frustration and/or negative evaluations |
| 3 | **Anger expression-out (*AX-O*)** | Measures how often angry feelings are expressed in verbally or physically aggressive behaviour |
| 4 | **Anger expression-in (*AX-I*)** | Measures how often angry feelings are experienced but not expressed (suppressed) |
| 5 | **Anger control-out (*AC-O*)** | Measures how often a person controls the outward expression of angry feelings |

*DOI: http://dx.doi.org/10.5772/intechopen.104589*

| | STAXI-2 scale/subscale | Description of scale/subscale |
|---|---|---|
| 6 | **Anger control-in (*AC-I*)** | Measures how often a person attempts to control angry feelings by calming down or cooling off |
| 7 | **Anger expression index (AX Index)** | Provides a general index of anger expression based on responses to the *AX-O*, *AX-I*, *AC-O*, & *AC-I* items |

**Table 1.**
*Brief overview of the STAXI-2 scales and subscales.*

It calculates the experience and expression of anger and is a 57-item self-report questionnaire. It consists of six scales and an anger expression index. It is a widely used scale for assessment, with the following dimensions:

State anger (S-Ang): the intensity of angry feelings at the time of completion;
Trait anger (T-Ang): a disposition to experience anger;
Anger Expression-Out (Ax-O): the expression of angry feelings out;
Anger Expression-In (AX-I): the suppression of angry feelings;
Anger Control-Out (AC-O): the prevention of anger expression toward other people or objects;
Anger Control-In (AC-I): the control of suppressed anger and
Anger Expression Index (AX-index): an overall index of the frequency of anger expression, regardless of direction.

## 6. Results

The maximum number of patients was 36–50 years. Seventy-eight out of 171 (46%) patients belonged to this age group in this study.

It has been noticed that hypertensive men reported more anger than hypertensive women. It is a randomized trial, and a separate analysis of anger between men and women has not been attempted. However, these findings were observed.

Sixty-four participants (28 females and 36 males) out of 171 had a positive family history of hypertension. Furthermore, it was observed that people with a family history of hypertension were more likely to suppress their anger.

This table shows the analysis of different variables done at the end of the study period—6 months. As seen in this table depicting the intervention arm—except state anger & its subgroups, all other anger variables & systolic and diastolic BP have a statistically significant reduction with the p-value <0.001 with a 95% confidence interval (**Table 2**).

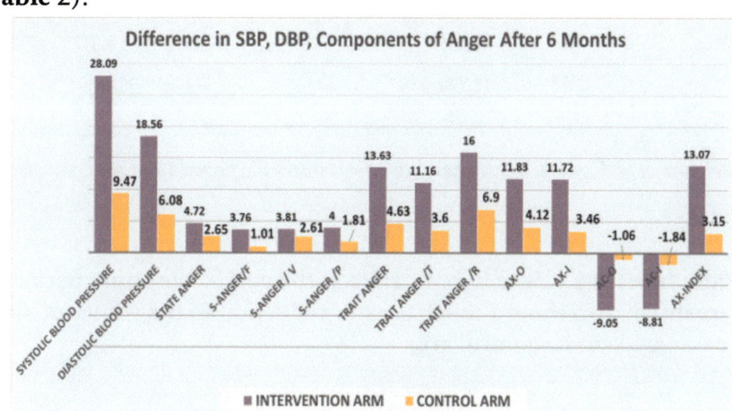

| | Group | Mean | Std. deviation | Std. error mean | Mean difference | 95% confidence interval of the difference | | P-value |
|---|---|---|---|---|---|---|---|---|
| | | | | | | Lower | Upper | |
| S_ang_diff | T | 4.72 | 9.505 | 1.025 | 2.062 | −0.414 | 4.539 | 0.102 |
| | C | 2.66 | 6.629 | 0.719 | | | | |
| S_ang_F_diff | T | 3.77 | 12.669 | 1.366 | 2.756 | −0.835 | 6.346 | 0.132 |
| | C | 1.01 | 11.048 | 1.198 | | | | |
| S_Ang_V_diff | T | 3.81 | 9.444 | 1.018 | 1.202 | −1.419 | 3.824 | 0.367 |
| | C | 2.61 | 7.838 | 0.850 | | | | |
| S_ang_P_diff | T | 4.00 | 10.993 | 1.185 | 2.188 | −0.551 | 4.927 | 0.117 |
| | C | 1.81 | 6.580 | 0.714 | | | | |
| T_Ang_diff | T | 13.63 | 8.609 | 0.928 | 8.993 | 6.473 | 11.512 | 0.000 |
| | C | 4.64 | 8.066 | 0.875 | | | | |
| T_Ang_T_diff | T | 11.16 | 9.483 | 1.023 | 7.563 | 4.937 | 10.189 | 0.000 |
| | C | 3.60 | 7.824 | 0.849 | | | | |
| diff_T_Ang_R | T | 16.00 | 9.239 | 0.996 | 9.106 | 6.362 | 11.85 | 0.000 |
| | C | 6.89 | 8.931 | 0.969 | | | | |
| Diff_AX_O | T | 11.84 | 11.699 | 1.262 | 7.72 | 4.492 | 10.947 | 0.000 |
| | C | 4.12 | 9.559 | 1.037 | | | | |
| Diff_AX_I | T | 11.72 | 10.125 | 1.092 | 8.262 | 5.598 | 10.926 | 0.000 |
| | C | 3.46 | 7.273 | 0.789 | | | | |
| Diff_AC_O | T | 9.05 | 12.362 | 1.333 | −7.988 | −11.125 | −4.851 | 0.000 |
| | C | 1.06 | 7.908 | 0.858 | | | | |
| Diff_AC_I | T | 13.91 | 12.043 | 1.299 | 10.754 | 7.664 | 13.845 | 0.000 |
| | C | 3.15 | 8.002 | 0.868 | | | | |
| Diff_AX_Index | T | 13.91 | 12.043 | 1.299 | 10.754 | 7.664 | 13.845 | 0.000 |
| | C | 3.15 | 8.002 | 0.868 | | | | |
| Diff_SBP | T | 31.20 | 14.839 | 1.609 | 20.474 | 16.299 | 24.648 | 0.000 |
| | C | 10.73 | 12.538 | 1.368 | | | | |
| Diff_DBP | T | 18.12 | 16.151 | 1.742 | 12.81 | 8.352 | 17.269 | 0.000 |
| | C | 5.31 | 13.220 | 1.434 | | | | |

**Table 2.**
*Change in variables in both groups w.r.t. anger after 6-months study period (Test used: unpaired* t*-test).*

This slide shows the values in both arms at the end of the study period. The values in the intervention arm show a much greater reduction in the values of all the variables compared to the control arm.

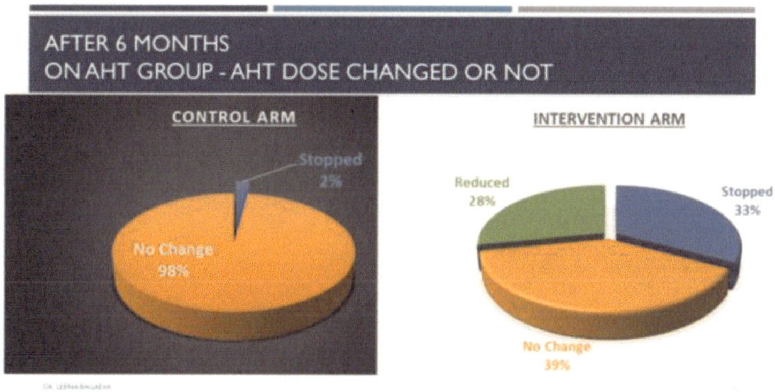


In both arms, the patients who were on standard antihypertensive treatment (AHT), in the control arm, 98% of patients continued with the same dose of their medicines at the end of the study period. However, standard AHT was stopped completely in the intervention group in 33% of patients. And in 28% of patients, the dose of AHT was reduced.

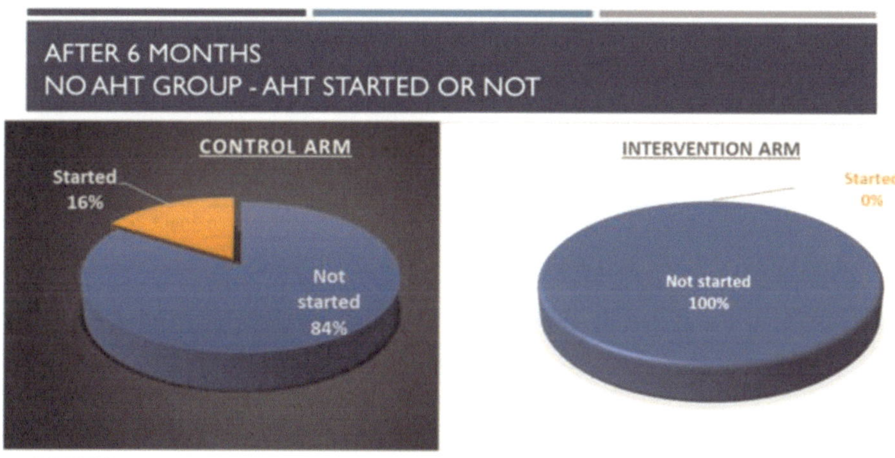


At the end of the study period, in both the arms, the patients who were not on standard AHT, in the control arm, 16% patients had to be prescribed standard AHT. Whereas in the intervention arm, the BP of all patients was maintained on the indicated homoeopathic medicine.

No statistical difference was found in rural and urban participants in both control and intervention arms with respect to anger and blood pressure variables (**Tables 3** and **4**).

The family history of hypertension was analyzed in female participants of the study, as shown in the above table, and it has been correlated with various anger components (**Table 5**).

The result suggests that women with a positive family history of hypertension scored higher on trait anger and angry temperament. Still, they tended to suppress their outward expression of anger than participants with negative F/H of HT. It correlates with higher blood pressure values. In expressing anger, cultural standards define what is appropriate and appear to determine such expressions' physiological consequences.

In the group analysis of male participants in the study, as shown in the above table, the results suggest that even men with a positive family history of

| Group statistics—Control group | | | | | | | | | |
|---|---|---|---|---|---|---|---|---|---|
| | Residence | *N* | Mean | Std. deviation | Std. error mean | *t* | Sig. (2-tailed) | 95% confidence interval of the difference | |
| | | | | | | | | Lower | Upper |
| S_ang_diff | U | 44 | 2.00 | 5.104 | 0.769 | −0.949 | 0.346 | −4.229 | 1.498 |
| | R | 41 | 3.37 | 7.955 | 1.242 | | | | |
| S_ang_F_diff | U | 44 | 0.55 | 10.498 | 1.583 | −0.401 | 0.689 | −5.761 | 3.827 |
| | R | 41 | 1.51 | 11.720 | 1.830 | | | | |
| S_Ang_V_diff | U | 44 | 1.68 | 5.960 | 0.899 | −1.135 | 0.260 | −5.306 | 1.450 |
| | R | 41 | 3.61 | 9.426 | 1.472 | | | | |
| S_ang_P_diff | U | 44 | 0.64 | 3.629 | 0.547 | −1.726 | 0.088 | −5.245 | 0.371 |
| | R | 41 | 3.07 | 8.580 | 1.340 | | | | |
| T_Ang_diff | U | 44 | 4.00 | 8.286 | 1.249 | −0.750 | 0.455 | −4.809 | 2.175 |
| | R | 41 | 5.32 | 7.869 | 1.229 | | | | |
| T_Ang_T_diff | U | 44 | 3.14 | 7.899 | 1.191 | −0.564 | 0.575 | −4.353 | 2.431 |
| | R | 41 | 4.10 | 7.810 | 1.220 | | | | |
| diff_T_Ang_R | U | 44 | 5.95 | 8.291 | 1.250 | −1.005 | 0.318 | −5.803 | 1.908 |
| | R | 41 | 7.90 | 9.570 | 1.495 | | | | |
| Diff_AX_O | U | 44 | 3.09 | 8.610 | 1.298 | −1.026 | 0.308 | −6.254 | 1.997 |
| | R | 41 | 5.22 | 10.477 | 1.636 | | | | |
| Diff_AX_I | U | 44 | 3.36 | 5.879 | 0.886 | −0.124 | 0.901 | −3.356 | 2.961 |
| | R | 41 | 3.56 | 8.597 | 1.343 | | | | |
| Diff_AC_O | U | 44 | −0.77 | 7.090 | 1.069 | 0.344 | 0.732 | −2.839 | 4.025 |
| | R | 41 | −1.37 | 8.780 | 1.371 | | | | |
| Diff_AC_I | U | 44 | 2.77 | 6.971 | 1.051 | −0.452 | 0.653 | −4.260 | 2.683 |
| | R | 41 | 3.56 | 9.050 | 1.413 | | | | |
| Diff_AX_Index | U | 44 | 2.77 | 6.971 | 1.051 | −0.452 | 0.653 | −4.260 | 2.683 |
| | R | 41 | 3.56 | 9.050 | 1.413 | | | | |
| Diff_sys_BP | U | 44 | 10.91 | 10.465 | 1.578 | 0.139 | 0.889 | −5.098 | 5.866 |
| | R | 40 | 10.53 | 14.620 | 2.312 | | | | |
| Diff_dia_BP | U | 44 | 6.16 | 8.271 | 1.247 | 0.614 | 0.541 | −3.960 | 7.498 |
| | R | 41 | 4.39 | 17.082 | 2.668 | | | | |

**Table 3.**
*To check if there is a significant difference in anger variables in the control group based on residence (rural/urban) of participants.*

hypertension have higher trait anger and anger temperament. Still, they tend to suppress their outward expression of anger compared to participants with negative F/H of HT. Besides, they try to resolve their anger by calming down or cooling off (**Table 6**).

| | Residence | N | Mean | Std. deviation | Std. error mean | *t* | Sig. (2-tailed) | Mean difference | 95% confidence interval of the difference | |
|---|---|---|---|---|---|---|---|---|---|---|
| | | | | | | | | | Lower | Upper |
| S_ang_diff | U | 48 | 4.46 | 10.057 | 1.452 | −0.286 | 0.775 | −0.594 | −4.721 | 3.532 |
| | R | 38 | 5.05 | 8.880 | 1.441 | | | | | |
| S_ang_F_diff | U | 48 | 2.08 | 14.510 | 2.094 | −1.393 | 0.167 | −3.811 | −9.252 | 1.629 |
| | R | 38 | 5.89 | 9.642 | 1.564 | | | | | |
| S_Ang_V_diff | U | 48 | 3.67 | 10.134 | 1.463 | −0.162 | 0.872 | −0.333 | −4.435 | 3.768 |
| | R | 38 | 4.00 | 8.624 | 1.399 | | | | | |
| S_ang_P_diff | U | 48 | 4.21 | 12.129 | 1.751 | 0.196 | 0.845 | 0.471 | −4.302 | 5.245 |
| | R | 38 | 3.74 | 9.520 | 1.544 | | | | | |
| T_Ang_diff | U | 48 | 13.79 | 9.455 | 1.365 | 0.197 | 0.844 | 0.371 | −3.368 | 4.109 |
| | R | 38 | 13.42 | 7.525 | 1.221 | | | | | |
| T_Ang_T_diff | U | 48 | 11.92 | 10.388 | 1.499 | 0.827 | 0.411 | 1.706 | −2.396 | 5.809 |
| | R | 38 | 10.21 | 8.237 | 1.336 | | | | | |
| diff_T_Ang_R | U | 48 | 15.17 | 10.188 | 1.471 | −0.939 | 0.350 | −1.886 | −5.878 | 2.106 |
| | R | 38 | 17.05 | 7.888 | 1.280 | | | | | |
| Diff_AX_O | U | 48 | 11.46 | 11.417 | 1.648 | −0.336 | 0.738 | −0.857 | −5.936 | 4.221 |
| | R | 38 | 12.32 | 12.184 | 1.976 | | | | | |
| Diff_AX_I | U | 48 | 11.71 | 10.462 | 1.510 | −0.013 | 0.990 | −0.029 | −4.426 | 4.369 |
| | R | 38 | 11.74 | 9.822 | 1.593 | | | | | |
| Diff_AC_O | U | 48 | −7.75 | 13.096 | 1.890 | 1.094 | 0.277 | 2.934 | −2.398 | 8.266 |
| | R | 38 | −10.68 | 11.326 | 1.837 | | | | | |
| Diff_AC_I | U | 48 | 12.42 | 12.836 | 1.853 | −1.295 | 0.199 | −3.373 | −8.552 | 1.807 |
| | R | 38 | 15.79 | 10.833 | 1.757 | | | | | |

| | Residence | $N$ | Mean | Std. deviation | Std. error mean | $t$ | Sig. (2-tailed) | Mean difference | 95% confidence interval of the difference | |
|---|---|---|---|---|---|---|---|---|---|---|
| | | | | | | | | | Lower | Upper |
| Diff_AX_Index | U | 48 | 12.42 | 12.836 | 1.853 | −1.295 | 0.199 | −3.373 | −8.552 | 1.807 |
| | R | 38 | 15.79 | 10.833 | 1.757 | | | | | |
| Diff_sys_BP | U | 47 | 33.43 | 14.764 | 2.154 | 1.551 | 0.125 | 4.978 | −1.407 | 11.364 |
| | R | 38 | 28.45 | 14.656 | 2.377 | | | | | |
| Diff_dia_BP | U | 48 | 18.60 | 18.252 | 2.634 | 0.313 | 0.755 | 1.104 | −5.907 | 8.116 |
| | R | 38 | 17.50 | 13.244 | 2.148 | | | | | |

**Table 4.**
*To check if there is a significant difference in anger variables in the treatment group based on residence (rural/urban) of participants.*

| | F/H of HT | Mean | Standard deviation | Standard error mean | *t* | Sig. (2-tailed) | Mean difference | 95% confidence interval of the difference | |
|---|---|---|---|---|---|---|---|---|---|
| | | | | | | | | Lower | Upper |
| S_ang_diff | 0.00 | 4.91 | 9.053 | 1.530 | −0.193 | 0.848 | −0.493 | −5.604 | 4.617 |
| | 1.00 | 5.41 | 11.064 | 2.129 | | | | | |
| S_ang_F_diff | 0.00 | 1.03 | 17.049 | 2.882 | −1.282 | 0.205 | −4.749 | −12.157 | 2.658 |
| | 1.00 | 5.78 | 10.112 | 1.946 | | | | | |
| S_Ang_V_diff | 0.00 | 4.23 | 10.138 | 1.714 | 0.058 | 0.954 | 0.154 | −5.171 | 5.48 |
| | 1.00 | 4.07 | 10.720 | 2.063 | | | | | |
| S_ang_P_diff | 0.00 | 2.91 | 8.936 | 1.510 | −0.927 | 0.358 | −2.715 | −8.576 | 3.146 |
| | 1.00 | 5.63 | 14.055 | 2.705 | | | | | |
| T_Ang_diff | 0.00 | 7.14 | 7.945 | 1.343 | −2.514 | 0.015 | −6.116 | −10.982 | −1.251 |
| | 1.00 | 13.26 | 11.206 | 2.157 | | | | | |
| T_Ang_T_diff | 0.00 | 5.89 | 7.955 | 1.345 | −2.572 | 0.013 | −6.114 | −10.869 | −1.359 |
| | 1.00 | 12.00 | 10.770 | 2.073 | | | | | |
| diff_T_Ang_R | 0.00 | 9.60 | 7.997 | 1.352 | −1.938 | 0.057 | −4.993 | −10.146 | 0.16 |
| | 1.00 | 14.59 | 12.239 | 2.355 | | | | | |
| Diff_AX_O | 0.00 | 5.31 | 10.220 | 1.728 | −1.711 | 0.092 | −4.315 | −9.36 | 0.729 |
| | 1.00 | 9.63 | 9.332 | 1.796 | | | | | |
| Diff_AX_I | 0.00 | 4.57 | 7.770 | 1.313 | −2.143 | 0.036 | −5.206 | −10.067 | −0.346 |
| | 1.00 | 9.78 | 11.345 | 2.183 | | | | | |
| Diff_AC_O | 0.00 | −1.83 | 9.790 | 1.655 | 3.044 | 0.003 | 7.949 | 2.725 | 13.173 |
| | 1.00 | −9.78 | 10.703 | 2.060 | | | | | |
| Diff_AC_I | 0.00 | 4.69 | 11.029 | 1.864 | −3.07 | 0.003 | −8.425 | −13.916 | −2.935 |
| | 1.00 | 13.11 | 10.293 | 1.981 | | | | | |
| Diff_AX_Index | 0.00 | 4.69 | 11.029 | 1.864 | −3.07 | 0.003 | −8.425 | −13.916 | −2.935 |
| | 1.00 | 13.11 | 10.293 | 1.981 | | | | | |

*00, negative family history; 1.00, positive family history.*

**Table 5.**
*Comparison of positive and negative F/H of HT in control and treatment groups: (females).*

| | fam_hist | Mean | Standard deviation | Standard error mean | Sig. (2-tailed) | Mean difference | Std. error difference | 95% confidence interval of the difference | |
|---|---|---|---|---|---|---|---|---|---|
| | | | | | | | | Lower | Upper |
| S_ang_diff | 0.00 | 2.03 | 5.990 | 0.737 | 0.110 | −2.262 | 1.405 | −5.048 | 0.523 |
| | 1.00 | 4.29 | 8.527 | 1.332 | | | | | |
| S_ang_F_diff | 0.00 | 1.06 | 7.510 | 0.924 | 0.262 | −2.305 | 2.043 | −6.356 | 1.746 |
| | 1.00 | 3.37 | 13.619 | 2.127 | | | | | |

| | fam_hist | Mean | Standard deviation | Standard error mean | Sig. (2-tailed) | Mean difference | Std. error difference | 95% confidence interval of the difference | |
|---|---|---|---|---|---|---|---|---|---|
| | | | | | | | | Lower | Upper |
| S_Ang/V_diff | 0.00 | 2.03 | 6.762 | 0.832 | 0.233 | −1.823 | 1.520 | −4.837 | 1.191 |
| | 1.00 | 3.85 | 8.893 | 1.389 | | | | | |
| S_ang_P_diff | 0.00 | 1.67 | 6.587 | 0.811 | 0.287 | −1.602 | 1.495 | −4.567 | 1.364 |
| | 1.00 | 3.27 | 8.829 | 1.379 | | | | | |
| T_Ang_diff | 0.00 | 7.03 | 9.628 | 1.185 | **0.012** | **−4.628** | **1.806** | −8.208 | −1.048 |
| | 1.00 | 11.66 | 8.111 | 1.267 | | | | | |
| T_Ang_T_diff | 0.00 | 4.94 | 8.891 | 1.094 | **0.012** | **−4.670** | **1.818** | −8.276 | −1.065 |
| | 1.00 | 9.61 | 9.542 | 1.490 | | | | | |
| diff_T_Ang/R | 0.00 | 9.88 | 10.864 | 1.337 | 0.081 | −3.536 | 2.006 | −7.513 | 0.441 |
| | 1.00 | 13.41 | 8.675 | 1.355 | | | | | |
| Diff_AX_O | 0.00 | 6.82 | 13.070 | 1.609 | 0.093 | −4.060 | 2.395 | −8.809 | 0.689 |
| | 1.00 | 10.88 | 10.159 | 1.587 | | | | | |
| Diff_AX_I | 0.00 | 6.85 | 10.366 | 1.276 | 0.130 | −2.956 | 1.935 | −6.793 | 0.880 |
| | 1.00 | 9.80 | 8.600 | 1.343 | | | | | |
| Diff_AC_O | 0.00 | −3.27 | 10.885 | 1.340 | 0.055 | 4.337 | 2.234 | −0.093 | 8.767 |
| | 1.00 | −7.61 | 11.783 | 1.840 | | | | | |
| Diff_AC_I | 0.00 | 6.55 | 11.707 | 1.441 | **0.022** | **−5.308** | **2.286** | −9.840 | −0.776 |
| | 1.00 | 11.85 | 11.139 | 1.740 | | | | | |
| Diff_AX_Index | 0.00 | 6.55 | 11.707 | 1.441 | **0.022** | **−5.308** | **2.286** | −9.840 | −0.776 |
| | 1.00 | 11.85 | 11.139 | 1.740 | | | | | |

**Table 6.**
*Comparison of positive and negative F/H of HT in control and treatment groups: (males).*

Table of associated illnesses these participants suffered from (**Table** 7):
It shows the list of associated ailments these patients had along with EHT.

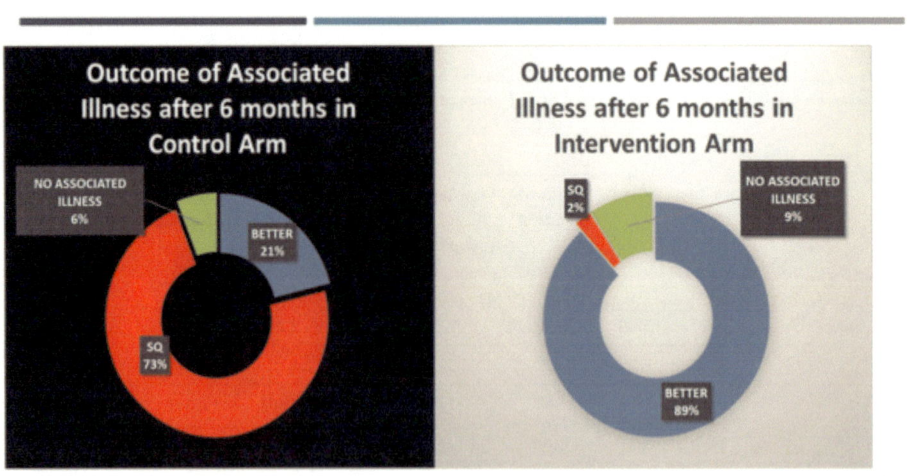

| Number | Associated illness | No. of patients | Total % |
|---|---|---|---|
| 1 | Alcoholism | 4 | 2.34 |
| 2 | Allergic dermatitis | 6 | 3.51 |
| 3 | Allergic rhinitis | 4 | 2.34 |
| 4 | Acid-peptic disorder | 34 | 19.88 |
| 5 | Benign paroxysmal postural vertigo | 1 | 0.6 |
| 6 | Cholelithiasis | 2 | 1.17 |
| 7 | Chronic obstructive pulmonary disease | 6 | 3.51 |
| 8 | Chronic suppurative otitis media | 1 | 0.6 |
| 9 | Climacteric complaints | 6 | 3.51 |
| 10 | Dysthymia | 4 | 2.34 |
| 11 | Diabetes mellitus | 36 | 21.05 |
| 12 | Dyslipidaemia | 6 | 3.51 |
| 13 | Epilepsy | 2 | 1.17 |
| 14 | Fibromyalgia | 12 | 7.02 |
| 15 | Frozen shoulder | 4 | 2.34 |
| 16 | Generalised anxiety disorder | 8 | 4.68 |
| 17 | Hypothyroidism | 12 | 7.02 |
| 18 | Hyperthyroidism | 1 | 0.6 |
| 19 | Hyperuricaemia | 8 | 4.68 |
| 20 | Irritable bowel syndrome | 2 | 1.17 |
| 21 | Malnutrition | 4 | 2.34 |
| 22 | Menstrual irregularities | 12 | 7.02 |
| 23 | Migraine | 2 | 1.17 |
| 24 | Obesity | 4 | 2.34 |
| 25 | Osteo-arthritis knees | 8 | 4.68 |
| 26 | Psoriasis | 2 | 1.17 |
| 27 | Rheumatoid arthritis | 4 | 2.34 |
| 28 | Urolithiasis | 6 | 3.51 |
| 29 | Urinary tract infection—recurrent | 2 | 1.17 |
| 30 | Vitiligo | 2 | 1.17 |

**Table 7.**
*Associated illnesses seen in patients along with essential hypertension.*

At the end of the study period:

About 89% of patients had relief in the symptoms of their comorbidities in the treatment group with the curative effect of the similimum, but 73% of patients' symptoms of associated illnesses were status quo in the control arm.

A Pearson's correlation test was done to determine whether there is a linear correlation between anger variables and systolic and diastolic BP. Unfortunately, in this study (like many others in the past), we could not find a significant correlation (**Table 8**).

(To check whether there is a correlation of anger variables with blood pressure)

| | | S_ang_PostHomRx | S_Ang_F_Post | S_Ang_V_Post | S_Ang_P_Post | T_AngPost | T_Ang_T_Post | T_Ang_R_Post | AX_O_Post | AX_I_Post | AC_O_Post | AC_I_PostHomRx | AX_Index_Post | Post_sys_BP | Post_dia_BP |
|---|---|---|---|---|---|---|---|---|---|---|---|---|---|---|---|
| S_ang_PostHomRx | Pearson Correlation | 1 | | | | | | | | | | | | | |
| | Sig. (2-tailed) | | | | | | | | | | | | | | |
| S_Ang_F_Post | Pearson Correlation | 0.951** | 1 | | | | | | | | | | | | |
| | Sig. (2-tailed) | 0 | | | | | | | | | | | | | |
| S_Ang_V_Post | Pearson Correlation | 0.613** | 0.526** | 1 | | | | | | | | | | | |
| | Sig. (2-tailed) | 0 | 0 | | | | | | | | | | | | |
| S_Ang_P_Post | Pearson Correlation | 0.594** | 0.506** | 0.985** | 1 | | | | | | | | | | |
| | Sig. (2-tailed) | 0 | 0 | 0 | | | | | | | | | | | |
| T_AngPost | Pearson Correlation | 0.269* | 0.311** | 0.115 | 0.07 | 1 | | | | | | | | | |
| | Sig. (2-tailed) | 0.012 | 0.004 | 0.29 | 0.52 | | | | | | | | | | |
| T_Ang_T_Post | Pearson Correlation | 0.236* | 0.276* | 0.107 | 0.072 | 0.922** | 1 | | | | | | | | |
| | Sig. (2-tailed) | 0.028 | 0.01 | 0.328 | 0.51 | 0 | | | | | | | | | |
| T_Ang_R_Post | Pearson Correlation | 0.279* | 0.341** | 0.102 | 0.036 | 0.848** | 0.636** | 1 | | | | | | | |
| | Sig. (2-tailed) | 0.009 | 0.001 | 0.349 | 0.74 | 0 | 0 | | | | | | | | |
| AX_O_Post | Pearson Correlation | -0.006 | -0.014 | 0.171 | 0.211 | 0.518** | 0.515** | 0.294** | 1 | | | | | | |
| | Sig. (2-tailed) | 0.959 | 0.895 | 0.115 | 0.051 | 0 | 0 | 0.006 | | | | | | | |
| AX_I_Post | Pearson Correlation | 0.302** | 0.354** | 0.033 | 0.019 | 0.461** | 0.363** | 0.474** | 0.135 | 1 | | | | | |
| | Sig. (2-tailed) | 0.005 | 0.001 | 0.759 | 0.861 | 0 | 0 | 0 | 0.214 | | | | | | |
| AC_O_Post | Pearson Correlation | 0.11 | 0.136 | 0.153 | 0.151 | -0.21 | -0.276* | 0.017 | -0.577** | 0.131 | 1 | | | | |
| | Sig. (2-tailed) | 0.313 | 0.206 | 0.161 | 0.166 | 0.052 | 0.1 | 0.879 | 0 | 0.229 | | | | | |
| AC_I_PostHomRx | Pearson Correlation | 0.087 | 0.066 | 0.164 | 0.134 | 0.093 | 0.024 | 0.215* | -0.213* | 0.083 | 0.757** | 1 | | | |
| | Sig. (2-tailed) | 0.423 | 0.545 | 0.131 | 0.218 | 0.392 | 0.827 | 0.047 | 0.049 | 0.446 | 0 | | | | |
| AX_Index_Post | Pearson Correlation | 0.016 | 0.034 | 0.176 | 0.183 | 0.352** | 0.379** | 0.155 | 0.675** | 0.262* | -0.881** | -0.781** | 1 | | |
| | Sig. (2-tailed) | 0.885 | 0.753 | 0.102 | 0.091 | 0.001 | 0 | 0.154 | 0 | 0.015 | 0 | 0 | | | |
| Post_sys_BP | Pearson Correlation | -0.112 | -0.12 | -0.003 | 0.024 | 0.033 | 0.049 | 0.017 | 0.135 | -0.040 | -0.178 | -0.163 | 0.172 | 1 | |
| | Sig. (2-tailed) | 0.306 | 0.272 | 0.977 | 0.83 | 0.765 | 0.657 | 0.874 | 0.214 | 0.712 | 0.101 | 0.133 | 0.113 | | |
| Post_dia_BP | Pearson Correlation | -0.047 | 0.087 | 0.178 | 0.184 | 0.044 | 0.012 | 0.072 | 0.166 | -0.049 | 0.046 | 0.012 | 0.042 | 0.738** | 1 |
| | Sig. (2-tailed) | 0.666 | 0.54 | 0.102 | 0.089 | 0.69 | 0.911 | 0.511 | 0.127 | 0.655 | 0.675 | 0.91 | 0.699 | 0 | |

Mild

Moderate

Severe

*Correlation of variables in each group.*

**Table 8.**
*Post-test correlations between variables in TREATMENT group.*

## 7. Discussion

The predictive importance of stress resulting in anger was seen only in the subgroup of participants with high genetic susceptibility to hypertension, defined as having one or more hypertensive parents. It is also important to emphasize that although a family history of hypertension was an important predictor of alterations in BP status on its own, high trait anger greatly potentiated this increased risk of developing elevated BP.

High-stress responsivity itself may have a possible genetic basis. In addition, there is a possible lack of generalizability to older persons because the sample was restricted to 18–65 years. It indicates that any adverse effects of increased life stress or decreased stress buffers would be most evident among those who are both high-stress responders and have a genetic susceptibility to hypertension and heart disease.

This study was conducted at charitable hospitals and in a plastics factory, where patients belonged to the low-income group. Hence, only 18% of patients had middle or high SES. Although employment itself does not seem to be a risk factor, there is some evidence that the combination of jobs and a family may increase hypertension and CHD incidence in women. In two studies, the Framingham study [90, 91] and the Minnesota Heart Survey, [92] working women reported greater levels of stress than working men or homemakers. A similar observation was found in the female participants in the present study. Many study participants were rotational factory shift workers, including working days, afternoon, and night shifts. Blood pressure elevation effects appear to be mainly mediated by maladaptive or unhealthy coping behaviors such as excessive consumption (food, cigarettes or bidis, gutka, and alcohol) and physical inactivity. These inconclusive results may have resulted partly from lifestyle differences in the study populations and have been strongly influenced by different perceptions of overwork and stress. It was found that psychological stress was associated with age, sex, and socioeconomic status. In addition, higher stress levels at work were found but lower levels of financial stress among persons with high versus low levels of income or education in both men and women. It was observed that blood pressure was explicitly related to job control (lower control linked to higher pressure) and perceived stress on the job. Participants with higher socioeconomic status and women were more stressed by low job control than men and people with lower socioeconomic status (SES). Women and young adults reported higher psychological stress levels, particularly at work, which raised age-and sex-related job strain issues with high demand and low control at work [34, 35].

A correlation between anger and hypertension (**Table 8**) was examined. The finding that none of the anger measures was associated with resting BP in this study is consistent with literature reviews on anger and hypertension [93–95]. In addition, previous reviews have found only low and inconsistent associations between trait anger and HT [96–98].

All homeopathic medicines alter the state of mind and disposition in their peculiar way [99]. Therefore, the changes in the patient's state of mind and disposition must be considered and matched with the particular homeopathic remedy that can produce a similar state in a healthy human being. As a result, permanent relief from the disease can occur. Furthermore, this ability to make distinctions among patients and superficially similar disease processes – that is, to "individualize" every case – is the natural result of the concern for the whole person, which lies at the core of homeopathic practice."

The study results also showed a reduction in anger in the control group, which was statistically significant but not as much as the reduction of anger variables in the treatment group, suggesting rapport building, up-front collaborative agenda-setting, and acknowledging social and emotional concerns as done during homeopathic case taking may help improve quality of care and efficiency. The consultation process's therapeutic benefits on health outcomes in conventional medicine and CAM have been depicted in various studies [78, 80]. These contextual effects include not the treatment's active components but are inherent within the whole treatment package such as the doctor–patient relationship, rapport-building and relationship maintenance, empathic response to social and emotional cues and mindfulness [100–105]). Research into homeopathic consultation has identified contextual factors such as empathy and empowerment [106], which may mediate the homeopathic therapeutic effect. Homeopathy consultations involve a complete exploration of the patient's emotional, spiritual, and physical wellbeing to enable the whole person's treatment, not just the illness.

Our consultation process was standardized in that specific topics were covered (e.g., detailed clinical history, current symptoms and medication, assessment of emotional and mental states, etc.) to identify the relevant information to prescribe. The consultations' content varied between patients and between consultations; homeopathic intervention was individualized and patient-centered and led by the patient's narratives.

The findings confirm previous work demonstrating that therapeutic benefits arise from inquiries within the homeopathic interview which includes communication skills, empathy, hopefulness, enablement, and narrative competence [82–84].

Homeopathic consultation necessitates a detailed understanding of the patient and is a unique and personalized approach. Therefore, the placebo effects of the homeopathic consultation may be specific to this therapy, possibly dependent on the process of the collaborative and highly individualized consultation imperative to find a homeopathic remedy and the associated symbolic meaning response for that patient [102].

During regular follow-ups every 2 weeks, there was no adverse reaction reported to homeopathic medicine in any study participants in the intervention group, proving the safety of the individualized medicine prescribed to the patients.

## 8. Conclusion

1. The results suggest the usefulness of the individualized homoeopathic treatment in the management of anger and the EHT in the population.

2. During regular follow-ups every 2 weeks, no adverse reaction to the homoeopathic medicine was found in any intervention group study participants, proving the safety of the individualized medicine prescribed to the patients.

3. STAXI-2 instrument was successfully used to measure the various anger variables in the study participants.

It was found that all the variables in both the groups were statistically not significantly different except the trait anger (T-Ang), angry temperament (T-Ang/T), and angry reaction (T-Ang/R), which were higher in the treatment group in comparison with the control group.

4. Convincing evidence did not emerge for the existence of strong linear relationships between anger and blood pressure.

5. A significant correlation between high blood pressure and suppressed anger was found in male and female participants with a positive family history of HTN.

6. The study results also showed a reduction of anger in the control group, which was statistically significant but not as much as the reduction of the anger variables in the treatment group, suggesting rapport building, up-front collaborative agenda-setting, and acknowledging social and emotional concerns as done during homoeopathic case taking might help improve quality of care and efficiency.

## 9. Limitations and future directions

1. Study needs replication with a larger sample size over a longer duration.

2. Presence of "Social desirability bias" – cannot be denied in a self-reporting scale-like STAXI-2.

3. Ambulatory BP monitoring is not used, so there can be misdiagnosed cases of white-coat hypertension or cases of masked HT that could have been missed.

4. Lack of generalizability to population older than 65 years of age.

5. Anger variables were not analysed separately for man and women as this being a randomized controlled trial, the number of male and female participants was unequal.

6. A double-blind, randomized controlled trial without using conventional anti-hypertensives is highly recommended.

## Author details

Leena S. Bagadia[1,2]* and Arun More[3]

1 Maharashtra University of Health Sciences, Nashik, India

2 Department of Forensic Medicine and Toxicology, Smt. CMP Homoeopathic Medical College, Mumbai, India

3 Organization Rural Health Progress Trust, India

*Address all correspondence to: leenabagadia@gmail.com

## References

[1] Inoue N. Stress and atherosclerotic cardiovascular disease. Journal of Atherosclerosis and Thrombosis. 2014;**21**(5):391-401

[2] Laugero KD, Gomez F, Manalo S, Dallman M. Corticosterone infused intracerbroventricularly inhibits energy storage and stimulates the hypothalamo-pituitary axis in adrenalectomized rats drinking sucrose. Endocrinology. 2002; **143**:4552-4562

[3] Scheuer DA, Bechtold AG, Shank SS, Akana SF. Glucocorticoids act in the dorsal hindbrain to increase arterial pressure. American Journal of Physiology. 2004;**286**:H458-H467

[4] Scheuer DA, Bechtold AG. Activation of dorsal hindbrain glucocorticoid receptors enhances the arterial pressure response to acute stress. Journal FASEB. 2004;**18**:A675-A679

[5] Sparrenberger F et al. Does psychosocial stress cause hypertension? A systematic review of observational studies. Journal of Human Hypertension. 2009;**23**(1):12-19

[6] Spruill TM. Chronic psychosocial stress and hypertension. Current Hypertension Reports. 2010;**12**(1):10-16

[7] Steptoe A. Psychosocial factors in the development of hypertension. Annals of Medicine. 2000;**32**(5):371-375

[8] Chobanian AV et al. Seventh report of the joint national committee on prevention, detection, evaluation, and treatment of high blood pressure. Hypertension. 2003;**42**(6):1206-1252

[9] The sixth report of the Joint National Committee on prevention, detection, evaluation, and treatment of high blood pressure. Archives of Internal Medicine. 1997;**157**(21):2413-2446

[10] The fifth report of the Joint National Committee on detection, evaluation, and treatment of high blood pressure (JNC V). Archives of Internal Medicine. 1993; **153**(2):154-183

[11] Grimsrud A, Stein DJ, Seedat S, Williams D, Myer L. The association between hypertension, depression and anxiety disorders: Results from a nationally-representative sample of South African adults. South African Medical Journal. 2009;**4**(5):358-366

[12] Barcelo A. Diabetes and hypertension in the Americas. West Indian Medical Journal. 2000;**49**:262-265

[13] Shapiro PA. Cardiovascular disorder. In: Sadock BJ, Sadock VA, editors. Kaplan and Sadock's Comprehensive Textbook of Psychiatry Psychosocial Factors Affecting Medical Condition. 8th ed. Philadelphia, PA: Lippincott Williams and Wilkins; 2004. pp. 430-2142

[14] Kubzansky LD, Kawachi I. Going to the heart of the matter: Do negative emotions cause coronary heart disease? Journal of Psychosomatic Research. 2000;**2000**(48):323-337

[15] Pickering TG, Gerin W. Cardiovascular reactivity in the laboratory and the role of behavioural factors in hypertension: A critical review. Annual Behavioural Medicine. 1990;**12**:3-16

[16] Brosschot JF, Gerin W, Thayer JF. The perseverative cognition hypothesis: A review of worry, prolonged stress-related physiological activation, and

health. Journal of Psychosomatic Research. 2006;**60**(2):113-124

[17] Gerin W, Davidson KW, Christenfeld NJ, Goyal T, Schwartz JE. The role of angry rumination and distraction in blood pressure recovery from emotional arousal. Psychosomatic Medicine. 2006;**68**(1):64-72

[18] Gerin W, Davidson KW, Schwartz AR, Christenfeld N. The role of emotional regulation in the development of hypertension. In: International Congress Series, Vol. 1241. Elsevier; 2002. pp. 91-97

[19] Ohira T, Hozawa A, Iribarren C, Daviglus ML, Matthews KA, Gross MD, et al. Longitudinal association of serum carotenoids and tocopherols with hostility: The CARDIA Study. American Journal of Epidemiology. 2008;**167**:42-50

[20] Dash SL, Swain PK, Sundaram KR. Hypertension: Epidemiology in an Indian tribal population. J.A.P.I. 1986;**34**: 567

[21] Kumar P, Chaudhary V. Epidemiological study of hypertension in a rural community of western Rajasthan. Indian Heart Journal. 1991;**43**(1):43-45

[22] Tuomisto MT. Intra-arterial blood pressure and heart reactivity to behavioural stress in normotensives, borderline and mild hypertensive men. Health Psychology. 1997;**16**(6):554-565

[23] Light KC. Hypertension and the reactivity hypothesis: The next generation. Psychosomatic Medicine. 2001;**63**(5):744-746

[24] Landesbergis PA, Schnoall PL, Warren K, Pickering TG, Schwrtz JE. Association between ambulatory blood pressure and alternative formulations of job strain. Scandinavian Journal of Work Environmental Health. 1994;**20**:349-363

[25] Rose G, Sivik T, Delimar N. Gender, psychological wellbeing, and somatic cardiovascular risk factors: Erratum. Integrative Physiological and Behavioural Science. 1996;**31**(3):274

[26] Ohlin B, Berglund G, Rosvall M, Nilsson PM. Job strain in men, but not in women, predicts a significant rise in blood pressure after 6.5 years of follow-up. Journal of Hypertension. 2007;**25**: 525-531

[27] Adler NE, Ostrove JM. Socioeconomic status and health: What we know and what we don't. Annals of the New York Academy of Sciences. 1999;**896**:3-15

[28] Albert MA, Glynn RJ, Buring J, Ridker PM. Impact of traditional and novel risk factors on the relationship between socioeconomic status and incident cardiovascular events. Circulation. 2006;**114**:2619-2626

[29] Seeman T, Merkin SS, Crimmins E, et al. Education, income and ethnic differences in cumulative biological risk profiles in a national sample of US adults: NHANES III (1988–1994). Social Science and Medicine. 2008;**66**:72-87

[30] Steptoe A, Marmot M. Psychosocial, haemostatic, and inflammatory correlates of delayed post-stress blood pressure recovery. Psychosomatic Medicine. 2006:531-537

[31] Sorlie PD, Rogot E. Mortality by employment status in the national longitudinal mortality study. American Journal of Epidemiology. 1990;**132**:983

[32] Adelmann PK, Antonucci TC, Crohan SE, Coleman LM. A causal analysis of employment and health in

midlife women. Women Health. 1990; **16**:5

[33] Repetti RL, Matthews KA, Waldron I. Employment and women's health. American Psychology. 1989;**44**:1394

[34] de Smet P, Sans S, Dramaix M, Boulenguez C, de Backer G, Ferrario M, et al. Gender and regional differences in perceived job stress across Europe. European Journal of Public Health. 2005; **15**(5):536-545. DOI: 10.1093/eurpub/cki028

[35] Kidwai R. Demographic factors, social problems, and material amenities as predictors of psychological distress: A cross-sectional study in Karachi, Pakistan. Social Psychiatry and Psychiatric Epidemiology. 2014;**49**(1): 27-39. DOI: 10.1007/s00127-013-0692-0

[36] Cottington EM, Matthews KA, Talbott E, Kuller LH. Occupational stress suppressed anger and hypertension. Psychosomatic Medicine. 1986;**48**(3): 249-260

[37] Williams JE, Nieto FJ, Sanford CP, Couper DJ, Tyroler HA. The association between trait-anger and incident stroke risk: The atherosclerosis risk in communities (ARIC) study. Stroke. 2002;**33**:13-20

[38] Spielberger CD, Jacobs G, Russell S, Crane R. Assessment of anger: The State-Trait Anger Scale. In: Butcher JN, Spielberger CD, editors. Advances in Personality Assessment (Vol. 2). Hillsdale, NJ: Lawrence Erlbaum; 1983. pp. 161-189

[39] Borteyrou X, Bruchon- Schweitzer M, Spielberger CD. The French adaptation of the STAXI-2. C.D. Spielberger's State-trait-anger expression inventory. Encephale. 2008;**34**(3): 249-255

[40] Player MS, King DE, Mainous AG, Geesey MA. Psychological factors and progression from pre-hypertension to hypertension or coronary heart disease. Annals of Family Medicine. 2007;**5**:403-411

[41] Rutledge T, Hogan BE. A quantitative review of prospective evidence linking psychological factors with hypertension development. Psychosomatic Medicine. 2002;**64**(5):758-766

[42] Borde-Perry WC, Campbell KL, Murtaugh KH, Gidding S, Falkner B. The association between hypertension and other cardiovascular risk factors in young adult African Americans. Journal of Clinical Hypertension. 2002;**4**(1):17-22

[43] Addotta K. Anger! 2006. Retrieved from: www.kipaddotta.com/mental-health/anger.html

[44] Chapter 2, Verse 63, Bhagwad Geeta

[45] DiGiuseppe R, Tafrate RC. Understanding Anger Disorders. USA: Oxford University Press; 2007

[46] Quinn CA, Rollock D, Vrana SR. A test of Spielberger's state-trait theory of anger with adolescents: Five hypotheses. Emotion. 2014;**14**(1):74

[47] Kisac I. Universite ogrencilerinin bazi degiskenlere gore surekli ofke ve ofke ifade Duzeyleri [PhD thesis]. Unpublished. Ankara: Hacettepe University Sosyal Bilimler Enstitusu; 1997

[48] Kassinove H, Tafrate RC. Anger management: The Complete Treatment Guidebook for Practitioners. California: Impact Publishers, Inc.; 2002

[49] Dey BK, Rahman A, Bairagi A, Roy K. Stress and anger of rural and urban adolescents. Psychology. 2014:177-184

[50] Naser A, Afshoon F, Mohammadi HR, Tavasoli E, Fard MR, Khalili A. Comparing the dimensions of aggression in adolescent athletes and non-athletes divorced families. European Journal of Experimental Biology. 2014;**4**(1):452-455

[51] Sharma N, Maqbool M. Relationship between body mass index and anger among graduate students. Indian Journal of Health and Wellbeing. 2014;**5**(6):723-725

[52] Balkaya F, Sahin NH. Cok Boyutlu ofke olcegi. Turk Psikiyatri Dergisi. 2003;**14**:192-202

[53] Berkowitz L. Aggression: Its Causes, Consequences, and Control. New York: McGraw-Hill; 1993

[54] Deffenbacher JL. Anger reduction: Issues, assessment, and intervention strategies. In: Siegman AW, Smith TW, editors. Anger, Hostility, and The Heart. Hillsdale, NJ: Erlbaum; 1994. pp. 239-269

[55] Eckhardt CI, Deffenbacher JL. Diagnosis of anger disorders. In: Kassinove H, editor. Anger Disorders: Definition, Diagnosis, and Treatment. Washington, DC: Taylor & Francis; 1995. pp. 27-48

[56] Spielberger CD, Johnson EH, Russell SF, Crane RJ, Jacobs GA, Worden TJ. The experience and expression of anger: Construction and validation of an anger expression scale. In: Chesney MA, Rosenman RH, editors. Anger and Hostility in Cardiovascular and Behavioural Disorders. Washington, DC: Hemisphere; 1985. pp. 5-30

[57] Bell IR, Koithan M. A model for homeopathic remedy effects: Low dose nanoparticles, allostatic cross-adaptation, and time-dependent sensitization in a complex adaptive system. BMC Complementary and Alternative Medicine. 2012;**12**(1):1-21

[58] Bhattacharyya SS, Mandal SK, Biswas R, Paul S, Pathak S, Boujedaini N, et al. In vitro studies demonstrate anticancer activity of an alkaloid of the plant *Gelsemium sempervirens*. Experimental Biology and Medicine (Maywood). 2008;**233**(12):1591-1601

[59] Chikramane PS, Suresh AK, Bellare JR, Kane SG. Extreme homeopathicdilutions retain starting materials: A nanoparticulate perspective. Homeopathy. 2010;**99**(4):231-242

[60] Upadhyay RP, Nayak C. Homeopathy emerging as nanomedicine. International Journal of High Dilution Research. 2011;**10**(37):299-310

[61] Ives JA, Moffett JR, Arun P, Lam D, Todorov TI, Brothers AB, et al. Enzyme stabilization by glass-derived silicates in glass-exposed aqueous solutions. Homeopathy. 2010;**99**(1):15-24

[62] Karatsoreos IN, McEwen BS. Psychobiological allostasis: Resistance, resilience and vulnerability. Trends in Cognitive Science. 2011;**15**(12):576-584

[63] McEwen BS. Central effects of stress hormones in health and disease: Understanding the protective and damaging effects of stress and stress mediators. European Journal of Pharmacology. 2008;**583**(2–3):174-185

[64] Van Wijk R, Wiegant FA. Postconditioning hormesis and the homeopathic Similia principle: Molecular aspects. Human & Experimental Toxicology. 2010;**29**(7):561-565

[65] Van Wijk R, Wiegant FA. Postconditioning hormesis and the similia principle. Frontiers in Bioscience (Elite Ed). 2011;**3**:1128-1138

[66] Khuda-Bukhsh AR, Bhattacharyya SS, Paul S, Dutta S, Boujedaini N, Belon P. Modulation of signal proteins: A plausible mechanism to explain how a potentized drug secale cor 30C diluted beyond Avogadro's limit combats skin papilloma in mice. Evidence-Based Complementary and Alternative Medicine. 2011;**2011**:286320

[67] Bellavite P, Ortolani R, Pontarollo F, Pitari G, Conforti A. Immunology and homeopathy. 5. The rationale of the 'Simile'. Evidence-Based Complementary and Alternative Medicine. 2007;**4**(2):149-163

[68] Bertani S, Lussignoli S, Andrioli G, Bellavite P, Conforti A. Dual effects of ahomeopathic mineral complex on carrageenan-induced oedema in rats. British Homeopathic Journal. 1999;**88** (3):101-105

[69] Malarczyk E, Pazdzioch-Czochra M, Graz M, Kochmanska-Rdest J, Jarosz-Wilkolazka A. Nonlinear changes in the activity of the oxygen-dependent demethylase system in *Rhodococcus erythropolis* cells in the presence of low and very low doses of formaldehyde. Nonlinear Biomedical Physics. 2011;**5**(1): 9

[70] Hyland ME, Lewith GT. Oscillatory effects in a homeopathic clinical trial: An explanation using complexity theory, and implications for clinical practice. Homeopathy. 2002;**91**(3):145-149

[71] Bell IR, Schwartz GE. Enhancement of adaptive biological effects by nanotechnology preparation methods in homeopathic medicines. Homeopathy. 2015;**104**(02):123-138

[72] Bell IR, Howerter A, Jackson N, Aickin M, Bootzin RR. Nonlinear dynamical systems effects of homeopathic remedies on multiscale entropy and correlation dimension of slow wave sleep EEG in young adults with histories of coffee-induced insomnia. Homeopathy. 2012;**101**(3): 182-192

[73] Iavicoli I, Calabrese EJ, Nascarella MA. Exposure to nanoparticles and hormesis. Dose Response. 2010;**8**(4): 501-517

[74] Wiegant F, Van Wijk R. The similia principle: Results obtained in a cellular model system. Homeopathy. 2010;**99**(1): 3-14

[75] Bell IR, Howerter A, Jackson N, Brooks AJ, Schwartz GE. Multi-weekresting EEG cordance change patterns from repeated olfactory activation with two constitutionally-salient homeopathic remedies in healthy young adults. The Journal of Alternative and Complementary Medicine. 2012;**18** (5):445-453

[76] Bellavite P, Signorini A. The Emerging Science of Homeopathy. Complexity, Biodynamics, and Nanopharmacology. 2nd ed. Berkeley: North Atlantic Books; 2002

[77] Bellavite P. Complexity science and homeopathy: A synthetic overview. Homeopathy: The Journal of the Faculty of Homeopathy. 2003;**92**(4):203-212

[78] Koithan M, Bell IR, Niemeyer K, Pincus D. A complex systems science perspective for whole systems of CAM research. Forsch Komplementar med Klass Naturheilkd. 2012;**19**(Suppl. 1): 7-14

[79] Pincus D, Metten A. Nonlinear dynamics in biopsychosocial resilience. Nonlinear Dynamics, Psychology, and Life Sciences. 2010;**14** (4):353-380

[80] Bell IR, Koithan M, Pincus D. Research methodological implications of nonlinear dynamical systems models for whole systems of complementary and alternative medicine. Forsch Komplementarmed Klass Naturheilkd. 2012;**19**(Suppl. 1):15-21

[81] Munir Ahmed R. Handbook of Advanced Teaching of Fundamentals of Homeopathy. Bengaluru: RGUHS; 2017. pp. 69-70

[82] Ahmad S. Homoeopathic Management of Hypertension. New Delhi: B. Jain Publishers (P) Ltd.; 1999 pp. 1, 6, 18-20

[83] Goldstein IB, Shapiro D, Thananopavarn C, Sambhi MP. Comparision of drug and behavioural treatment of essential hypertension. Health Psychology. 1982;**1**:7-26

[84] Lubrosky L, Crits-Christoph MS, Brady JP, et al. Behavioural versus pharmacological treatments for essential hypertension—A needed comparison. Psychosomatic Medicine. 1982;**44**:202-213

[85] Wadden TA, Stunkard AJ. Possible dangers in the pharmacological treatment of mild essential hypertension (letter). New England Journal of Medicine. 1982;**307**:1523-1524

[86] Dunbar JM, Stunkard AJ. Adherence to diet and drug regimens. In: Levy R, Rifkind R, Diennis B, Ernst N, editors. Nutrition, Lipids, and Coronary Heart Disease. New York: Ravn Press; 1979

[87] Dragioti E, Tsartsalis D, Kallikazaros I. Impact of anti-hypertensive medication on psychological status and quality of life in essential hypertension. European Psychiatry. 2015;**30**:615. DOI: 10.1016/S0924-9338(15)30489-2 Abstracts of the 23rd European Congress of Psychiatry Article: 0615

[88] Digby B. The Homoeopathic Family Guide. ALM Process, Homoeoforce. Bergvlei. 1997. pp. 5, 7

[89] Siervo M, Lara J, Chowdhury S, Ashor A, Oggioni C, Mathers JC. Effects of the dietary approach to stop hypertension (DASH) diet on cardiovascular risk factors: A systematic review and meta-analysis. British Journal of Nutrition. 2015;**113**(1):1-5

[90] Haynes SG, Feinleib M. Women, work and coronary heart disease: Prospective findings from the Framingham heart study. American Journal of Public Health. 1980;**70**:133

[91] Haynes SG, Feinleib M, Kannel WB. The relationship of psychosocial factors to coronary heart disease in the Framingham Study III. Eight-year incidence of coronary heart disease. American Journal of Epidemiology. 1980;**111**:37

[92] Sorensen G, Pirie P, Folsom A, Luepker R, Jacobs D, Gillium R. Sex differences in the relationship between work and health: The Minnesota Heart Survey. Journal of Health and Social Behaviour. 1985, 1985;**26**:379

[93] Mills J, Schneider RM, Dimsdale JE. Anger assessment and reactivity to stress. Journal of Psychosomatic Research. 1989, 1989;**33**:379-382

[94] Knight RG, Paulin JM, Wall-Manning HJ. Self reported anger intensity and blood pressure. British Journal of Clinical Psychology. 1987, 1987;**26**:5-6

[95] Friedman R, Schwartz JE, Schnall PL, Landsbergis PA, Pieper C, Gerin W, et al. Psychological variables in hypertension: Relationship to casual ambulatory blood pressure.

Psychosomatic Medicine. 2001, 2001;**63**: 19-31

[96] Suls J, Wan CK, Costa PT. Relationship of trait anger to resting blood pressure: A metaanalysis. Health Psychology. 1995;**14**:444-456

[97] Jorgensen RS, Johnson BT, Kolodziej ME, Schreer GE. Elevated blood pressure and personality: A meta-analytic review. Psychology Bulletin. 1996;**1996**(120): 293-320

[98] Mann SJ. The mind-body link in ssential hypertension: Time for a new paradigm. Alternative Therapy Health Medicine. 2000, 2000;**6**:39-45

[99] Hahnemann S. Organon of the Medical Art. 6th ed. Redmond, WA: Birdcage Books; 1843

[100] Di Blasi Z, Harkness E, Ernst E, Georgiou A, Kleijnen J. Influence of context effects on health outcomes: A systematic review. Lancet. 2002;**357**:757

[101] Walach H. Placebo and placebo effects—A concise review. Focus on Alternative and Complementary Therapies. 2003;**8**:178-187

[102] Moerman D, Jonas W. Deconstructing the placebo effect and finding the meaning response. Annals of Internal Medicine. 2002;**136**:471-476

[103] Hyland M. A tale of two therapies: Psychotherapy and complementary and alternative medicine and the human effect. Clinical Medicine. 2005;**5**:361-367

[104] Mercer SW. Practitioner empathy, patient enablement and health outcomes of patients attending the Glasgow Homeopathic Hospital: A retrospective and prospective comparison. Wiener Medizinische Wochenschrift. 2005;**155**: 498-501

[105] Hartog C. Elements of effective communication rediscoveries from homeopathy. Patient Education and Counceling. 2009;**77**:172-178

[106] Thompson T, Weiss M. Homeopathy—What are the active ingredients? An exploratory study using the UK Medical Research Council's framework for the evaluation of complex interventions. BMC Complementary and Alternative Medicine. 2006;**6**:37

Chapter 5

# The Influence of Anger and Imagery on the Maintenance and Treatment of PTSD

*Tony McHugh and Glen Bates*


## Abstract

Research on post-traumatic stress disorder (PTSD) has burgeoned since its introduction in DSM-III in 1980. PTSD is conceptualised as a disorder of recovery and has been regarded as intrusion-driven, disordered, anxiety. However, recently there has been a call for explanatory theories of PTSD that better capture the complexity of the condition. Problematic anger is now recognised as an important aspect of PTSD in most sufferers. It is a key predictor of the development, maintenance and severity of PTSD and may be the principal impediment to successful treatment. Nevertheless, the psychological mechanisms underlying the relationship between PTSD and anger are not well understood. This chapter reviews evidence that imagery is an important mechanism within this relationship and is fundamental to the experience of traumatic stress reactions. Imagery is directly related to the prevalence of intrusions in PTSD and is highly correlated with posttraumatic anger. Further, visual imagery with angry content has profound psycho-physiological effects, magnifies the intensity of experienced anger and, ultimately, mediates the experience of PTSD itself. This review elucidates the linkages between angry imagery and PTSD symptomatology and offers propositions for adapting imagery-based PTSD interventions to the treatment of anger-affected PTSD.


**Keywords:** imagery, anxiety, anger, PTSD, treatment

## 1. Introduction

Interest in PTSD as a clinical phenomenon burgeoned following its formal introduction in the third edition of the Diagnostic and Statistical Manual of Mental Disorders in 1980 [1]. Today, the PTSD literature is vast and "internationalised" [2]. Based on available estimates [3] and publication trends [4] more than 20,000 articles on PTSD have thusfar been produced.

Post DSM-III, research has driven many advances in conceptualising how PTSD develops, how it is experienced, prolonged and effectively treated. That work has resulted in detailed explication of the disorder's phenomenology, extensive theorising about its aetiology and clinically important descriptive and explanatory models of PTSD associated with best practice treatment.

Despite this progress, there remain many uncertainties, controversies, prominent points of disagreement and critical knowledge gaps about PTSD. For example, there is ongoing debate over which experiences may be considered traumatic [5] and the nature of the stressor(s) required to meet diagnostic criteria. Moreover, DSM 5 [6] and ICD 11 [7] differ in how they derfine the construct of complex PTSD. There is also uncertainty about how to best treat PTSD. This is most evident when PTSD is complicated by psychiatric comorbidities such as anxiety, substance abuse and depressive disorders that require decisions to be made about treatment sequencing. Practitioners have expressed concern about sub-optimal implementation and translation of evidence-based psychological treatments for PTSD [8]. This has led to calls for further examination of transdiagnostic protocols [9] and personalised approaches for treating PTSD to enhance treatment outcome efficacy [10].

Another significant problem relates to the influence of dysfunctional anger in PTSD. Dysfunctional anger there is associated with increased morbidity and mortality. For example, through physical ill-health via conditions like cardio-vascular [11] and hypertensive disease, especially stroke [12]. The ruminative processes and negative self, other and world-appraisals associated with dysfunctional anger can impair the capacity to reason, and diminish problem-solving and goal-setting ability [13, 14]. Anger can also be a sign of unsuccessful attempts to deal with the experience of a traumatic event.

Sufferers of enduring PTSD often experience unrelenting, intense and distressing anger and significant impairment in interpersonal functioning. Those experiences are associated with degraded interpersonal relatedness [15], disparagement of others, and failure in relationship and family functioning [16]. When anger is extreme this can produce social alienation [17]. This leaves a trail of hurt and damage that most disconcertingly has a strong nexus to aggression [18, 19], violence [20] and suicidality [21].

Current and ex-serving military personnel are troublingly prone to experiencing problematic anger associated with their combat service and are considered the angriest veterans yet encountered [22, 23]. However, while dysfunctional anger is best documented in military personnel and veterans with PTSD [24, 25], it has been identified as a problem across a range of PTSD-affected populations. Such populations include those occupationally at risk for PTSD, like first responders [26], crime victims and perpetrators, those injured in workplace and road traffic accidents [27] and survivors of disasters [28], terrorism, atrocities, torture and political oppression [26, 29, 30].

PTSD has been characterised as a disorder of recovery requiring efficacious application of better psychological theories and treatments if better treatment outcomes are to be achieved [31, 32]. Highly pertinent to this objective, anger is not only strongly related to the maintenance of PTSD but plays a critical causal role. Upper-end estimates suggest 40% of PTSD score variance can be attributed to anger [33] and that reductions in anger lead not only to reductions in PTSD symptoms but caseness [34, 35]. Anger is also associated with poorer prognosis, high treatment dropout and is, perhaps, the principal impediment to the successful treatment of PTSD. This has been recognised in comprehensive reviews of anger [9] and anger in PTSD [34] and treatment studies, such as those focused on combat veterans [35].

Anger has emerged as an important aspect of the experience of PTSD that warrants further attention. However, there remains a need for nuanced explanatory models which capture the psychological mechanisms underlying the relationship between anger and PTSD. Accordingly, this chapter seeks to make clear why and how those phenomena are joined. Specifically, it seeks to elucidate the role of imagery as a psychological mechanism underlying the relationship of anger and PTSD in an integrated (visual-linguistic) cognitive model. These core objectives are pursued by reviewing the dominant theories of anger and anger in PTSD, and imagery. The limits of existing explanations of the influence of anger on PTSD and the role of imagery in that relationship are considered. A model of anger in PTSD is proposed that emphasises the role of imagery. This provides a platform for developing a fuller description and theoretical account of the aetiology and maintenance of PTSD. This platform permits identification of conditions required for better adapting imagery-based PTSD interventions to the treatment of anger-affected PTSD. It also suggests directions for future research on the role of anger and anger-Influenced imagery in PTSD.

## 2. The relationship between PTSD and anger

Anger is strongly associated with other dysphoric and aversive emotions. When dysfunctional it is closely associated with psychiatric conditions. Research shows that individuals with anxiety disorders experience greater anger severity, aggression, hostility and anger-related impairment, compared to those without them [9]. Anger is also often prominent in chronic pain conditions (particularly complex regional pain syndromes and fibromyalgia) [36] and psychotic spectrum disorders [9]. It is further associated with personality disorders, especially borderline, narcissistic, paranoid and antisocial types [37].

Anger's strongest link is, however, with PTSD. Sufferers of PTSD experience greater anger compared to individuals with subthreshold PTSD [38] and those without it [9]. They also have greater difficulty with anger control, compared to individuals suffering social or generalised anxiety or panic and obsessive-compulsive disorders [9, 39]. This has been identified in clinical samples like combat veterans [24] and non-clinical student samples [38].

The anger-PTSD association reflects several influences. Initially, there is the effect of anger's base-rate prevalence. Although it is not well understood clinically, anger, along with anxiety and depression, forms the "big three" [40], "unholy trinity" or "FAD" (fear-anger-depression) [41] of negative affect, but is considered the predominant emotion in treatment contexts [42]. Moreover, negative affects rarely occur alone. Typically, they share a content overlap and are recursively interdependent in their dysphoric effects. Consequently, beyond the direct impact of its high base-rate, anger also has a significant indirect association with PTSD through its strong relationship with other primary emotions [43].

Anger is more intertwined with other negative affects than any other emotion and comorbid aversive emotions are the norm in PTSD. Prominent, high impact emotions in PTSD that share an intimate relationship with anger include horror and disgust [44] and "responsibility emotions", such as guilt and shame [45, 46]. Shame-proneness is thought to be related to anger arousal, resentment and irritability and associated with indirect/non-expression of anger [47]. The angriest people have strong underlying feelings of guilt and shame [48]. Tournier observed that "Irritation-aggressiveness: this is the law of unconscious and repressed guilt [... and ...] those affected by guilt may be understandably irritable and at times, explode in anger or rage" (page 150) [49].

Considered one of the "moral emotions" [50], anger is a response to perceived failure to meet responsibility [51] and social norms [52] and is concerned with norm enforcement [53]. Exposure to potentially traumatising events (PTEs), and particularly extreme and malevolent interpersonal PTEs, almost inevitably raises issues of causality and intense meaning-related issues around responsibility and failure by commission or omission. This is provided for in hypothetical constructs that seek to explain trauma-related responses associated with anger. For example, the core symptoms of posttraumatic embitterment disorder [54] include: negativity, helplessness, blame of self and others, non-specific somatic symptoms, phobic avoidance of persons or situations related to the PTE, intrusions, phantasies of revenge and aggression. Additionally, in betrayal-based moral injury [55], anger is directed at another person who is perceived as having perpetrated a betrayal resulting in the injury or worse of associates.

Importantly, it is the relationship anger has with PTSD that is critical. This was highlighted almost 30 years ago by Lasko, Gervis, Kuhne, Orr and Pitman [56], who observed "increased aggression in war veterans is more appropriately regarded as a property of PTSD, rather than a direct consequence of military combat" (page 373). That observation was elaborated upon in the first meta-analysis undertaken in relation to anger and PTSD by Orth & Wieland in 2006. They concluded that "anger and hostility are substantially related to PTSD among samples who have experienced all possible types of traumatic events, not only in individuals with combat-related PTSD" (page 704) [57].

## 3. Anger in PTSD and the role of imagery: Insights, theories and models

Imagery has emerged as a fundamental cognitive process which is intimately involved in all emotional responses and an important feature of the experience of many forms of psychopathology [58]. It is also integral to interventions aimed at ameliorating negative emotional states and appears to be an important mechanism where anger is associated with PTSD [34].

### 3.1 Imagery in the stress and trauma literature

Mental imagery is the quasi-perceptual, subjectively-influenced, cognitive representation and recollection of perceptual experience in working memory in the absence of the originating stimulus [59, 60]. Although all five senses can generate imagery, its predominant form is visual [61]. Importantly, while all senses can be involved, the visual domain is most typically engaged in the application of imaginal treatments of PTSD. Referred to by a variety of names-including visual imagination [62], pictures in the mind [63] and seeing in the mind's eye [64]—visual imagery is less visually acute than perception. However, it preserves the perceptible properties of the stimulus and ultimately gives rise to the subjective experience of perception [60]. Henceforth, the term imagery refers to visual imagery. As imagery is more affectively-valenced than thought [58, 65], it imbues emotional memory with an intensity consistent with the original experience [66]. Thus mental images can be experienced as "realer than real" [62] and even influence the ability to experience emotion [67].

Imagery has an especially important relationship with negative emotion [68, 69] and psychopathology. Its role is well-documented in psychotic, dissociative, mood, substance-related, psychosomatic and anxiety disorders [58, 70, 71]. Imagery's strongest connection to negative, disordered emotion is however, among the anxiety disorders, notably specific phobia, social anxiety and stress disorders [72]. Imagery is implicated in various forms of specific phobia, including the imagery of the feared stimuli central to snake, spider and vomiting phobias [73, 74]. It is also a key factor in social anxiety disorder [75] especially where it pertains to negative imagery of the self [76]. Its relationship to PTSD is axiomatic, intrusive imagery being accepted as a core symptom, risk factor and severity-moderator [77].

The role of imagery in PTSD has been investigated overwhelmingly by reference to the affect of fear. This dates to the late nineteenth century, when Pierre Janet proposed that posttraumatic syndromes driven by intrusive recollections were experienced as disordered anxiety [78, 79], An anxiety-based conception of trauma response is evident in the early posttraumatic stress case descriptions and constructs (e.g., nostalgia and railway spine). It is also emphasised in the early-to-mid twentieth century constructs of shell shock, combat exhaustion and compensation neuroses [80]. Subsequently, the diagnostic and classificatory systems of psychiatry—in ICD-9 [81] and DSM-III [1], formalised this anxiety-based definition of PTSD and ICD 10 [82], and DSM-IV [83] in turn, reiterated it. Highly effective, anxiety-focused treatments have, consequently, been designed and implemented consistent with this anxiety-based conceptualisation of PTSD. Those treatments are summarised and discussed shortly for their implications.

Notwithstanding the advances made in PTSDs treatment, the historical focus on fear as its primary emotion may have impeded a fuller understanding of the disorder [84]. This is demonstrated in the growing recognition that PTSD is associated with emotions other than anxiety [85]. Fifty percent or more of PTSD's affective experience is estimated to relate to anger directly or in conjunction with disgust, guilt and shame [31, 86].

The relocation of PTSD to the Trauma and Stressor Related Disorders section of DSM 5 [6] from its previous location in the Anxiety Disorders section of DSM-III [1] and V [83] indicates the disorder's ongoing conceptual evolution. There is, of course, no barrier to exploring PTSD as strongly-anger related because of an association with imagery: the worth of that will be proven by the data.

These classificatory changes, however, remain contentious [87]. Proponents of major theories of PTSD such as the emotional processing model of PTSD understand it as an anxiety disorder [80, 88, 89] and the view that PTSD is an anxiety disorder is tenacious [80]. Irrespective of this, the insistence that the distress of all who experience PTSD is, without exception, anxious, has obscured evidence that the distress of a substantial group of sufferers is not primarily anxious in nature.

Research of anger in PTSD related to imagery has received less attention than that focused on anxiety in PTSD. Nonetheless, various studies suggest imagery and anger share an important relationship in the presence of PTSD. Higher levels of anger are associated with greater responsivity to imagery, while visual intrusions not only compound, but elicit, anger [57, 90]. Two reviews have explored the underlying relationship between imagery and anger as an aspect of negative emotion or in its own right. The first, by Holmes and Mathews [58] identified three overarching explanatory themes for the impact of imagery on negative emotion (anger included). The first centred on imagery's direct effect on the brain's emotional systems (whereby, imagery stimulates and is stimulated by, emotional and physiological arousal). The second noted its similar impact to real events (imagining an act engages the same neurological motor and sensory programs involved in carrying it out). The final theme was the capacity of imagery to reactivate feeling states such that attempts to avoid or suppress imagery result in unwanted and unintentional increases in its frequency and intensity. The second review by McHugh and colleagues [34] identified neurological, psychopathological and affective lines of evidence for the relationship of anger and imagery. They also formulated an imagery-informed model for better understanding the relationship of anger to PTSD, while detailing imagery's powerful effect on anger in PTSD.

Research has further identified imagery's role in eliciting angry mood and physiological reactivity [43]. Angry imagery has a particularly powerful effect on human physiological responses [91] and can generate responses greater than those derived from anger-provoking events themselves [92]. This link is evidenced by imagery's role in successful treatments for problematic anger across a range of populations [13, 93, 94].

Anger research shows that imagery impacts anger irrespective of imagery ability or repetition [95]. Consistent with this, high-intensity, emotional distress in PTSD promotes the experience of intrusions [59]. Posttraumatic intrusion repetition in turn increases imagery capacity [96] and vividness [97], in a circular affect-imagery relationship. Anger is not exempt from this and imagery's association with anger and anger in PTSD may not be dose-dependent. Thus, any level of imagery may be potent in its capacity to escalate anger. Finally, in PTSD, there is evidence that visual intrusions are both a cause and consequence of posttraumatic anger [57, 90, 98] and PTSD sufferers with high imagery control have fewer intrusions and less anger than those with low imagery control [99].

### 3.2 Theoretical models of anger and anger in PTSD

Several theoretical perspectives on the aetiology and maintenance of anger are potentially applicable to better understanding anger in PTSD. These theories are detailed in **Table 1**.

Of these theories, many are foundational psychological theories. Among them, social learning theory [100] understands behavioural modelling as crucial to the development of learned anger through the propensity of individuals to imitate behaviour observed in significant others (e.g., parents). In this theory three regulatory systems control behaviour—contingencies, feedback loops and cognitive function. It is proposed that anger can exist as a means for dealing with distress and is more likely to occur during affective distress and when some contingency exists for anger alleviation. The result is a circular problem of aversion, distress and anger.

Social learning theory fits well with the conditioning model of PTSD proposed by Keane and colleagues [107]. A social-interactionist learning theory, it was derived from conditioning theories of pathological anxiety, such as classic Pavlovian fear conditioning and Mowrer's two factor model [31]. Consistent with such theories, it posits that unconditioned stimuli (e.g., traumatic events associated with military experiences) automatically evoke unconditioned emotional (fear) responses. The intensity of this response generates avoidant protective responses. Warzone and combat-situations are quintessential stress environments. In combat life and death contingencies motivate highly-charged anger and emotional information processing that can become distorted and predictive of later anger in PTSD [108]. These reactions are often facilitated by pre-combat military training that mobilises the supposed "strength" of anger to avoid the dysphoric "weakness" of anxiety. This training dehumanises enemy combatants and operationalises the military imperative to negate and eliminate their threat. This renders military personnel more likely to respond to (objective) stress and trauma with anger, thereby precluding or impeding the development of other salient emotions such as anxiety and remorse [107].

| Theory | Content |
|---|---|
| Social learning theory [100] | Understands behavioural modelling is crucial to new learning. It emphasises the individual propensity to imitate behaviour observed in significant others, especially parents. According to it, three regulatory systems are thought to control behaviour: (1) contingencies, (2) feedback and (3) cognitive function. It proposes anger can serve as a habit to deal with distress and is more likely to occur when there is affective distress and some contingency exists for angry problem alleviating (e.g., as in anxiousness and anger) and the result is a circular problem of aversion, distress and anger. |
| Information processing theory [101, 102] | Asserts that the manner in which individuals perceive phenomena plays a role in maintaining emotions. Problem anger is often be associated with threat identification and unless corrective information is applied, misinterpretation ensues. Past events, thoughts, feelings and behavioural responses and meanings, are all stored in a "memory network". |
| Appraisal theory [103, 104] | Proposes that it is the perception of an event, not the event itself which is the key determinant of angry affect. It further emphasises that appraisals are not only necessary, but sufficient causal factors for the experience of anger. |
| Primary/ secondary emotion taxonomy [43] | Suggests overcontrol of (primary) anger around concern about the consequences of its expression and uncontrolled expression of (secondary) anger are both potent causes of dysfunction. |
| Contextual model of anger [105] | Emphasises the experience of anger reflects the role of:<br>1. Situational factors; like, disrespectful treatment, unfairness/injustice, frustration/ interruption, annoying traits in others and irritations.<br>2. Distal factors; such as embeddedness (via issues that may be personal., familial or social), interrelatedness (with other emotions and past experiences) transformationalism (from isolated instances of anger to chronic anger problemsand severe acts of aggression) and<br>3. Ambient factors; for example, those relating to the environment (incl. weather). |
| Neo-Associationist Theory [106] | Proposes anger involves a constellation of inter-related physiological, motoric and cognitive "responses". These are associated with the inclination to defend against or attack a target. |

**Table 1.**
*Major explanatory theories of anger.*

The programmatic nature of pre-combat training makes anger in PTSD difficult to de-operationalise and anger can become associated with a multitude of seemingly trivial day-to-day occurrences. These are not directly associated with the original traumatic experience but are subjectively interpreted as if they were and are associated with extreme levels of distress. What is not as readily understood is the significant function anger can play in the avoidance of such affects. This is specifically accommodated in Greenberg and Paivio's [43] primary-secondary emotion taxonomy and Beck's model of anxiety [109] which both emphasise the tendency to replace incapacitating distress with anger's action-orientation. Anger thus becomes a costly camouflage for other primary emotions.

Two more anger theories with significant potential utility in explaining anger in PTSD, are the information processing theory of anger [101] and the appraisal theory of anger [103, 104]. The information processing theory asserts that the perception of potential cues to anger is critical in maintaining angry affect. It proposes that problem anger is associated with threat identification and unless corrective information is applied, misinterpretation ensues. It also proposes that past events, thoughts, feelings and behavioural responses and meanings, are all stored in a latent "memory network" ready for activation. The appraisal theory of anger proposes event perception, and not the actual event, is the key determinant of anger, and that appraisals are not only necessary, but sufficient, causal factors for the experience of anger. This is particularly the case for perceptions of responsibility, culpability and entitlement [51, 110]. Neither of these theories have been explicitly investigated for their specific utility in explaining anger in PTSD populations. Nonetheless, they are consistent with established PTSD theories. Thus, the potential utility of the information processing theory of anger is suggested by both the information processing theory [111] and the conditioning model [107] of PTSD and the threat identification and misinterpretation they identify as occurring after exposure to military PTEs. The potential utility of the appraisal theory of anger is suggested by the warning signal hypothesis [112, 113] and the cognitive vulnerabilities model of PTSD [114]. Euphemistic of notions of neuroticism, the latter emphasises the impact of a negative attributional style for past and current-events and looming cognitive style for future-events on PTSD. This functions as a danger schema for predicting future threat and is strongly connected to perceptions about trauma and PTSD symptoms.

Two anger models have been explicitly investigated in relation to anger in PTSD. The first theory, the primary, secondary and instrumental emotion taxonomy developed by Greenberg and Paivio [43] holds that primary emotions, like fear and shame, are fundamental, direct and initial reactions to events and situations. Secondary emotions, by definition, are responses to thoughts or feelings, rather than the situation (e.g., anger in response to hurt, fear or guilt). Their theory posits that anger can be experienced as preferential to underlying, aversive, dysphoric states.

This taxonomy has been applied to research on veterans [115] and female crime victims [18]. The data support the view that anger deflects sufferers from intrusion-activated fear to a state less associated with feelings of vulnerability. This is consistent with the assertion by Riggs, Dancu, Gershuny, Greenberg and Foa that, in PTSD, anger and dissociation are both processes of disengagement or avoidance of the traumatic memory and fear network [18]. It is also consistent with Forbes and colleagues [22] finding that angry veterans with PTSD believe they are misunderstood and maltreated and tend to blame others for their mixed-emotion distress. These processes, are avoidant in nature. Although they may afford temporary relief from anxious distress through the pseudo-positivity of anger, they inhibit habituation. This prevents disconfirmatory or safety-related cues being incorporated into the trauma memory network to modify its associations and interpretations [18, 115, 116].

The neo-associationist memory network theory [106] extends the insights of the information processing and appraisal theories of anger. It proposes that anger involves a constellation of inter-related physiological, motoric and cognitive "responses". Associated with the inclination to defend against or attack a target, research on veterans with PTSD shows that associative networks connect negative affect with anger-related feelings, thoughts, intrusive memories and aggressive behavioural inclinations [117].

In addition to the PTSD-focused research on anger theories, studies of survivor mode [35, 118] have been undertaken in relation to anger in PTSD. This is a dysregulation model of anger in PTSD and not an anger theory per se. It views anger as governed by higher-order cognitive perceptual processes and emotional functions. It is the only PTSD specific, anger model designed and researched with PTSD in mind. It emphasises the importance of anger-related schemata in interpreting the self, others and the world. Such schemata reset anger activation-inhibition patterns toward a cognitive set revolving around mis-perceived threat. This invokes an unrecognised,

| Danger | Emotions/states | Contrariness | Injustice | Diminishment | Expectations |
|---|---|---|---|---|---|
| Perceived: | Feelings/sensations of: | Perceived: | Perceived: | Perceived: | Unmet/misplaced: |
| Risk (physical and psychological) to self/significant others | (Dis)tress | Disagreement | Unfairness | Dismissal | Rights |
| threat of attack to self/significant others | worry, fear | challenging | wrongdoing | diminishment | wants |
| other's failure to see risk or danger to self or significant others | insecurity | individualism | moral transgression | disrespected | desires |
| vulnerability (physical and psychological) | tension | "non-team" | malfeasance | devalued | needs |
| recklessness | jealousy, envy | behaviour | plotting | shamed | entitlements |
| impulsivity | hatred | norm exception | culpability | humiliation | standards |
| carelessness | annoyance | defiance | persecution | blame | norms |
| mistakes | vengefulness | disloyalty | discrimination | betrayal | (esp. of others) |
| other's (pre)caution failure | guilt and shame | "passivity" | revenge | exploitation | |
| bullying | embarrassment | indifference | overreaction | duplicity | |
| intimidation | disgust | ambivalence | insensitivity | criticism | |
| coercion | loss, grief and despair | disengagement | "sloth" | rejection | |
| malevolence | depression | selfishness | | neglect | |
| | helplessness | rejection | | abandonment | |
| | hopelessness | deceit | | intolerance | |
| | powerlessness | disloyalty | | | |
| | sadness and sorrow | disobedience | | | |
| | fatigue | dishonesty | | | |
| | remorse, regret | "stupidity" | | | |
| | disappointment | deviance | | | |
| | suspicion & paranoia | perversity | | | |
| | perfectionism | demanding | | | |

**Table 2.**
*Perceptions, cognitions, emotions and constructs associated with anger in PTSD.*

peremptory, all-consuming threat-anger action program that is enacted automatically in response to the merest or ambiguous, cues.

Studies of these three perspectives are few and their propositions around the mechanisms likely to contribute to anger in PTSD are not well-established. Taken together, their propositions emphasise anger's threat perception and appraisal-tendencies and its interconnectedness with other emotions (especially anxiety, guilt, shame and disgust). They also underscore that anger is linked to meaning making around responsibility and culpability associated with the conduct of the individuals or others. This is particularly true for behaviours with questionable morality, injustice or malevolence, diminishment and the self-focused expectations and behaviours of others.

Such a theoretical synthesis is supported by the testimony of individuals with PTSD involving prominent anger. McHugh [4] reported on the accounts of post-traumatic anger in a sample of 500 treatment seeking current and ex-serving military personal and first responders with PTSD. The sample was comprised primarily of police but also included ambulance officers, fire services personnel and other emergency services workers. The content of their intrusions and their recollections, cognitions and associated negative emotions, states of being and action tendencies are described in **Table 2**.

That testimony demonstrates the plethora of phenomena that can underlie the experience of anger in PTSD. It also conveys both the mental busyness of those with, enduring, angry PTSD and the powerful avoidant role anger plays in distracting from contemplation of crucial underlying issues.

In summary, theories and explanatory models of anger and anger in PTSD provide potentially important clinical understandings. Research suggest that frameworks such as the neo-associationist and primary/secondary taxonomy have direct clinical relevance to anger in PTSD. To date, however, research of anger has been limited in comparison to other affects such as anxiety and depression [52, 119] and there has been little attention given to anger in PTSD. Furthermore, empirical research focusing on the involvement of imagery in the facilitation, exacerbation and prolongation of anger in PTSD has thus far been negligible. Consequently, despite the involvement of imagery in emotional, cognitive and memory processes in PTSD, there is a dearth of theories and explanatory models of the relationship of imagery and anger in PTSD. There is therefore a clear need for multi-representational descriptive and explanatory theories and models.

### 3.3 The sequential impacts of anger and imagery on PTSD: a summary understanding

Drawing on the theoretical models of anger and PTSD described in the preceding sections, this section outlines a conceptual understanding of imagery's role in the sequential processing of anger in PTSD. **Figure 1** lays out a hypothetical sequential processing map of how anger develops in response to trauma-related cues and triggers.

As shown in **Figure 1**, PTSD is considered to involve disordered information processing along the lines of the information processing and appraisal literatures. Such disordered processing is strongly associated with the experience of dysphoric and aversive emotional states. Typically, this involves anxiety, emotions of responsibility (e.g., guilt and shame) and emotions of repugnance (e.g., horror or disgust). As argued by Greenberg and Paivio [43], in this context anger emerges as a primary, secondary or substituted affect associated with such primary emotions.

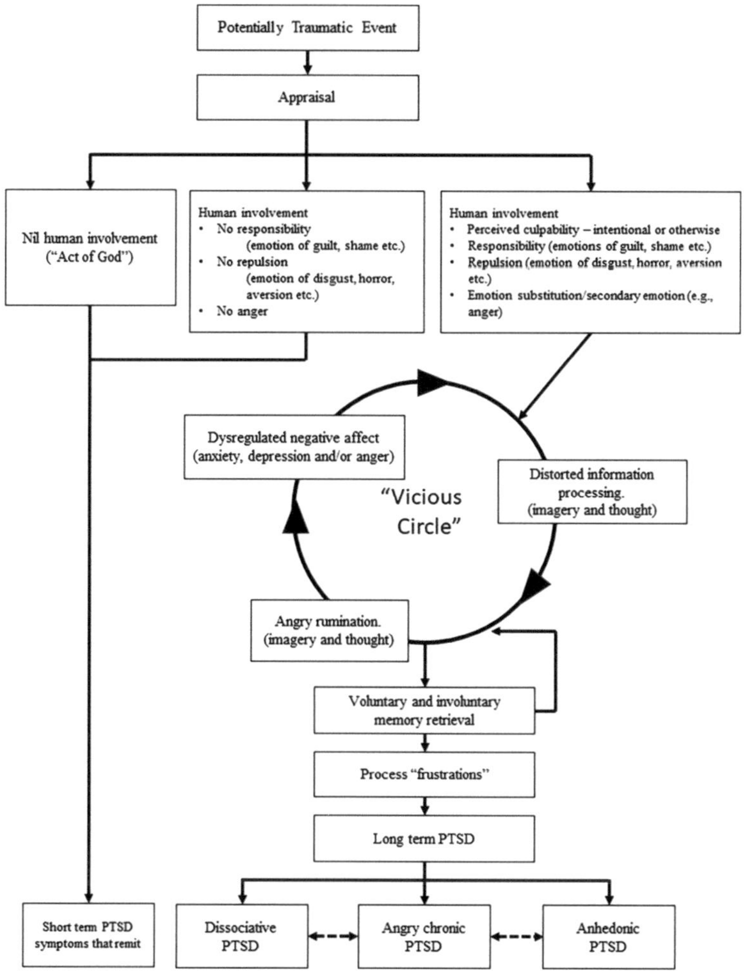


**Figure 1.**
*Sequential processing map of the hypothetical development of in response to trauma-related cues and triggers.*

Anger is particularly evident where the PTE has involved human culpability and, above all, where there is malevolence or morally dubious behaviour. That is provided for in trauma typologies [4, 34, 120]. The impact and chronicity of PTSD is thus intimately associated with the event perpetrator's intention, the event's meaning and its moral status [121–123]. Under such circumstances, information processing demands are significant, and cognition becomes laboured and prone to be "affected by affect". Where such demands apply, consistent with Beck's cognitive model [109] imagery is likely to be invoked in a vicious circle where processing becomes automated due to the effect of priming or the encoding of information and schematic processing via mental maps. These maps interpret tasks and the environment in which they occur out of conscious memory. Such schematic pattern analysis and interpretive maps are likely to drive and respond to priming (**Figure 1**). This part of the framework is consistent with appraisal-focused theories of PTSD.

The encoding of information in memory, increases the capacity to recall the event and related information from cuing, intentionally or otherwise [124]. This robustly exacerbates angry responses to post-priming trivial events [125, 126] and repetitive anger episodes lead to automaticity and secondary episodes that occur within 10–20 min of the first [126]. Anger episode duration increases with repetition and intensity. Primed by via repeated provocation (imagined or real) anger escalates in a non-linear fashion and significantly outlasts event duration (**Figure 1**). Thus provoked, anger can escalate even when the provocation remains constant (e.g., via a constant low-level annoying sound) and the sequence of escalation proceeds via reproaches, insults and threats [126]. Priming, perceived or actual provocation and externally-located causation are associated with rumination. That rumination may be verbal or imaginal in nature [34].

Other important anger moderating and mediating factors include disruption of anger due to fear, the presence/absence of distraction possibilities and apology [126, 127]. The duration and, concomitantly, rate of anger decline is influenced by the inability to control and cease rumination. Importantly, when anger occurs the form of revenge fantasies, rumination can have a half-life of more than a couple of weeks [128].

Because of the content of the intrusions and recollections involved in PTSD (**Table 3**) or the process repetition of the memory, poorly controlled verbal or imagery-based cognition increases the intensity of PTSD symptoms and associated anger. Appraisal theories of PTSD and anger suggest anger is likely to be prolonged

| | |
|---|---|
| *Cognitive Therapy for PTSD* [129] | In CT-PTSD, the individual is assisted to modify unhelpful responses which result from biased or distorted thoughts and memories associated with or arising from their traumatic experience (s). It seeks to modify excessively negative appraisals, correct autobiographical memory disturbance and address cognitive distortions and problematic behaviours, as well as any subsequent maladaptive or unhelpful beliefs individuals may develop about themselves, others and the world. It does so on the basis that PTSD remains persistent when individuals process the trauma in a way that leads to a sense of serious, current stress and danger which leads to involuntary re-experiencing of aspects of the trauma. |
| *Prolonged exposure* [88] | In PE, the individual is supported to gradually confront their memories of their traumatic experience and situational reminders of that experience that are otherwise avoided. This involves assisting them to change the way they think and feel about the traumatic experience and develop more helpful ways of coping, through education about common reactions to trauma, breathing retraining, behavioural exposure (to feared situations that clients avoided due to trauma-related fear), imaginal and processing (discussion of thoughts and feelings related to the exposure exercises) |
| *Eye movement desensitisation and reprocessing* [130] | In EMDR, the individual is required to focus on particular images, thoughts and bodily sensations related to the traumatic experience while simultaneously being sensorily stimulated. Most commonly, this is done by having the client move their eyes back and forth across their visual field (e.g., by tracking the movement of the therapist's finger). This process may be repeated many times. It is proposed that this dual attention protocol facilitates the processing of the traumatic memory into existing knowledge and memory networks and assists the individual to process the trauma. Although the precise operational mechanisms involved are not known, over time, EMDR has increasingly included treatment components comparable with CBT interventions. |
| *Cognitive processing therapy* [131] | In CPT, the individual is assisted to identify unhelpful thoughts and beliefs ("stuck points") and subsequently challenge and replace them with rational alternatives. This is done via an adaptation of standard cognitive therapy approaches. CPT has a smaller exposure component than PE that is typically restricted to writing an account of the traumatic experience. CPT also helps to address associated problems such as depression, guilt and anger. |

**Table 3.**
*Evidence-based treatments for PTSD.*

where rumination is poorly controlled and potentially distracting factors and apology are absent. That perspective aligns with the cognitive vulnerabilities model of PTSD [114] and multi-representational theories of PTSD; such as the Dual Representation Theory of PTSD [129] and Schematic, Propositional, Analogue, Associative, and Representational Systems model of PTSD [132].

In this sequential model, anger can be ignited by the recollection of what happened, who caused or permitted it to happen and what occurred afterward. Anger can also emanate from the ruminative replaying of unfinished business in dreams or involuntary or, often unwitting, voluntary daytime recollections [133]. Shown in **Figure 1**, irrespective of the source or intentionality, the resulting distress intensifies avoidance.

The pressure to avoid is associated with deliberate and unwittingly attempts to suppress intrusions. This is especially the case for aversive negative-emotion-influenced autobiographical imagery. Such imagery is typically experienced with a greater sense of reality (e.g., as measured by vividness), compared to non-emotional or semantic imagery [58]. Attempted suppression of intrusive phenomena is, however, almost always ineffective. This is well accounted for by Ironic Process Theory/the Zeigarnik Effect [134–136]. Efforts to suppress mental content, images included, can paradoxically lead to increased (re)occurrence of that specific content. Thus, rather than its intended outcome, avoidance leads to perverse, counter-intentional and unwitting rebounds [137] and even increases intrusions and imagery [138].

In an apparent case of the "greater the emotion, the greater the PSTD", symptoms are magnified when the dysphoric emotions associated with PTSD reach sufficient intensity thresholds. Anger can be either or both an initiator or potentiator of to this symptom escalation. Imagery is never far from such increases and the relationships among PTSD, anger and imagery are anything but coincidental [4].

## 4. A guideline for the evidence based psychological treatment of anger in PTSD

Treatments for PTSD with a high level of supporting evidence (i.e., randomised controlled trials with substantial sample sizes, systematic reviews and meta-analysis) are listed in **Table 3**. These treatments comprise: trauma-focused cognitive therapy, prolonged exposure, eye movement desensitisation and reprocessing and cognitive processing therapy. Collectively, the interventions fall under the rubric of trauma-focused cognitive-behavioural therapy, meaning they directly focus on recollections, cues and triggers of the PTE and its associated cognitions and emotions [139].

All these interventions require practitioners to pay deliberate, detailed attention to the provision of psychoeducation to assist clients to develop and maintain a personal model of recovery. They also require clinicians to help clients to develop skills to manage the maladaptive cognitions and affects which arise in the context of PTSD. Ultimately, they necessitate clinicians assisting clients to reprocess memories of causal traumatising events that they most likely, will have been avoiding. Finally, treatment aids the (re) development of functional abilities relating to everyday events based on the restoration of homeostatic mechanisms, habituation to emotion and new learning [88].

As well as exposure, imagery underpins various PTSD treatment interventions, including imagery rescripting and reprocessing therapy [140] and the treatment of post-traumatic nightmares via imagery rehearsal [141]. Imaginal exposure is, however, by far the most researched of these intervention techniques and its efficacy has been demonstrated across a broad sweep of trauma-exposed populations. Over 50 randomised controlled trials with substantial sample sizes [142, 143], multiple meta-analyses [144] and systematic reviews [145] support the use of imaginal exposure. It has deep historical roots in the treatment of pathological anxiety and has demonstrated treatment superiority across the range of anxiety disorders. It considered the most important advance in the psychological treatment of anxious distress in the last 70 years [146].

The utility of exposure in the treatment of PTSD characterised by fear, of course, does not explain whether, how or why it will ameliorate anger in PTSD. Effectively treating anger in PTSD, requires understanding of its aetiology and maintaining factors and its best practice treatment. This review has detailed the former; the latter is, however, yet to be established. To begin to address this gap the following prototypical guidelines are suggested for the effective application of evidence-supported imagery interventions to PTSD where anger is the predominant emotion.

### 4.1 Know and observe the limits of imagery-based interventions in the context of PTSD

Whether in the psychological or physical treatment realm, no intervention is, or can be, effective without exception. Thus while exposure is the gold standard treatment for PTSD [147, 148] and the archetypal example of imagery-focused approach to PTSD treatment, not all PTSD presentations respond well to it. For example, a study of active US military personnel with PTSD ($N$ = 326) randomly allocated to massed exposure (10 daily treatment sessions delivered over 2 weeks) or spaced exposure (10 treatment sessions delivered over 8 weeks) treatments identified classes of responders. These classes comprised rapid responders, steep linear responders, gradual responders, non-responders and symptom exacerbation [88]. Similar responder typologies emerged in a study of individuals with PTSD associated with multiple interpersonal traumata and previous attempts at treatment ($N$ = 73) [149]. Participants received an intensive phase of treatment (12 daily 90-minute sessions over 4 days) followed by a booster phase (4 weekly 90-minute booster sessions). While 71% were classed as treatment responders, cluster analysis demonstrated four treatment response trajectories. These were: fast responders (13%), slow responders (26%), partial responders (32%), and non-responders (29%).

The reasons for variations in treatment response to exposure have been ongoingly reviewed. Research has identified the impact on response to exposure treatment of symptom profiles. For example, those associated with PTSD's numbing symptom cluster [150], residual sleep problems [151] and emotional dysregulation [152] and ruminative and absorption processes [34]. Other studies have demonstrated that specific brain regions are involved in a differential response to or discriminated between responders and non-responders to exposure treatment. These include the bilateral superior frontal gyrus and pre-supplementary motor area [153] and pre-treatment hippocampal volumes [154]—and pre-treatment hormone levels, as measured in cortisol [155].

Importantly, a variety of imagery-related characteristics can mediate or moderate the efficacy of exposure in the treatment of PTSD. Although PTSD, anger and imagery share a connection, exposure and other imagery-based treatments may be unsuited to the certain presentations of anger in PTSD due to the appraisals and the presence of other negative affects [4]. This is because of the effect of the event types and the associated appraisals. To illustrate, PTSD-related anxiety classically revolves around issues of danger and risk. In contrast, in PTSD-associated anger (as noted in section 2, page 4), those appraisals, their underlying assumptions and the emotions that arise extend well beyond issues of danger and risk. As depicted in **Table 3**, those issues relate to wrong and injustice, diminishment, annoyance around expectations, disgust, guilt and shame and other non-anxiety-based affects. Such issues and associated anger are highly likely to be present in the face of horrific, macabre or morally-questionable behaviours associated with PTEs.

Given this, it is possible that the application of exposure, to problematic anger may not produce image decay and emotional habituation—the active mechanism involved in the remediation of the anxiety associated with PTSD. Instead, this may induce or exacerbate the frequency, intensity and duration of angry affect. This is because anger control is not about habituation and holding an angry image in the mind's eye until it decays. Rather, it is related to image control. Importantly, PTSD sufferers with high imagery control are known to have fewer intrusions and less anger than those with low imagery control [99]. While what constitutes imagery control in anger is opaque, imagery elimination and suppression are unviable alternatives to the unmitigated experience of imagery. Arguably, imagery control is characterised by the ability to down-regulate, disconnect from or relinquish imagery.

At different times, imagery may have little effect on anger in PTSD or have a large, singular and direct effect on anger. Arguably, any such effect may also be indirect and multiply determined in its interaction with other cognitive mechanisms, like thought-based appraisals. Furthermore, the motivations for angry responding may also possess a utilitarian social value (e.g., in relation to social justice and protection of the weak). Consequently, activating/invoking angry mentation via imaginal exposure may not produce the sought-after reduction in angry affect. This is greatest in PTSD, where anger interferes with the development of the treatment alliance that is so important in the successful treatment of PTSD [156] and, is perhaps, the principal impediment to the successful treatment of PTSD. Comprehensive reviews [9, 34] and treatment studies [35] having recognised its impact and metanalyses demonstrate its interference in exposure tasks [39]. Anger's impact on treatment is particularly notable in combat veterans [157], but is also likely to affect populations subject to malevolent interpersonal trauma (e.g., childhood and pernicious adult sexual assault [158]).

As Meichenbaum [13] incisively observed, intense anger is not easy to work with and clients with angry presentations may become more so during treatment and direct anger and aggression toward clinicians. He further noted that such angry clients are often highly impatient, easily frustrated, unrealistic about treatment goals, typically noncompliant with treatment and treatment resistant. In the face of such anger, clinician effectiveness is subject to significant challenge. Consequently, in worst case scenarios, clinicians are liable to be rendered impassive in the face of significant client anger. This may partially account for the all-too-often failure of clinicians to follow evidence based practice [8, 159] and to divert from protocols when faced with difficult-to-treat anger [160]. This is of concern as it is likely to produce sub-optimal implementation and translation of evidence-based psychological treatments of PTSD.

### 4.2 Recognise the influence of individual differences and circumstances on imagery

To be effective, exposure must be applied while cognisant of individual differences in the capacity to image in a person-appropriate manner. Group characteristics, such as ethnicity influence the capacity to experience imagery. Notably, imagery is greater among the peoples of East Asia [161] and indigenous cultures, like those of Australia, which utilise imagery in practical day-to-day tasks [162]. There are also gender differences in the capacity to utilise imagery [163]. Women have a superior ability to generate and maintain images [164] and experience more vivid images than men [165, 166]. They also react more strongly to unpleasant affective images, while men react more strongly to pleasant affective images [167]. Finally, the experience of imagery reduces with age [164, 168–170] and there is unequivocal evidence that imagery capacity degrades with age [171, 172].

The efficacy of exposure is also influenced by innate differences in imagery capacity. There are various abilities or traits related to the capacity to image. These include absorption, thinness of reality-imagination boundaries and imagery vividness [173]. Some types of imagery are personality based [174]. The style of imagery-based information processing is also affected by cognitive style and appraisal tendencies. This involves the balance between reflective thinking and thought-based information processing, known as verbalising style [175, 176]. Individuals with a higher capacity for visual imagery experience more visual and other sensory details when remembering or imagining past and future events [177].

Many abilities and personality traits influence the capacity to image. Imagery vividness has been associated with angry personality-based obsessionality [178] and individuals with high trait anger have been shown to have greater reactivity to angry imagery in the absence of enhanced imagery ability [95]. Imagery absorption is another dispositional trait that is highly correlated with the tendency to image and the intensity of the imagery experience [179, 180]. Under conditions of significant stress, absorption can become an imagery-based coping mechanism.

Greater imagery control is associated with greater internal locus of control [181], while extraversion and introversion are associated with imagery fluency [182]. The latter is consistent with the long-standing interpretation that extraverts are verbalisers and introverts are imagers [175, 176]. Importantly, this appears to be mediated by stress levels and Stricklin and Penk [183] found that, among incarcerated female offenders, extroverts reported more vivid imagery than introverts under high-distress. In contrast, introverts reported more vivid imagery than extroverts under low-distress.

The suitability of imagery to the remediation of anger is PTSD is also likely to vary according to situational circumstances. This is well illustrated from workplace injuries, where compensation and treatment claims involving psychological injuries are more difficult to administer and likely to become complicated where their aftermath possesses certain characteristics. These include a workplace climate which fails to promote workplace health and wellbeing or where the risk of injury is poorly managed or increased by inappropriate work practices. It can also involve the failure of the insurer to promptly approve best practice treatment for the injuries and worker perception(s) that the employer and/or insurer do not adequately care for them or where the event is associated with the injury involved horror, disgust human malevolence or culpable negligence [147]. In such circumstances, a sense of injustice motivates angry psychological distress in workers. Anger is associated with what happened and who allowed it to happen and/or failed to respond to their needs after an injury they neither expected nor caused. This powerful sense of wrong and the restorative justice required to address can instigate blazing and righteous anger and consequent revenge fantasises in those who perceive themselves unduly treated in the workplace [128]. This can lead to the targeting of health service providers and compensatory health and legal systems by individuals with traumatic injuries [184].

The Contextual Model of Anger (see **Table 1**) heavily emphasises the importance of the interaction of several contributing factors. First is the anger derived from situational factors involving the experience of perceived or objective disrespectful conduct, unfairness, injustice, being wronged, thwarting of goal attainment and annoying behaviour of others. The second anger causing factor relates to ambient factors. For example, those relating to the environment, such as noise odour and temperature. Over time, through repetitious exposure and associative tendencies these factors become compounded in a third, distal factor. This involves embeddedness (via issues that may be personal, familial or social), interrelatedness (with other emotions and past experiences) and transformationalism (from isolated instances of anger to chronic anger problems and severe acts of aggression).

Novaco proposes that anger involves regulatory deficits in three psychological domains These include a cognitive domain (justification, attentional focus, rumination, hostile attitude and suspicion); an arousal domain (intensity, duration, somatic activation and irritability) and a behavioural domain (impulsive reactions, verbal aggression, physical confrontation and indirect expression of anger). The more deficits, characteristics and domains activated the greater the anger. Thus, in a study of veterans with PTSD and high levels of anger in multi-year anger treatment trial, Chemtob and others [35] described individuals who displayed high intensity regulatory deficits in all three domains of anger as "ball of rage patients".

### 4.3 Apply evidence-supported and anger-specific treatments to anger in PTSD

There is strong evidence of the general effectiveness of anger treatment. Bushman and colleagues have written extensively about this and have emphasised the utility of anger regulation interventions, such as cognitive therapy (especially distancing, behavioural distancing and language moderation), skills training and relaxation training [185, 186]. Meta-analyses by Tafrate [187], Edmondson and Conger [188], Beck and Fernandez [189], DiGiuseppe and Tafrate [190], Del Vecchio and O'Leary [191] and Henwood and others [192] and Lee and DiGiuseppe [193] report effect sizes as measured by Cohen's d [194] ranging from 0.64 to 1.16. Notably, Glancy and Saini [195] in their systematic review of meta-analyses of psychological treatments of anger and aggression, observed there are strong effect sizes for "classical" CBT approaches (skills training and problem solving) but lesser effect sizes for "variants", like acceptance and commitment therapy. They found multi-component interventions to be most effective (d = .93), followed by skills training (d = .85) and cognitive interventions alone (d = .83). They reported a trend for manualised treatments to produce larger effects than non-manualised treatments (d = .85 v. 76) The number of sessions also has a positive and significant relationship to the magnitude of the effect size, although the modal number of sessions is 8.5 and range of sessions provided is from 3 to 40. They further noted that such outcomes been established for clients of diverse backgrounds. This included forensic clients, violent recidivists, batterers, adults with intellectual and learning disabilities or serious mental illness, aggressive drivers and military personnel and veterans.

In comparison to the treatment of anger per se, the development of treatment strategies for anger in PTSD is in its formative stages and few interventions for anger and aggression in PTSD have been elaborated [196]. The CBT approaches identified in these reviews and meta-analyses have implicit applicability to anger in PTSD, provided they are nuanced for the impact of traumatisation. Research on PTSD associated anger demonstrates that cognitive therapy and skills training are effective in treatment of dysfunctional anger. These appear most effective when delivered individually or by group and face-to-face or remotely (e.g., by teleconferencing) [197].

Two studies have examined treatment approaches with solid face validity with promising results. The first by Mackintosh and colleagues [22], investigated the roles of anger regulation skills (i.e., relaxation training) and therapeutic alliance in reducing anger symptoms in contemporary ($N$ = 109) US veterans. It identified that gains in calming skills predicted significantly larger reductions in anger symptoms. This finding has intuitive merit, for it is not possible that, apart from situations involving Schadenfreude, an individual can be simultaneously calm and angry. It also fits well with the above-identified effectiveness literature on the treatment of anger.

The other study used self-instruction training (SIT) which is an intervention with intuitive validity in the treatment of anger in PTSD [13, 198]. The aim of SIT is to enhance coping in face of adverse events by the use of pre-rehearsed self-talk instruction. Cash and colleagues [199], in an Australian contemporary serving combat personnel population, established a cognitive skills training set centred around self-instruction training. They used SIT targeted at negating the operation of schema modes [200], and reported impressive anger and PTSD symptom reduction effects (they reported effect sizes of 1.6 as measured by Cohen's d) pre to post-treatment. This efficacy of SIT for anger in PTSD fits with the long-demonstrated history of the efficacy of SIT, including for individuals with overlapping comorbidities, like anxiety, mood and substance abuse disorders [13]. It is also supported by the reviews and metanalyses cited at the start of this sub-section of the review.

Although such studies do not explicitly argue in favour of the use of imagery, it is clearly possible for it be involved in their implementation. Imagery may also be utilised in other treatment strategies for anger regulation, such as cognitive therapy, and treatment methods, such distancing and behavioural rehearsal. The best practice use of imagery in treatments of anger and anger in PTSD is yet to be determined. For example, the style of SIT deployed by Cash and colleagues emphasised a coping approach that sought to tolerate challenging situations. Their approach stands in contrast to the imaginal reliving of hierarchically organised provocative situations and experiences in stress-related anger studies by Novaco on populations as diverse as incarcerated individuals with intellectual disabilities and police [201]. The relative merits of these approaches-with their competing emphases on coping versus habituation-for reducing or exacerbating anger in PTSD, require explication. This is also the case for other treatments of anger involving imagery. This may require existing anger treatments to be finessed for the impact of trauma when applying them to anger in PTSD.

### 4.4 Locate anger work within a phased PTSD treatment model

All treatments for PTSD are recommended for delivery via a staged sequence. This has been agreed for some time among theoreticians and researchers and long argued from diverse theoretical paradigms, including eclectic, psychodynamic and integrative perspectives (see **Table 4**).

A stage intervention sequence requires clinicians to provide an explanatory model of posttraumatic stress and how it best treated. A treatment roadmap is also needed that outlines the shared and individual responsibilities of clinician and client. Such an approach, provides a psychologically reassuring treatment structure for clients and enables them to build a personal model of recovery. A comprehensive staged model of treatment has been articulated by Keane and Kaloupek [208]. It involves six stages of treatment: (1) emotional and behavioural stabilisation, (2) education and

| Eclectic [202] | Psychodynamic [203] | Psychodynamic [204–206] | Integrative approaches [207] |
|---|---|---|---|
| Encounter/ Education Phase | Psycho-physiological Assessment Phase | Initial Exploration and development of therapeutic relationship Phase | Education and Affect Regulation Phase |
| Skill building & client empowerment Phase | Behaviour therapy Phase | Working through Phase and event re-appraisal Phase | Self-harming/limiting behaviour reduction via cognitive interventions Phase |
| Exploring trauma & its impact | Dynamic therapy | Development of new adaptive actions | Trauma focussed work |
| Evaluation & integration Phase | Existential therapy | Working Through (Marmar/ Lindy) Practice of adaptive actions until automatic Horowitz | Self-awareness and self-acceptance Phase |
| Termination Phase | Termination Phase | Termination & Loss Phase | |

**Table 4.**
*Staged treatment models and theoretical treatment orientations.*

information, (3) arousal management, (4) exposure treatment, (5), cognitive restructuring and (6) relapse prevention and maintenance. A space for exposure is provided in its fourth stage. This is preceded by an arousal management treatment stage, where any anger-focused work required may be given focus.

It has long been recognised that, where posttraumatic anger is intense, more treatment will typically be needed before the implementation of exposure treatment [209]. Anger is particularly associated with enduring PTSD resulting from events characterised by culpability, issues of existential meaning (or in its simple form, moral injury [210]. It is also associated with intense primary (e.g., shame and guilt) responsibility and/or repugnance-related (e.g., horror and disgust) emotions. In prolonged PTSD anger is further connected to strong overarching concerns with atonement or revenge that manifest as psychopathology [116]. This almost inevitably requires treatment of greater frequency and duration.

### 4.5 An algorithm for the use of imagery-focused treatment in PTSD

Taking the treatment requirements, and the literature on which they are based, into account, a phased decision sequence can be proposed for imagery-focused treatment of PTSD with or without anger. When the primary presenting emotion is:

- anxiety experienced as worry or fear—use imaginal and behavioural exposure augmented by trauma-informed anger-work for any irritability that may arise in conduct of that exposure work

- anger secondary to anxiety or a sense of danger—use behavioural and imaginal exposure preceded by trauma-anger-work focused on coping in the moment not reliving past experiences and addressing the avoidant, emotion substitution and camouflaging impact of the presenting anger and

- a non-fear-based affect-and especially where there are issues of responsibility (guilt and shame), repugnance (horror, disgust or repulsion), wrong or injustice or a sense of diminishment, and expectations that run contrary to a "team ethic" or the needs of others—use trauma-informed anger-work that takes account of thought, appraisal, language and imagery inputs and utilises evidence-based anger interventions.

## 5. Directions for future research

Over a decade ago, Shalev noted that the US Institute of Medicine judged the scientific evidence for the treatment of PTSD as below the level expected for such a common, disabling disorder. He observed significant progress was being made in the disorder's treatment, but was limited by an apparent treatment-ceiling-effect and a need for more efficacious application of better psychological theories [32]. Consistent with this view, the need to broaden the focus of enquiry in PTSD beyond anxiety-based models was simultaneously identified in comprehensive reviews [31, 211].

As shown in this review, anger may be the predominant emotion for a majority of PTSD presentations [31] and it has vast costs that heavily impact on individuals, partners, families and communities. Yet, research on anger remains surprisingly sparse, with the most recent estimates suggesting it may equal as little 0.6 % of all PTSD publications [4]. There is an unequivocal need to increase research on anger in PTSD. This section suggests directions for future work.

An initial objective of research on PTSD must be to explicitly recognise the importance of anger to PTSD. Anger has been described as forgotten [212], unrecognised [9] and misunderstood [213] and the rate of research of anger in PTSD is lower than the level that might be reasonably expected on account of wide-ranging deleterious impacts. Explicit acknowledgement of anger's importance for prolonging PTSD, and as a factor influencing treatment outcome, will facilitate research on enhancing treatment protocols for treatment resistant clients. This proposition is supported by the work of various PTSD researchers who have illuminated the problem of anger, including Pitman and others [209], Elbogen, Johnson and Beckham [20], Forbes, McHugh and Chemtob [214], Morland and others [23, 197], Rona and colleagues [108] and Worthen and associate [215].

A second important research objective is to better understand the nature of anger and its relationship to imagery in PTSD. Despite its importance, the phenomenology of dysfunctional anger and imagery in anger in PTSD is not well described. Clearer identification of imaginal and linguistic cognitive processes and their relationship to anger-related PTSD in an integrated (visuo-linguistic) cognitive model of anger in PTSD would be another important step in research on anger in PTSD.

Research that identifies how anger in PTSD interacts with the characteristics of the PTE will be important in identifying differences in maintaining factors of PTSD after specific PTEs. It will also be useful to understanding the relationship between anger and cumulative trauma (e.g., due to vocation and occupation), the impact of perpetration versus experience of PTEs and the respective impact of exposure to PTEs versus how individuals are cared for post event.

The minting of PTSD in DSM-III created a research impetus that led to critical advances in knowledge of the disorder. That research impetus continues and DSM 5 has identified a dissociative PTSD subtype, sub-syndromal/prodromal PTSD and even a PTSD genotype [31, 211]. There is potentially significant value in exploring the possibility of an angry PTSD subtype to clearly identify individuals for whom anger is the primary emotional and evolve treatments to assist them.

A third area for further inquiry relates to the linkages between anger and other trauma-related emotions. This review has shown that anger can occur in PTSD as a primary or secondary emotion connected to anxiety, responsibility-related emotions (especially shame and guilt) [43] and repugnance-related affects (like disgust and horror) [4, 44]. Understanding how anger is linked to other emotions and to symptom maintenance will aid the further refinement of treatment interventions for anger in PTSD. A full comprehension of the nature of anger in PTSD also requires a deeper understanding of the many cognitive processes associated with anger in PTSD. The application of imagery-based interventions to anger in the context of PTSD may be differentially efficacious depending on the cognitions, appraisals and affective causal pathways involved.

Based on the central argument of this review, a specific set of imagery-related research objectives could be pursued. As part of this, it will be important to establish what it is about visual imagery that promotes or hinders the efficacy of imaginal exposure in PTSD in the presence of anger. This exploration of imagery as a mechanism underlying anger's relationship to PTSD and the treatment of the disorder, will aid the development of a fuller account of the aetiology and maintenance of PTSD and offer new possibilities for enhanced treatment outcomes. Research is needed on psychological phenomena such as control, voluntary and involuntary experience of intrusions, the impact of content and process-related imagery and distress, cognitive style as expressed in the balance between imagery and linguistic-cognition and the association between personal style and imagery.

The dearth of theories and explanatory models about the role of imagery in anger in PTSD and any other mechanisms which may underlie their relationship are compelling grounds for testing and developing models and theories about different aspects of imagery in its interaction with anger in PTSD. So that imagery is integrated into descriptive and explanatory models with other important influences, like cognitive style and personality, it is important that such theories operate at multi-representational levels of explanation, are well operationalised and easily testable. Finally, it is important that focus be applied to the role of anger in PTSD as an explanation for the non-response to proven imagery-based treatments, like exposure. As part of this, any the means by imagery may reduce the treatment interference of anger must be investigated.

## 6. Conclusion

This review has elucidated the linkages between anger in PTSD and advanced various propositions underscoring the role of imagery as an underlying mechanism in their relationship. Based on that exposition, guidelines and an algorithm for the efficacious treatment of anger in PTSD have been proposed. That algorithm and those guidelines underscore the importance of appreciating the limits of imagery-based interventions in the context of PTSD and recognising the influence of individual differences and circumstances on imagery in PTSD. They also stress the need to apply evidence-supported anger-specific treatments to anger in PTSD and locate anger-work within a phased PTSD treatment model. This represents the first articulation of such guidance and it is, accordingly, best understood as prototypical in nature.

PTSD is a disorder of recovery and there are significant, positive treatment outcomes associated with evidence-based, gold standard psychological interventions like exposure treatment. This particularly the case where anxiety is the predominant emotion experienced by those with PTSD. Many individuals, however, are likely to be troubled by enduring PTSD characterised by posttraumatic anger. A significant minority of this group are either slow or fail to benefit from the receipt of first rank PTSD treatments, like imaginal exposure. This group is the logical target for increased conceptual and empirical research and descriptive and explanatory theoretical models of anger in PTSD and its treatment are much required. It is also important, given the imagery-based connections between anger and PTSD identified in this review, that such theoretical models attend to the role of imagery. Poor imagery control is the law of poor anger control. This is particularly so in anger in PTSD.

To better account for and treat anger in PTSD, the theoretical models developed need to be multi-representational in nature and attend to affective, physiological, behavioural and account for both linguistic and imaginal cognitive processes. Such an approach is entirely consistent with the observation of Aaron T Beck that "effective cognitive therapy depends greatly on moving beyond purely verbal exchanges to encouraging patients and therapists to resort to their auditory or visual imagery capacities" (page 107) [216].

## Author details

Tony McHugh[1] and Glen Bates[2*]

1 University of Melbourne, Parkville, Australia

2 Swinburne University of Technology, Hawthorn, Australia

*Address all correspondence to: gbates@swin.edu.au

## References

[1] American Psychiatric Association. Diagnostic and Statistical Manual of Mental Disorders (DSM III). 3rd ed. Washington DC: American Psychiatric Association; 1980

[2] Fodor KE, Unterhitzenberger J, Chou C-Y, Kartal D, Leistner S, Milosavljevic M, et al. Is traumatic stress research global? A bibliometric analysis. European Journal of Psychotraumatology. 2014;**5**(1):23269

[3] Bedard M, Greif JL, Buckley TC. International publication trends in the traumatic stress literature. Journal of Traumatic Stress: Official Publication of The International Society for Traumatic Stress Studies. 2004;**17**(2):97-101

[4] McHugh AF. I'm hurt, annoyed and see things: Anger in PTSD and the role of visual imagery [PhD Thesis]. 2015

[5] Haslam N. Concept creep: Psychology's expanding concepts of harm and pathology. Psychological Inquiry. 2016;**27**(1):1-17

[6] American Psychiatric Association. Diagnostic and Statistical Manual of Mental Disorders (DSM V). 5th ed. Washington DC: American Psychiatric Association; 2013

[7] World Health Organization (WHO). International Statistical Classification of Diseases and Related Health Problems (11th ed). 2019. Geneva: World Health Organization; Available from: https://icd.who.int/

[8] van Minnen A, Hendriks L, Olff M. When do trauma experts choose exposure therapy for PTSD patients? A controlled study of therapist and patient factors. Behaviour Research and Therapy. 2010;**48**(4):312-320

[9] Cassiello-Robbins C, Barlow DH. Anger: The unrecognized emotion in emotional disorders. Clinical Psychology: Science and Practice. 2016;**23**(1):66

[10] Forbes D, Bisson JI, Monson CM, Berliner L. Effective Treatments for PTSD. 3rd ed. New York: Guilford Press; 2020. p. 578

[11] Burg MM, Soufer R. Post-traumatic stress disorder and cardiovascular disease. Current Cardiology Reports. 2016;**18**(10):1-7

[12] Perkins JD, Wilkins SS, Kamran S, Shuaib A. Post-traumatic stress disorder and its association with stroke and stroke risk factors: A literature review. Neurobiology of Stress. 2021;**2021**:100332

[13] Meichenbaum D. Anger control problems. In: Freeman A, Felgoise SH, Neza AM, Nezu CM, Reinecke MA, editors. Encyclopedia of Cognitive Behavior Therapy. Boston MA: Springer; 2005. pp. 23-26

[14] Paunovic N. Cognitive factors in the maintenance of PTSD. Behaviour Therapy. 1998;**27**(4):167-178

[15] Beckham J, Moore S, Reynolds V. Interpersonal hostility and violence in Vietnam combat veterans with chronic posttraumatic stress disorder: A review of theoretical models and empirical evidence. Aggression and Violent Behavior. 2000;**5**(5):451-466

[16] Taft CT, Schumm JA, Panuzio J, Proctor SP. An examination of family adjustment among Operation Desert Storm veterans. Journal of Consulting and Clinical Psychology. 2008;**76**(4):648

[17] Forbes D, Creamer M, Allen N, Elliott P, McHugh T, Debenham P, et al. The MMPI-2 as a predictor of symptom change following treatment for posttraumatic stress disorder. Journal of Personality Assessment. 2002;**79**(2):321-336

[18] Riggs DS, Dancu CV, Gershuny BS, Greenberg D, Foa EB. Anger and post-traumatic stress disorder in female crime victims. Journal of Traumatic Stress. 1992;**5**(4):613-625

[19] Taft CT, Street AE, Marshall AD, Dowdall DJ, Riggs DS. Posttraumatic stress disorder, anger, and partner abuse among Vietnam combat veterans. Journal of Family Psychology. 2007;**21**(2):270

[20] Elbogen EB, Johnson SC, Beckham JC. Anger, aggression, and violence. In: Moore B, Penk W, editors. Treating PTSD in Military Personnel: A Clinical Handbook. New York: Guilford Press; 2011. pp. 305-325

[21] Cowlishaw S, Metcalf O, Little J, Hinton M, Forbes D, Varker T, et al. Cross-lagged Analyses of Anger and PTSD Symptoms among Veterans in Treatment: Psychological Trauma, Theory, Research, Practice, and Policy. US: Educational Publishing Foundation; 2021

[22] Mackintosh MA, Morland LA, Frueh BC, Greene CJ, Rosen CS. Peeking into the black boxmechanisms of action for anger management treatment. Journal of Anxiety Disorders. 2014;**28**(7):687-695

[23] Moreland LA, Love AR, Mackingtosh MA, Greene CJ, Rosen CS. Treating anger and aggression in military populations: Research updates and clinical implications. Clinical Psychology: Science and Practice. 2012;**19**(3):305

[24] Jakupcak M, Conybeare D, Phelps L, Hunt S, Holmes HA, Felker B, et al. Anger, hostility, and aggression among Iraq and Afghanistan war veterans reporting PTSD and subthreshold PTSD. Journal of Traumatic Stress: Official Publication of the International Society for Traumatic Stress Studies. 2007;**20**(6):945-954

[25] O'Toole BI, Marshall RP, Grayson DA, Schureck RJ, Dobson M, Ffrench M, et al. The Australian Vietnam veterans health study: III. Psychological health of Australian Vietnam veterans and its relationship to combat. International Journal of Epidemiology. 1996;**25**(2):331-340

[26] Evans S, Giosan C, Patt I, Spielman L, Difede J. Anger and its association to distress and social/occupational functioning in symptomatic disaster relief workers responding to the September 11, 2001, World Trade Center disaster. Journal of Traumatic Stress. 2006;**19**(1):147-152

[27] Ehlers A, Mayou RA, Bryant B. Psychological predictors of chronic posttraumatic stress disorder after motor vehicle accidents. Journal of Abnormal Psychology. 1998;**107**(3):508

[28] Forbes D, McHugh A. Anger-the Missing Piece in the 5 Essential Elements Approach. Psychiatry, 2021;**84**(4):367-372

[29] Mearns J, Mauch TG. Negative mood regulation expectancies predict anger among police officers and buffer the effects of job stress. The Journal of Nervous and Mental Disease. 1998;**186**(2):120-125

[30] Dunnegan SW. Violence, trauma and substance abuse. Journal of Psychoactive Drugs. 1997;**29**(4):345-351

[31] Friedman MJ. PTSD and related disorders. In: Stein D, Friedman MJ, Blanco C, editors. Post-traumatic Stress

Disorder. Hoboken, NJ: Wiley Blackwell; 2011. pp. 1-34

[32] Shalev AY. Posttraumatic stress disorder and stress-related disorders. Psychiatric Clinics. 2009;**32**(3):687-704

[33] Novaco RW, Chemtob CM. Anger and combat-related posttraumatic stress disorder. Journal of Traumatic Stress. 2002;**15**(2):123-132

[34] McHugh T, Forbes D, Bates G, Hopwood M, Creamer M. Anger in PTSD: Is there a need for a concept of PTSD-related posttraumatic anger? Clinical Psychology Review. 2012;**32**(2):93-104

[35] Chemtob CM, Novaco RW, Hamada RS, Gross DM, Smith G. Anger regulation deficits in combat-related posttraumatic stress disorder. Journal of Traumatic Stress. 1997;**10**(1):17-36

[36] McHugh T. Assessing and Treating Angry PTSD. Melbourne: Australian Psychological Society; 2021

[37] Fernandez E, Johnson SL. Anger in psychological disorders: Prevalence, presentation, etiology and prognostic implications. Clinical Psychology Review. 2016;**46**:124-135

[38] Jakupcak M, Tull MT. Effects of trauma exposure on anger, aggression, and violence in a nonclinical sample of men. Violence and Victims. 2005;**20**(5):589-598

[39] Olatunji BO, Ciesielski BG, Tolin DF. Fear and loathing: A meta-analytic review of the specificity of anger in PTSD. Behavior Therapy. 2010;**41**(1):93-105

[40] Frisch MB. Quality of Life Therapy: Applying a Life Satisfaction Approach to Positive Psychology and Cognitive Therapy. New York: John Wiley & Sons; 2005

[41] Zuckerman DM, Prusoff BA, Weissman MM, Padian NS. Personality as a predictor of psychotherapy and pharmacotherapy outcome for depressed outpatients. Journal of Consulting and Clinical Psychology. 1980;**48**(6):730

[42] Fernandez E. Anxiety, Depression, and Anger in Pain: Research Findings and Clinical Options. Dallas, TX: Advanced Psychological Resource; 2002

[43] Greenberg LS, Paivio SC. Working with Emotions in Psychotherapy. New York: Guilford Press; 1997

[44] Steel Z, Hilbrink D. Dealing with horror. In: Frame T, editor. Moral Injury: Unseen Wounds in an Age of Barbarism. Sydney: UNSW Press; 2015

[45] Clifton EG, Feeny NC, Zoellner LA. Anger and guilt in treatment for chronic posttraumatic stress disorder. Journal of Behavior Therapy and Experimental Psychiatry. 2017;**54**:9-16

[46] Norman S, Allard C, Browne K, Capone C, Davis B, Kubany E. Trauma Informed Guilt Reduction Therapy: Treating Guilt and Shame Resulting from Trauma and Moral Injury. Cambridge MA: Academic Press; 2019

[47] Hoglund CL, Nicholas KB. Shame, guilt, and anger in college students exposed to abusive family environments. Journal of Family Violence. 1995;**10**(2):141-157

[48] Tangney JP, George M, Wagner P, Fletcher C, Gramzow R. Shamed into anger? The relation of shame and guilt to anger and self-reported aggression. In: Parrot WG, editor. Emotions in Social Psychology Essential Readings.

New York: Psychology Press; 2001. pp. 285-294

[49] Tournier P. Guilt and Grace: A Psychological Study. Michigan: Harper & Row; 1962

[50] Hutcherson CA, Gross JJ. The moral emotions: A social–functionalist account of anger, disgust, and contempt. Journal of Personality and Social Psychology. 2011;**100**(4):719

[51] Lemerise EA, Dodge KA. The development of anger and hostile interactions. In: Lewis M, Haviland JM, editors. Handbook of Emotions. New York: Guilford Press; 1993

[52] Digiuseppe R, Tafrate RC. A comprehensive treatment model for anger disorders. Psychotherapy: Theory, Research, Practice Training. 2001;**38**(3):262

[53] Fessler DM. Madmen: An evolutionary perspective on anger and men's violent responses to transgression. In: Potegal M, Stemmler G, Speilbeger C, editors. International Handbook of Anger. New York: Springer; 2010. pp. 361-381

[54] Linden M, Schippan B, Baumann K, Spielberg R. Post-traumatic embitterment disorder (PTED). Differentiation of a specific form of adjustment disorders. Der Nervenarzt. 2004;**75**(1):51-57

[55] Litz BT, Lebowitz L, Gray MJ, Nash WP. Adaptive Disclosure: A New Treatment for Military Trauma, Loss, and Moral Injury. New York: Guilford Press; 2017

[56] Lasko NB, Gurvits TV, Kuhne AA, Orr SP, Pitman RK. Aggression and its correlates in Vietnam veterans with and without chronic posttraumatic stress disorder. Comprehensive Psychiatry. 1994;**35**(5):373-381

[57] Orth U, Wieland E. Anger, hostility, and posttraumatic stress disorder in trauma-exposed adults: A meta-analysis. Journal of Consulting and Clinical Psychology. 2006;**74**(4):698

[58] Holmes EA, Mathews A. Mental imagery in emotion and emotional disorders. Clinical Psychology Review. 2010;**30**(3):349-362

[59] Kosslyn SM. Reflective thinking and mental imagery: A perspective on the development of posttraumatic stress disorder. Development and Psychopathology. 2005;**17**(3):851-863

[60] Kosslyn SM, Thompson WL, Ganis G. The Case for Mental Imagery. New York: Oxford University Press; 2006

[61] Pearson DG, Deeprose C, Wallace-Hadrill SM, Heyes SB, Holmes EA. Assessing mental imagery in clinical psychology: A review of imagery measures and a guiding framework. Clinical Psychology Review. 2013;**33**(1):1-23

[62] Richardson A. Individual differences in visual imagination imagery. In: Kunzendorf R, Wallace B, editors. Individual Differences in Conscious Experience. Philadelphia: Benjamins; 2000. pp. 125-146

[63] Libby LK, Eibach RP. The role of visual imagery in social cognition. In: The Oxford Handbook of Social Cognition. Oxford University Press; 2013. pp. 147-166

[64] Thomas N. Mental Imagery [Internet]. Stanford Encyclopedia of Philosophy. 2014. Available from: https://plato.stanford.edu/entries/mental-imagery/

[65] Holmes EA, Mathews A. Mental imagery and emotion: A special relationship? Emotion. 2005;**5**(4):489

[66] Kunzendorf RG, Hartmann E, Thomas L, Berensen L. Emotionally directing visual sensations: I. Generating images that contextualize emotion and become "symbolic.". Imagination, Cognition and Personality. 2000;**19**(3):269-278

[67] Suler JR. Imagery ability and the experience of affect by free associative imagery. Journal of Mental Imagery. 1985;**9**(1):101-110

[68] Bywaters M, Andrade J, Turpin G. Intrusive and non-intrusive memories in a non-clinical sample: The effects of mood and affect on imagery vividness. Memory. 2004;**12**(4):467-478

[69] Dadds M, Hawes D, Schaefer B, Vaka K. Individual differences in imagery and reports of aversions. Memory. 2004;**12**(4):462-466

[70] Hackmann A, Holmes E. Reflecting on imagery: A clinical perspective and overview of the special issue of memory on mental imagery and memory in psychopathology. Memory. 2004;**12**(4):389-402

[71] Holmes EA, Brewin CR, Hennessy RG. Trauma films, information processing, and intrusive memory development. Journal of Experimental Psychology: General. 2004;**133**(1):3

[72] Cuthbert BN, Lang PJ, Strauss C, Drobes D, Patrick CJ, Bradley MM. The psychophysiology of anxiety disorder: Fear memory imagery. Psychophysiology. 2003;**40**(3):407-422

[73] Pratt D, Cooper MJ, Hackmann A. Imagery and its characteristics in people who are anxious about spiders. Behavioural and Cognitive Psychotherapy. 2004;**32**(2):165-176

[74] Price K, Veale D, Brewin CR. Intrusive imagery in people with a specific phobia of vomiting. Journal of Behavior Therapy and Experimental Psychiatry. 2012;**43**(1):672-678

[75] Makkar SR, Grisham JR. Social anxiety and the effects of negative self-imagery on emotion, cognition, and post-event processing. Behaviour Research and Therapy. 2011;**49**(10):654-664

[76] Clark DM, Wells A. A cognitive model of social phobia. In: Heimberg G, editor. Social Phobia: Diagnosis, Assessment, and Treatment. New York: Guilford Press; 1995

[77] Laor N, Wolmer L, Wiener Z, Reiss A, Muller U, Weizman R, et al. The function of image control in the psychophysiology of posttraumatic stress disorder. Journal of Traumatic Stress: Official Publication of The International Society for Traumatic Stress Studies. 1998;**11**(4):679-696

[78] Van der Kolk BA, Brown P, Van der Hart O. Pierre Janet on post-traumatic stress. Journal of Traumatic Stress. 1989;**2**(4):365-378

[79] Weisaeth L. The history of psychic trauma. In: Friedman MJ, Keane TM, Resick PA, editors. Handbook of PTSD Science and Practise. New York: Guilford Press; 2014. pp. 38-59

[80] Zoellner LA, Rothbaum BO, Feeny NC. PTSD not an anxiety disorder? DSM committee proposal turns back the hands of time. Depression and Anxiety. 2011;**28**(10):853

[81] World Health Organization (WHO). International statistical classification

of diseases and related health problems (9th ed.). Geneva: World Health Organization; 1979.

[82] World Health Organization (WHO). International statistical classification of diseases and related health problems (10th ed.). Geneva: World Health Organization; 1992. Available from: https://icd.who.int/

[83] American Psychiatric Association. Diagnostic and Statistical Manual of Mental Disorders (DSM IV). 4th ed. Washington DC: American Psychiatric Association; 1994

[84] Gillihan SJ, Cahill SP, Foa EB. Psychological theories of PTSD. In: Friedman MJ, Keane TM, Resick PA, editors. Handbook of PTSD: Science and Practice. New York: Guilford Press; 2014. pp. 166-184

[85] Resick PA, Miller MW. Posttraumatic stress disorder: Anxiety or traumatic stress disorder? Journal of Traumatic Stress. 2009;**22**(5):384-390

[86] Øktedalen T, Hoffart A, Langkaas TF. Trauma-related shame and guilt as time-varying predictors of posttraumatic stress disorder symptoms during imagery exposure and imagery rescripting—A randomized controlled trial. Psychotherapy Research. 2015;**25**(5):518-532

[87] Hoge CW, Yehuda R, Castro CA, McFarlane AC, Vermetten E, Jetly R, et al. Unintended consequences of changing the definition of posttraumatic stress disorder in DSM-5: Critique and call for action. JAMA Psychiatry. 2016;**73**(7):750-752

[88] Brown LA, Zandberg LJ, Foa EB. Mechanisms of change in prolonged exposure therapy for PTSD: Implications for clinical practice. Journal of Psychotherapy Integration. 2019;**29**(1):6

[89] Foa EB, McLean CP. The efficacy of exposure therapy for anxiety-related disorders and its underlying mechanisms: The case of OCD and PTSD. Annual Review of Clinical Psychology. 2016;**12**:1-28

[90] vanOyen WC. Traumatic intrusive imagery as an emotional memory phenomenon: A review of research and explanatory information processing theories. Clinical Psychology Review. 1997;**17**(5):509-536

[91] Schwartz GE, Weinberger DA, Singer JA. Cardiovascular differentiation of happiness, sadness, anger, and fear following imagery and exercise. Psychosomatic Medicine. 1981;**43**(4):343-364

[92] Foster PS, Smith EW, Webster DG. The psychophysiological differentiation of actual, imagined, and recollected anger. Imagination, Cognition and Personality. 1999;**18**(3):189-203

[93] Arntz A, Tiesema M, Kindt M. Treatment of PTSD: A comparison of imaginal exposure with and without imagery rescripting. Journal of Behavior Therapy and Experimental Psychiatry. 2007;**38**(4):345-370

[94] Novaco RW. Anger and coping with stress. In: Wilson GT, editor. Cognitive Behavior Therapy. New York: Springer; 1978. pp. 135-173

[95] Slomine BS, Greene AF. Anger imagery and corrugator electromyography. Journal of Psychosomatic Research. 1993;**37**(6):671-676

[96] Rauch SA, Foa EB, Furr JM, Filip JC. Imagery vividness and perceived anxious arousal in prolonged exposure treatment

for PTSD. Journal of Traumatic Stress: Official Publication of The International Society for Traumatic Stress Studies. 2004;**17**(6):461-465

[97] Laor N, Wolmer L, Wiener Z, Sharon O, Weizman R, Toren P, et al. Image vividness as a psychophysiological regulator in posttraumatic stress disorder. Journal of Clinical and Experimental Neuropsychology. 1999;**21**(1):39-48

[98] Schützwohl M, Maercker A. Anger in former East German political prisoners: Relationship to posttraumatic stress reactions and social support. The Journal of Nervous and Mental Disease. 2000;**188**(8):483-489

[99] Laor N, Wolmer L, Wiener Z, Weizman R, Toren P, Ron S. Image control and symptom expression in posttraumatic stress disorder. The Journal of Nervous and Mental Disease. 1999;**187**:673-679

[100] Bandura A. Self-efficacy: Toward a unifying theory of behavioral change. Psychological Review. 1977;**84**(2):191

[101] Schultz D, Grodack A, Izard CE. State and trait anger, fear, and social information processing. In: Potegal M, Stemmler G, Spielberger C, editors. International Handbook of Anger. New York: Springer; 2010. pp. 311-325

[102] Van Kleef GA, De Dreu CK, Manstead AS. The interpersonal effects of emotions in negotiations: A motivated information processing approach. Journal of Personality and Social Psychology. 2004;**87**(4):510

[103] Berkowitz L, Harmon-Jones E. Toward an understanding of the determinants of anger. Emotion. 2004;**4**(2):107

[104] Cox DE, Harrison DW. Models of anger: Contributions from psychophysiology, neuropsychology and the cognitive behavioral perspective. Brain Structure and Function. 2008;**212**(5):371-385

[105] Novaco RW. Clinicians ought to view anger contextually. Behaviour Change. 1993;**10**(4):208-218

[106] Berkowitz L. On the formation and regulation of anger and aggression: A cognitive-neoassociationistic analysis. American Psychologist. 1990;**45**(4):494

[107] Keane T, Zimering R, Caddell J. A behavioral formulation of Postraumatic Stress Disorder in Vietnam veterans. The Behavior Therapist. 1985;**1**(8):9-12

[108] Rona RJ, Jones M, Hull L, MacManus D, Fear NT, Wessely S. Anger in the UK Armed Forces: Strong association with mental health, childhood antisocial behavior, and combat role. The Journal of Nervous and Mental Disease. 2015;**203**(1):15-22

[109] Beck AT, Emery G. Anxiety Disorders and Phobias: A Cognitive Perspective. New York: Basic Books; 1985

[110] Wranik T, Scherer KR. Why do I get angry? A componential appraisal approach. In: Potegal M, Stemmler G, Speilbeger C, editors. International Handbook of Anger. New York: Springer; 2010. pp. 243-266

[111] Creamer M, Burgess P, Pattison P. Reaction to trauma: A cognitive processing model. Journal of Abnormal Psychology. 1992;**101**(3):452

[112] Ehlers A. Understanding and Treating Unwanted Trauma Memories in Posttraumatic Stress Disorder. Zeitschrift für Psychologie/Journal of Psychology. 2010;**218**(2):141-145

[113] Ehlers A, Hackmann A, Michael T. Intrusive re-experiencing in post-traumatic stress disorder: Phenomenology, theory, and therapy. Memory. 2004;**12**(4):403-415

[114] Elwood LS, Hahn KS, Olatunji BO, Williams NL. Cognitive vulnerabilities to the development of PTSD: A review of four vulnerabilities and the proposal of an integrative vulnerability model. Clinical Psychology Review. 2009;**29**(1):87-100

[115] Feeny NC, Zoellner LA, Foa EB. Anger, dissociation, and posttraumatic stress disorder among female assault victims. Journal of Traumatic Stress. 2000;**13**(1):89-100

[116] Paivio SC, Pascual-Leone A. Emotion-Focused Therapy for Complex Trauma: An Integrative Approach. Washington DC: American Psychological Association; 2010

[117] Taft CT, Vogt DS, Marshall AD, Panuzio J, Niles BL. Aggression among combat veterans: Relationships with combat exposure and symptoms of posttraumatic stress disorder, dysphoria, and anxiety. Journal of Traumatic Stress. 2007;**20**(2):135-145

[118] Novaco RW, Chemtob CM. Anger and trauma: Conceptualization, assessment, and treatment. 1998;

[119] Kassinove H, Sukhodolsky DG. Anger disorders: Basic science and practice issues. Issues in Comprehensive Pediatric Nursing. 1995;**18**(3):173-205

[120] Tomb DA. The phenomenology of post-traumatic stress disorder. Psychiatric Clinics. 1994;**17**(2):237-250

[121] Chung H, Breslau N. The latent structure of post-traumatic stress disorder: Tests of invariance by gender and trauma type. Psychological Medicine. 2008;**38**(4):563-573

[122] Litz BT, Stein N, Delaney E, Lebowitz L, Nash WP, Silva C, et al. Moral injury and moral repair in war veterans: A preliminary model and intervention strategy. Clinical Psychology Review. 2009;**29**(8):695-706

[123] Rosen GM, Lilienfeld SO. Posttraumatic stress disorder: An empirical evaluation of core assumptions. Clinical Psychology Review. 2008;**28**(5):837-868

[124] McNally RJ. Remembering Trauma. USA: Belknap Press/Harvard University Press; 2003

[125] Mammen OK, Pilkonis PA, Kolko DJ, Groff A. Anger and Anger Attacks as Precipitants of Aggression: What We Can Learn from Child Physical abuse. Anger, Aggression and Interventions for Interpersonal Violence. 2007:283-311

[126] Potegal M. The temporal dynamics of anger: Phenomena, processes, and perplexities. In: Potegal M, Stemmler G, Spielberger C, editors. International Handbook of Anger. New York: Springer. 385-401

[127] Berkowitz L. Appraisals and anger: How complete are the usual appraisal accounts of anger? In: Potegal M, Stemmler G, Speilbeger C, editors. International Handbook of Anger. New York: Springer; 2010. pp. 267-286

[128] Tripp TM, Bies RJ. "Righteous" anger and revenge in the workplace: The fantasies, the feuds, the forgiveness. In: Potegal M, Stemmler G, Speilbeger C, editors. International Handbook of Anger. New York: Springer; 2010. pp. 413-431

[129] Brewin CR, Dalgleish T, Joseph S. A dual representation theory

of posttraumatic stress disorder. Psychological Review. 1996;**103**(4):670

[130] Shapiro E, Maxfield L. The efficacy of EMDR early interventions. Journal of EMDR Practice and Research. 2019;**13**(4):291-301

[131] Resick PA, Monson CM, Chard KM. Cognitive Processing Therapy for PTSD: A Comprehensive Manual. New York: Guilford Press; 2016

[132] Dalgleish T. Cognitive approaches to posttraumatic stress disorder: The evolution of multirepresentational theorizing. Psychological Bulletin. 2004;**130**(2):228

[133] Rubin DC, Berntsen D. The frequency of voluntary and involuntary autobiographical memories across the life span. Memory & Cognition. 2009;**37**(5):679-688

[134] James IA, Kendell K. Unfinished processing in the emotional disorders: The Zeigarnik effect. Behavioural and Cognitive Psychotherapy. 1997;**25**(4):329-337

[135] Wegner DM. Ironic processes of mental control. Psychological Review. 1994;**101**(1):34

[136] Wenzlaff RM. Intrusive thoughts in depression. Journal of Cognitive Psychotherapy. 2002;**16**(2):145-160

[137] Clark DA. Unwanted mental intrusions in clinical disorders: An introduction. Journal of Cognitive Psychotherapy. 2002;**16**(2):123-126

[138] Holmes EA. Intrusive, emotional mental imagery and trauma: Experimental and clinical clues. Imagination, Cognition and Personality. 2003;**23**(2):147-154

[139] Watkins LE, Sprang KR, Rothbaum BO. Treating PTSD: A review of evidence-based psychotherapy interventions. Frontiers in Behavioral Neuroscience. 2018;**12**:258

[140] Smucker MR. Imagery rescripting and reprocessing therapy. In: Freeman A, Felgoise SH, Nezu AM, Nezu CM, Reinecke MA, editors. Encyclopedia of Cognitive Behavior Therapy. Boston, MA: Springer; 2005. pp. 226-229

[141] Forbes D, Phelps A, McHugh T. Treatment of combat-related nightmares using imagery rehearsal: A pilot study. Journal of Traumatic Stress: Official Publication of The International Society for Traumatic Stress Studies. 2001;**14**(2):433-442

[142] Bryant RA, Moulds ML, Guthrie RM, Dang ST, Mastrodomenico J, Nixon RD, et al. A randomized controlled trial of exposure therapy and cognitive restructuring for posttraumatic stress disorder. Journal of Consulting and Clinical Psychology. 2008;**76**(4):695

[143] Tarrier N, Pilgrim H, Sommerfield C, Faragher B, Reynolds M, Graham E, et al. A randomized trial of cognitive therapy and imaginal exposure in the treatment of chronic posttraumatic stress disorder. Journal of Consulting and Clinical Psychology. 1999;**67**(1):13

[144] Powers MB, Halpern JM, Ferenschak MP, Gillihan SJ, Foa EB. A meta-analytic review of prolonged exposure for posttraumatic stress disorder. Clinical Psychology Review. 2010;**30**(6):635-641

[145] Cusack K, Jonas DE, Forneris CA, Wines C, Sonis J, Middleton JC, et al. Psychological treatments for adults with posttraumatic stress disorder: A systematic review and meta-analysis.

Clinical Psychology Review. 2016;**43**:128-141

[146] McNally RJ. Mechanisms of exposure therapy: How neuroscience can improve psychological treatments for anxiety disorders. Clinical Psychology Review. 2007;**27**(6):750-759

[147] Forbes D, Adler AB. Advancing anger research. In: Adler AB, Forbes D, editors. Anger at Work: Prevention, Intervention, and Treatment in High-risk Occupations. American Psychological Association; 2021

[148] Forbes D, Creamer M, Phelps A, Bryant R, McFarlane A, Devilly GJ, et al. Australian guidelines for the treatment of adults with acute stress disorder and post-traumatic stress disorder. Australian & New Zealand Journal of Psychiatry. 2007;**41**(8):637-648

[149] Hendriks L, de Kleine RA, Broekman TG, Hendriks G-J, van Minnen A. Intensive prolonged exposure therapy for chronic PTSD patients following multiple trauma and multiple treatment attempts. European Journal of Psychotraumatology. 2018;**9**(1):1425574

[150] Korte KJ, Allan NP, Gros DF, Acierno R. Differential treatment response trajectories in individuals with subclinical and clinical PTSD. Journal of Anxiety Disorders. 2016;**38**:95-101

[151] López CM, Lancaster CL, Gros DF, Acierno R. Residual sleep problems predict reduced response to prolonged exposure among veterans with PTSD. Journal of Psychopathology and Behavioral Assessment. 2017;**39**(4):755-763

[152] Gilmore AK, Lopez C, Muzzy W, Brown WJ, Grubaugh A, Oesterle DW, et al. Emotion dysregulation predicts dropout from prolonged exposure treatment among women veterans with military sexual trauma-related posttraumatic stress disorder. Women's Health Issues. 2020;**30**(6):462-469

[153] Zhutovsky P, Thomas RM, Olff M, van Rooij SJ, Kennis M, van Wingen GA, et al. Individual prediction of psychotherapy outcome in posttraumatic stress disorder using neuroimaging data. Translational Psychiatry. 2019;**9**(1):1-10

[154] Rubin M, Shvil E, Papini S, Chhetry BT, Helpman L, Markowitz JC, et al. Greater hippocampal volume is associated with PTSD treatment response. Psychiatry Research: Neuroimaging. 2016;**252**:36-39

[155] van Gelderen MJ, Nijdam MJ, de Vries F, Meijer OC, Vermetten E. Exposure-related cortisol predicts outcome of psychotherapy in veterans with treatment-resistant posttraumatic stress disorder. Journal of Psychiatric Research. 2020;**130**:387-393

[156] Forbes D, Parslow R, Creamer M, Allen N, McHugh T, Hopwood M. Mechanisms of anger and treatment outcome in combat veterans with posttraumatic stress disorder. Journal of Traumatic Stress: Official Publication of The International Society for Traumatic Stress Studies. 2008;**21**(2):142-149

[157] Stevenson VE, Chemtob CM. Premature treatment termination by angry patients with combat-related post-traumatic stress disorder. Military Medicine. 2000;**165**(5):422-424

[158] Andrews B, Brewin CR, Rose S, Kirk M. Predicting PTSD symptoms in victims of violent crime: The role of shame, anger, and childhood abuse. Journal of Abnormal Psychology. 2000;**109**(1):69

[159] Becker CB, Zayfert C, Anderson E. A survey of psychologists' attitudes towards and utilization of exposure therapy for PTSD. Behaviour Research and Therapy. 2004;**42**(3):277-292

[160] Boswell JF, Gallagher MW, Sauer-Zavala SE, Bullis J, Gorman JM, Shear MK, et al. Patient characteristics and variability in adherence and competence in cognitive-behavioral therapy for panic disorder. Journal of Consulting and Clinical Psychology. 2013;**81**(3):443

[161] Liang B, Kale SH. Cultural differences in imagery generation: The influence of abstract versus concrete thinking. Journal of Business Research. 2012;**65**(3):333-339

[162] Fallon F. Visual or symbolic, analytic or holistic: A comparison of the cognitive styles of South-East Asian and Australian Students. ISANA Proceedings. 2004:1-9

[163] Campos A. Gender differences in imagery. Personality and Individual Differences. 2014;**59**:107-111

[164] Kosslyn SM, Margolis J, Barrett A, Goldknopf E, Daly P. Age differences in imagery abilities. Child Development. 1990;**61**(4):995-1010

[165] Campos A, Pérez-Fabello MJ, Gómez-Juncal R. Gender and age differences in measured and self-perceived imaging capacity. Personality and Individual Differences. 2004;**37**(7):1383-1389

[166] Richardson JT. Gender differences in the vividness of visual imagery questionnaire: A meta-analysis. 1995

[167] Sabatinelli D, Flaisch T, Bradley MM, Fitzsimmons JR, Lang PJ. Affective picture perception: Gender differences in visual cortex? Neuroreport. 2004;**15**(7):1109-1112

[168] Giambra LM. Sex differences in daydreaming and related mental activity from the late teens to the early nineties. The International Journal of Aging and Human Development. 1980;**10**(1):1-34

[169] Giambra LM. Daydreaming characteristics across the life-span: Age differences and seven to twenty year longitudinal changes. Individual differences in conscious experience. 2000 Feb 15:147-206

[170] Giambra LM. The temporal setting, emotions, and imagery of daydreams: Age changes and age differences from late adolescent to the old-old. Imagination, Cognition and Personality. 2000;**19**(4):367-413

[171] Dror IE, Kosslyn SM. Mental imagery and aging. Psychology and Aging. 1994;**9**(1):90

[172] Dror IE, Kosslyn SM. Age degradation in top-down processing: Identifying objects from canonical and noncanonical viewpoints. Experimental Aging Research. 1998;**24**(3):203-216

[173] Rader CM, Kunzendorf RG, Carrabino C. The relation of imagery vividness, absorption, reality boundaries and synesthesia to hypnotic states and traits. In: Kunzendorf R, Spanos NP, Wallace B, editors. Hypnosis and Imagination. Amityville, New York: Routledge; 1996. pp. 99-121

[174] MacInnis DJ, Price LL. The role of imagery in information processing: Review and extensions. Journal of Consumer Research. 1987;**13**(4):473-491

[175] Riding R, Cheema I. Cognitive styles—An overview and

integration. Educational Psychology. 1991;**11**(3-4):193-215

[176] Riding R, Rayner S. Cognitive Styles and Learning Strategies: Understanding Style Differences in Learning and Behavior. London: David Fulton Publishers; 1998

[177] D'Argembeau A, Van der Linden M. Individual differences in the phenomenology of mental time travel: The effect of vivid visual imagery and emotion regulation strategies. Consciousness and Cognition. 2006;**15**(2):342-350

[178] Dyck DG, Moser CG, Janisse MP. Type A behavior and situation-specific perceptions of control. Psychological Reports. 1987;**60**(3):991-999

[179] Belicki K, Belicki D. Predisposition for nightmares: A study of hypnotic ability, vividness of imagery, and absorption. Journal of Clinical Psychology. 1986;**42**(5):714-718

[180] Roche SM, McConkey KM. Absorption: Nature, assessment, and correlates. Journal of Personality and Social Psychology. 1990;**59**(1):91

[181] Bryan BA. The Relationship of Locus of Control and Imagery Ability to College Students' Life Satisfaction. Ohio University; 1999

[182] Huckabee MW. Introversion-extraversion and imagery. Psychological Reports. 1974;**34**(2):453-454

[183] Stricklin AB, Penk ML. Vividness and control of imagery in personality types. Journal of Mental Imagery. 1980;**4**:111-114

[184] Fernandez E, Wasan A. The anger of pain sufferers: Attributions to agents and appraisals of wrongdoings. In: Potegal M, Stemmler G, Speilbeger C, editors. International Handbook of Anger. New York: Springer; 2010. pp. 449-464

[185] Bushman BJ. Does venting anger feed or extinguish the flame? Catharsis, rumination, distraction, anger, and aggressive responding. Personality and Social Psychology Bulletin. 2002;**28**(6):724-731

[186] Mischkowski D, Kross E, Bushman BJ. Flies on the wall are less aggressive: Self-distancing "in the heat of the moment" reduces aggressive thoughts, angry feelings and aggressive behavior. Journal of Experimental Social Psychology. 2012;**48**(5):1187-1191

[187] Tafrate RC. Evaluation of treatment strategies for adult anger disorders. In: Kassinove H, editor. Anger Disorders: Definition, Diagnosis, and Treatment. Oxfordshire: Taylor & Francis; 1995. pp. 109-129

[188] Edmondson CB, Conger JC. A review of treatment efficacy for individuals with anger problems: Conceptual, assessment, and methodological issues. Clinical Psychology Review. 1996;**16**(3):251-275

[189] Beck R, Fernandez E. Cognitive-behavioral therapy in the treatment of anger: A meta-analysis. Cognitive Therapy and Research. 1998;**22**(1):63-74

[190] DiGiuseppe R, Tafrate RC. Anger treatment for adults: A meta-analytic review. Clinical Psychology: Science and Practice. 2003;**10**(1):70

[191] Del Vecchio T, O'Leary KD. Effectiveness of anger treatments for specific anger problems: A meta-analytic review. Clinical Psychology Review. 2004;**24**(1):15-34

[192] Henwood KS, Chou S, Browne KD. A systematic review and meta-analysis

on the effectiveness of CBT informed anger management. Aggression and Violent Behavior. 2015;**25**:280-292

[193] Lee AH, DiGiuseppe R. Anger and aggression treatments: A review of meta-analyses. Current Opinion in Psychology. 2018;**19**:65-74

[194] Diener MJ. Cohen's d. In: Weiner IB, Craighead WE, editors. The Corsini Encyclopedia of Psychology. New York: John Wiley & Sons; 2010. pp. 1-1

[195] Glancy GD, Saini M. Forensic psychiatry and the law. Journal of American Academy of Psychiatry Law. 2009;**37**:438-441

[196] Taft CT, Creech SK, Kachadourian L. Assessment and treatment of posttraumatic anger and aggression: A review. Journal of Rehabilitation Research & Development. 2012;**49**(5):777-788

[197] Morland LA, Greene CJ, Rosen CS, Foy D, Reilly P, Shore J, et al. Telemedicine for anger management therapy in a rural population of combat veterans with posttraumatic stress disorder: A randomized noninferiority trial. The Journal of Clinical Psychiatry. 2010;**71**(7):855-863

[198] Meichenbaum D. Self-instructional training. In: Cognitive-Behavior Modification. New York: Springer; 1977. pp. 17-54

[199] Cash R, Varker T, McHugh T, Metcalf O, Howard A, Lloyd D, et al. Effectiveness of an anger intervention for military members with PTSD: A clinical case series. Military Medicine. 2018;**183**(9-10):e286-e290

[200] Frueh BC, Henning KR, Pellegrin KL, Chobot K. Relationship between scores on anger measures and PTSD symptomatology, employment, and compensation-seeking status in combat veterans. Journal of Clinical Psychology. 1997;**53**(8):871-878

[201] Novaco RW. Remediating anger and aggression with violent offenders. Legal and Criminological Psychology. 1997;**2**(1):77-88

[202] Wilson JP. The historical evolution of PTSD diagnostic criteria. In: Psychotraumatology. New York: Springer; 1995. pp. 9-26

[203] Shalev AY. Discussion: Treatment of prolonged posttraumatic stress disorder—learning from experience. Journal of Traumatic Stress. 1997;**10**(3):415-423

[204] Marmar CR, Foy D, Kagan B, Pynoos RS. An integrated approach for treating posttraumatic stress. In: Posttraumatic stress disorder: A clinical review. Baltimore, MD, US: The Sidran Press; 1994. pp. 99-132

[205] Horowitz MJ. Stress Response Syndromes: PTSD, Grief, Adjustment, and Dissociative Disorders. Northvale: Jason Aronson; 2011

[206] Lindy JD. An outline for the psychoanalytic psychotherapy of post-traumatic stress disorder. Trauma and Its Wake. 1986;**2**:195-212

[207] Briere JN, Scott C. Principles of Trauma Therapy: A Guide to Symptoms, Evaluation, and Treatment evaluation, and treatment (DSM-5 update). Newbury Park: Sage Publications; 2014

[208] Keane TM, Kaloupek DG. Validated treatments for post traumatic stress disorder. Clinical Psychologist. 1996;**49**:7-8

[209] Pitman RK, Altman B, Greenwald E, Longpre RE, Macklin ML,

Poire RE, et al. Psychiatric complications during flooding therapy for post-traumatic stress disorder. The Journal of Clinical Psychiatry. 1991;**52**:17-20

[210] Frame T. Moral Injury: Unseen Wounds in an Age of Barbarism. NewSouth Books; 2015

[211] Friedman MJ, Resick PA, Keane TM. In: Friedman MJ, Keane TM, Resick PA, editors. PTSD from DSM-III to DSM-5: Progress and Challenges. 2nd ed. New York: Guilford Press; 2014. pp. 3-20

[212] DiGiuseppe R, Tafrate RC. Understanding Anger Disorders. Oxford UK: Oxford University Press; 2007

[213] Tavris C. Anger: The Misunderstood Emotion. Manhattan: Simon and Schuster; 1989

[214] Forbes D, McHugh TF, Chemtob CM. Regulating anger in combat-related posttraumatic stress disorder. In: Fernandez E, editor. Treatments for Anger in Specific Populations: Theory, Application and Outcome. USA: Oxford University Press; 2013. pp. 52-83

[215] Worthen M, Rathod SD, Cohen G, Sampson L, Ursano R, Gifford R, et al. Anger problems and posttraumatic stress disorder in male and female National Guard and Reserve Service members. Journal of Psychiatric Research. 2014;**55**:52-58

[216] Singer JL. Imagery in Psychotherapy. American Psychological Association; 2006

Chapter 6

# Oxidative Stress and Cardiovascular Diseases: The Role of Mitochondria

*Imen Ghorbel, Mariem Chaâbane, Awatef Elwej, Fatma Ghorbel-Koubaa and Najiba Zeghal*

## Abstract

The redox status is determined by the balance between the production of reactive oxygen species (ROS) and their removal by the antioxidant defense system. Mitochondria, the center of oxidative metabolism and the principal site of ROS production, are crucial in health and also in the pathogenesis of many diseases. Mitochondrial dysfunction, resulting in a vicious cycle contributing to cellular damage and consequent cell death, has been proven to play a critical role in the pathogenesis of cardiovascular diseases. Previous studies have shown that mitochondrial transfer in cells plays a crucial role in regulating cardiovascular system development and maintaining normal tissue homeostasis. We review and evaluate in this chapter the evidence for mitochondrial dysfunction as a consequence of stress exposure and a contributing factor to cardiovascular diseases.

**Keywords:** oxidative stress, cardiovascular diseases, mitochondria

## 1. Introduction

Mitochondria, considered as integral players in cellular energy production, represent a critical nexus of biological, psychological, and social factors underlying the mechanisms implicated in stress response. Oxidative stress is identified as an imbalance between the production of reactive oxygen species (ROS), including free radicals, and the antioxidant defense status in the living organisms. Free radicals are any atom or group of atoms containing one or more unpaired electrons in their outer valence shell, while ROS regroup all the free radicals and non-radical reactive species deriving from molecular oxygen and they are commonly found in biological systems [1]. As a result of their impaired ability for ATP synthesis and for an increased production of ROS, mitochondria appear to be central hubs of the pathophysiological process contributing to many diseases [2]. Mitochondria are especially abundant in the cardiac tissue; hence, mitochondrial dysregulation and ROS production are thought to contribute significantly to cardiac pathology. Cardiovascular diseases (CVD) are the leading cause of death in the world and oxidative stress is one of the most significant risk factors.

Under physiological conditions, cardiac ROS signaling regulates heart development and cardiomyocyte maturation, cardiac calcium handling, excitation-contraction coupling, and vascular tone [3]. However, pathological conditions of unregulated ROS production can result in oxidative stress, proteins and lipids damage and cell death [4]. It has been demonstrated that autophagy can be a crucial mechanism for preventing the accumulation of ROS by removing damaged mitochondria [5]. In this selective chapter, we will discuss the role of mitochondria in oxidative stress-related heart disorders.

## 2. Mitochondria and oxidative stress

### 2.1 Mitochondria and physiological functions

Mitochondria are essential organelle which accommodate in their inner membrane large numbers of five oxidative phosphorylation complexes (complexes I–V). They are the only organelles containing their own genome – the mitochondrial DNA (mtDNA). The latter encodes proteins essential to electron flow through a series of protein complexes called the respiratory chain (also known as electron transport chain, or ETC) [6].

Perturbations in mitochondrial structure and function include impaired replication, alterations in mtDNA copy number, increased ROS production, mtDNA mutations and organelle damage [7].

Mitochondrial complex I, a key component of the ETC, aerobically oxidizes NADH in the ETC to generate ATP. The principal function of mitochondria is to use products of glycolysis, proteolysis, or lipolysis and oxygen through biochemical reactions leading to ATP formation [8]. The origin of heat in the human body is the free energy released during the chemical breakdown of molecules. In fact, the main mechanism of heat production and thermoregulation consists in uncoupling chemical reactions in the mitochondrial matrix from ATP synthesis, a phenomenon called "mitochondrial uncoupling". ATP hydrolysis by the $NA^+/K^+$ ATPase is also a substantial source of heat which is thought to contribute to thermogenesis [9]. Mitochondria have also emerged as major players in steroid hormone actions and to sequester $Ca^{2+}$ ions to contain that process, as well as to express genes in order to regulate important cell functions [7]. Disruption of mitochondrial homeostasis contributes to the pathogenesis of many disorders, including neurodegeneration, myocardial infarction, cancer, and metabolic diseases [10].

### 2.2 Stress exposure: implication for mitochondria function

ROS include many species such as superoxide ($O_2^{\bullet -}$) and hydroxyl ($OH^{\bullet}$) radicals, hydrogen peroxide ($H_2O_2$) and peroxynitrite ($ONOO^{\bullet -}$), the result of the reaction of superoxide with nitric oxide (NO) [11]. The excessive formation of ROS and the impairment of defensive antioxidant systems lead to oxidative stress. Under severe or prolonged exposure to a stressful condition, mitochondria become fragmented, increasing the risk of cell death [12]. Prolonged fragmentation leads to pronounced oxidative stress and mitochondrial DNA damage [13].

The initial formation of mitochondrial reactive oxygen and nitrogen species can also activate secondary sources of oxidants involving permeability transition pore [14]. The main endogenous process that generates ROS is oxidative phosphorylation [15]. Initial

ROS production can induce specific cell signaling pathways mediated by protein phosphorylation and transcriptional factors such as NO synthase and NRF2 (transcription factor nuclear factor erythroid 2), that could later provide a feed-back to downregulate ROS production [16, 17].

The regulation of mitochondrial ROS generation and their levels is exerted by a number of factors, such as the redox state of respiratory components and oxygen tension [18]. Mitochondria have unique redox-related enzymes and transporters such as glutaredoxin 2, which functions to catalyze reversible oxidation and glutathionylation of mitochondrial membrane proteins as well as protecting from oxidative stress and apoptosis [19]. Therefore, we suggest a strong connection between mitochondrial dysfunction and oxidative stress.

Biomarkers of oxidative stress include the products of lipid peroxidation, malondialdehyde (MDA) and protein oxidation (advanced oxidation protein products, AOPP) [20]. Extensive lipid peroxidation in biological membranes can lead to disturbances of structural integrity, a loss of fluidity, a decrease of membrane potential, and an increase of permeability to ions. Moreover, enzymes, such as catalase (CAT), superoxide dismutase (SOD) and glutathione peroxidase (GPx) also serve as biomarkers of oxidative insult. SOD is recognized as a primary line of defense mechanism in the antioxidant system by catalyzing the dismutation of superoxide radicals ($O_2^{\bullet -}$) into molecular oxygen ($O_2$) and $H_2O_2$. This latter is neutralized by the combined action of CAT and GPx in all vertebrates [21]. Some proteins, such as secretory IgA and heat shock proteins (HSPs), serve as indicators of immunity or resistance mechanisms to stress. An alteration in biomarkers can reflect the severity of deviation from normality or the degree of damage.

## 3. Stress associated cardiovascular diseases

High-energy stress imposes mitochondria to be more prone to injury. High-energy demanding tissues, such as the myocardium, are also more sensitive to mitochondrial dysregulation. The prevalence of cardiovascular diseases (CVD) is significantly increased in aging persons. CVD are a main cause of morbidity and mortality in the world and their incidence is closely correlated with age [22]. The cardiovascular system is a closed network containing arteries, veins and capillaries. Apoptosis is one of the most common patterns of programmed cell death in the cardiovascular system [23]. Bcl-2 is an anti-apoptotic protein mainly located in the nuclear and mitochondrial membrane, but the family member Bax, that promotes apoptosis, is mainly located in the cytoplasm [24]. The mechanism of mitochondrial transfer-induced anti-apoptosis might involve the decrease of Bax/Bcl-2 ratio and the inhibition of caspase-3 activity [25]. Thus, mitochondria have a critical role in oxidative stress related CVD (**Figure 1**).

Furthermore, chronic inflammation promotes intimal thickening and plaque formation which narrows the vascular lumen and compromises blood flow. Oxidative stress contributes to atherosclerotic plaque formation via induction of endothelial dysfunction, vascular inflammation, and accumulation of oxidized low-density lipoproteins [26].

CVD are characterized by increased levels of ROS formation due to an imbalance between pro-oxidative enzymes (xanthine oxidase, NADPH oxidase) and antioxidant enzymes such as catalase (CAT), superoxide dismutase (SOD) and glutathione peroxidase (GPx), resulting in a deviation of cellular redox environment from the

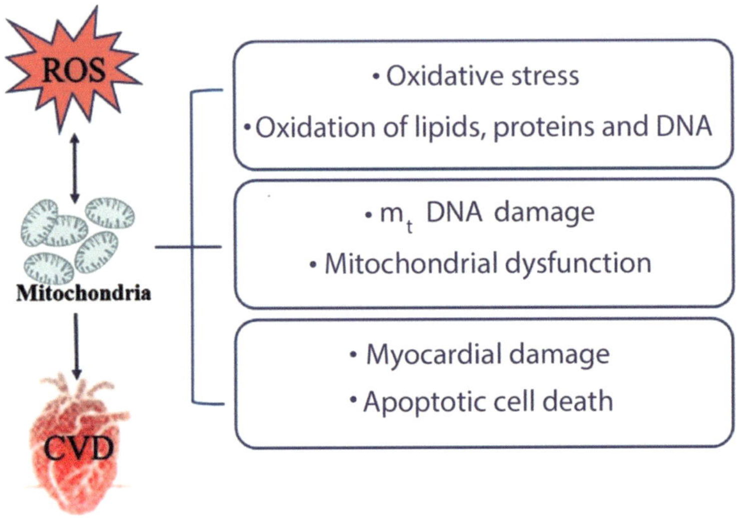


**Figure 1.**
*Oxidative stress and cardiovascular diseases: The role of mitochondria.*

normal [27]. NADPH oxidase (NOX) plays a crucial role in determining the redox state of the heart [28, 29]. Importantly, NOX enzymes have been implicated in the pathophysiology of many CVD, including atherosclerosis, hypertension and heart failure [30]. In the cardiomyocyte, ROS may be generated in the mitochondria at the ETC, by monoamine oxidase, by nicotinamide adenine dinucleotide phosphate, NOX and uncoupling of nitric oxide oxidase. Metabolic disorders increase mitochondrial protein acetylation, which directly contributes to mitochondrial dysfunction in cardiovascular diseases and heart failure [31]. Cardiac dysfunction associated with metabolic disorders such as diabetes, high blood pressure, and obesity causes the activation of mitochondria apoptotic signaling pathways and cardiomyocyte contractile dysfunction [32].

## 4. Conclusion

ROS are considered as one of the major causative factors leading to diseases pathogenesis. These data clearly demonstrated the role of mitochondria in oxidative stress-related heart disorders.

## Author details

Imen Ghorbel*, Mariem Chaâbane, Awatef Elwej, Fatma Ghorbel-Koubaa
and Najiba Zeghal
Animal Physiology Laboratory, Sfax Faculty of Sciences, University of Sfax, Sfax, BP, Tunisia

*Address all correspondence to: ghorbel21@gmail.com

## References

[1] Keshari AK, Verma AK, Kumar T, Srivastava R. Oxidative stress: A review. The International Journal of Science and Technoledge. 2015;**3**:155-162

[2] Szeto HH. Mitochondria-targeted peptide antioxidants: Novel neuroprotective agents. The AAPS Journal. 2006;**8**:521-531

[3] Burgoyne JR, Mongue-Din H, Eaton P, Shah AM. Redox signaling in cardiac physiology and pathology. Circulation Research. 2012;**111**:1091-1106

[4] Richardson AG, Schadt EE. The role of macromolecular damage in aging and age-related disease. Journal of Gerontology. 2014;**69**:28-32

[5] Kroemer G, Mariño G, Levine B. Autophagy and the integrated stress response. Molecular Cell. 2010;**40**:280-293

[6] Wallace DC. Mitochondrial DNA variation in human radiation and disease. Cell. 2015;**163**:33-38

[7] Picard M, McManus MJ. Mitochondrial Signaling and Neurodegeneration. Vol. 1. Cham: Springer International Publishing; 2016. pp. 107-137

[8] Anndrezza AC, Nierenberg NAA. Mitochondrial dysfunction: At the core of psychiatric disorders? Biological Psychiatry. 2018;**83**:718-719

[9] Rolfe DF, Brown GC. Cellular energy utilization and molecular origin of standard metabolic rate in mammals. Physiological Reviews. 1997;**77**:731-758

[10] Bock FJ, Tait SWG. Mitochondria as multifaceted regulators of cell death. Nature Reviews Molecular Cell Biology. 2020;**21**:85-100

[11] Noori S. An overview of oxidative stress and antioxidant defensive system. Open Access Scientific Reports. 2012;**1**:413

[12] Hoffmann A, Spengler D. The mitochondrion as potential interface in early-life stress brain programming. Frontiers in Behavioral Neuroscience. 2018;**12**:306

[13] Liesa M, Shirihai OS. Mitochondrial dynamics in the regulation of nutrient utilization and energy expenditure. Cell Metabolism. 2013;**17**:491-506

[14] Wenzel P, Mollnau H, Oelze M, Schulz E, Wickramanayake JM, Muller J, et al. First evidence for a crosstalk between mitochondrial and NADPH oxidase-derived reactive oxygen species in nitroglycerin-triggered vascular dysfunction. Antioxidants & Redox Signaling. 2008;**10**:1435-1447

[15] Cosentino F, Francia P, Camici GG, Pelicci PG, Luscher TF, Volpe M. Final common molecular pathways of aging and cardiovascular disease: Role of the p66Shc protein. Arteriosclerosis, Thrombosis, and Vascular Biology. 2008;**28**:622-628

[16] Cai H, Li Z, Davis ME, Kanner W, Harrison DG, Dudley SC. Akt-dependent phosphorylation of serine 1179 and mitogen-activated protein kinase kinase/extracellular signal-regulated kinase 1/2 cooperatively mediate activation of the endothelial nitric-oxide synthase by hydrogen peroxide. Molecular Pharmacology. 2003;**63**:325-331

[17] Sies H, Berndt C, Jones DP. Oxidative stress. Annual Review of Biochemistry. 2017;**86**:715-748

[18] Forrester SJ, Kikuchi DS, Hernandes MS, Xu Q, Griendling KK. Reactive oxygen species in metabolic and inflammatory signaling. Circulation Research. 2018;**122**:877-902

[19] Garcia J, Han D, Sancheti H, Yap LP, Kaplowitz N, Cadenas E. Regulation of mitochondrial glutathione redox status and protein glutathionylation by respiratory substrates. The Journal of Biological Chemistry. 2010;**285**:39646-39654

[20] Ghorbel I, Khemakhem M, Boudawara O, Marrekchi R, Jamouss K, Ben Amar R, et al. Effects of dietary extra virgin olive oil and its fractions on antioxidant status and DNA damage in the heart of rats co-exposed to aluminum and acrylamide. Food & Function. 2015;**9**:3098-3108

[21] Bruce A, Freeman D, James C. Biology of disease-free radicals and tissue injury. Laboratory Investigation. 1982;**47**:412-426

[22] Richardson AG, Schadt EE. The role of macromolecular damage in aging and age-related disease. Journals of Gerontology Series A: Biomedical Sciences and Medical Sciences. 2014;**69**:S28-S32

[23] Koyanagi M, Brandes RP, Haendeler J, Zeiher AM, Dimmeler S. Cell to-cell connection of endothelial progenitor cells with cardiac myocytes by nanotubes: A novel mechanism for cell fate changes? Circulation Research. 2005;**96**:1039-1041

[24] Zhou Z, Meng M, Ni H. Chemosensitizing effect of Astragalus polysaccharides on nasopharyngeal carcinoma cells by inducing apoptosis and modulating expression of Bax/Bcl-2 ratio and caspases. Medical Science Monitor. 2017;**23**:462-469

[25] Han H, Hu J, Yan Q, Zhu J, Zhu Z, Chen Y, et al. Bone marrowderived mesenchymal stem cells rescue injured H9c2 cells via transferring intact mitochondria through tunneling nanotubes in an in vitro simulated ischemia/reperfusion model. Molecular Medicine Reports. 2016;**13**:1517-1524

[26] Burtenshaw D, Kitching M, Redmond EM, Megson IL, Cahill PA. Reactive oxygen species (ROS), intimal thickening, and subclinical atherosclerotic disease. Frontiers in Cardiovascular Medicine. 2019;**6**:89. DOI: 10.3389/fcvm.2019.00089

[27] Sies H. Oxidative stress: A concept in redox biology and medicine. Redox Biology. 2015;**4**:180-183

[28] Cave AC, Brewer AC, Narayanapanicker A, Ray R, Grieve DJ, Walker S, et al. Nadph oxidases in cardiovascular health and disease. Antioxidants & Redox Signaling. 2006;**8**:691-728

[29] Griendling KK, Sorescu D, Ushio-Fukai M. NADPH oxidase: Role in cardiovascular biology and disease. Circulation Research. 2000;**86**:494-501

[30] Brandes RP, Weissmann N, Schröder K. NADPH oxidases in cardiovascular disease. Free Radical Biology & Medicine. 2010;**49**:687-706

[31] Horton JL, Martin OJ, Lai L, Riley NM, Richards AL, Vega RB, et al. Mitochondrial protein hyperacetylation in the failing heart. JCI Insight. 2016;**1**(2):e84897

[32] Li A, Zheng N, Ding X. Mitochondrial abnormalities: A hub in metabolic syndrome-related cardiac dysfunction caused by oxidative stress. Heart Failure Reviews. https://doi.org/10.1007/s10741-021-10109-6. [published online May 5, 2021]

Section 3

# Pathophysiology of Stress Disorders

Chapter 7

# Correlates of Mobbing among Medical Residents in a University General Hospital: The Experience from Greece and Review of Literature

*Panagiota Xaplanteri*

## Abstract

The term "mobbing" (moral harassment) in the workplace is defined as the systematic and persistent intimidation, the insult, the exclusion, and the unfair behavior toward a target person. There is little experience regarding mobbing in Greek hospitals, especially among medical residents. In this study, 92 medical residents from the University General Hospital of Patras, Greece (UGHP) were challenged to complete the Einarsen Negative Acts Questionnaire revised (NAQ-R) along with their demographic characteristics. Sector specialty of participants: Internal Medicine, Surgical, and Laboratory Sector. No statistically significant difference occurred relative to sex ($p = 0.14$), training ($p = 0.735$), the specialty years ($p = 0.478$), or years of work as a trainee in UGHP ($p = 0.052$). Statistically significant difference ($p = 0.0174$) occured with respect to: (a) age, where at age group 25–35 with regard to to age groups 35–35 and 45–55, and (b) Sector ($p = 0.0043$) with higher score in the Sector of Surgery, and lowest in the Laboratory Sector (mean = 45.4). Not much data are available regarding the mobbing phenomenon among medical residents worldwide. A review of the literature is also attempted in this study. This research is a pioneer in the Greek medical sector.

**Keywords:** mobbing, medical residents, university hospital, Negative Acts Questionnaire, moral harassment, workplace

## 1. Introduction

Smooth interpersonal relationships in the workplace environment are critical to the unobstructed function of an organization [1]. The term "mobbing" (moral harassment) in the workplace is defined as the systematic and persistent intimidation, the insult, the exclusion, and the unfair behavior toward a target person [2–4].

According to Pranjić et al. [5], the phenomenon of moral harassment in doctors has five dimensions. First, an attempt is made to underestimate their work with humiliation in front of colleagues or patients, bad criticism, and discipline implied by threats. The second dimension includes sarcasm and use of any form of violence to undermine the victim's personal integrity. The third dimension involves the isolation of the victim by concealing useful information and unjustified non-authorization or promotion. There is undue pressure through increased workload and deadlines that cannot be achieved. The fifth dimension aims to destabilize the victim through leakage of malicious rumors, continuous depreciation, and sudden removal of jurisdictions [5].

The causes of the phenomenon include competition, envy, diversity (gender, religion, sexuality, and social origin), and a workplace environment with a great deal of workload and simultaneous conflict of roles [6]. The phenomenon is associated with psychological stress and low job satisfaction and the consequences are detrimental to young doctors as revealed by many studies [2, 5, 7].

In Greece, despite that 13.2% of workers declare that they have been victims of mobbing, there is no relevant legislation. Only laws related to the assault of human dignity exist [8, 9]. The lack of clear legal framework makes it thus very difficult for the victim to take legal action against the offenders as he/she "bears the burden of proof" [2, 6, 10]. The recognition of the problem is often difficult, as the person is devastated psychologically and has no courage to defend himself/herself or is afraid of retaliation [1, 11–13].

The difficult situation of the victim is compounded by the current economic crisis in Greece. Under the hardship of finding a job, the need for survival becomes a priority increasing the tolerance of violence [14]. As a result, the phenomenon of mobbing is being added as a problem of the hospitals in the public sector together with the financial constraints, the pay cuts, and the brain drain [15, 16]. At the same time, there is increasing pressure to augment the efficiency of organizations, which creates a fertile ground for mobbing against young doctors [5, 13, 17–23].

In Greece, although there is increasing evidence that the phenomenon is present among young doctors, no such study is ever conducted in the medical residents of a University Hospital [18, 20]. Greek University Hospitals accept a plethora of patients with severe diseases. The University General Hospital of Patras accepts over 100,000 persons per year in the Emergency Sector, and over 40,000 hospitalized patients [24]. Because of the economic crisis, the brain drain of young doctors in Greece leads to fewer and fewer medical residents getting the job done in a difficult working environment with demanding working hours and reduced wages [15]. As a result, the outcomes of the present study are significant in order to delineate the working conditions of the remaining young doctors.

The University General Hospital of Patras was therefore selected for this study, as it receives a large number of patients from all over the Western Greece region; the amount of workload is consequently large. In addition, the number of medical residents was such in order to obtain a satisfactory sample size; this survey is a pioneer in the health sector in Greece.

The basic research hypothesis of the present study was that the phenomenon of mobbing among medical residents might be present at a considerable intensity in Greece. The following scientific questions are raised and addressed in this study: Is there a mobbing effect in medical residents? Are there independent associations between mobbing, genders, age, educational level sector the residents work in? On the basis of this hypothesis, the ultimate goal of this investigation was to demonstrate to what extent there is mobbing among medical residents.

## 2. Material and method

### 2.1 Study sample

Medical residents were asked to state their gender, age group, the sector where they work (Laboratory, Internal Medicine, and Surgery), and how many years they were specialized in total, but also in the present organization. The UGHP was chosen as it accepts a plethora of incidents from across the region of Western Greece and therefore the amount of workload is large. Written approval was obtained from the UGHP Ethics Committee (decision number 40/18.01.18). Moreover, a written statement was submitted by the researchers to the UGHP Ethics Committee safeguarding the anonymity of the participants; to ensure anonymity, each respondent was given an identical envelope in which he/she enclosed his/her answers. During the completion of the questionnaires, any questions of understanding were answered and the necessary clarifications were given.

The research population was 243 medical residents who, according to the records of the UGHP Human Resources Sector, were working on the organization at the time of the study; despite efforts to maximize participation, the sample of participants for the present study consisted of a total of 92 individuals (participation rate: 37.9%), from all specialties in the Laboratory, Internal Medicine and Surgery Sector. The remaining medical residents refused to participate with the most common justifications, the lack of time due to excessive workload (78%), or indifference (19%), being cautious about the reassurances of anonymity (3%). There were even aggressive behaviors towards the researcher of the present study.

### 2.2 Questionnaires

A questionnaire covering socio-demographic (gender, age, education), and work-related parameters (sector-specialty; total years of work as a medical resident; years of work as a medical resident especially at UGHP) was distributed to study participants. The Einarsen Negative Acts Questionnaire revised (NAQ-R) was used as the tool to measure exposure to mobbing in the workplace environment. This questionnaire has a high coefficient of internal coherence (Cronbach-alpha = 0.915). Kakoulakis et al. have validated it in Greek [4, 7]. The author of the present study requested and got written approval for the use of the questionnaire.

NAQ includes a total of 23 questions. Of these, questions 1, 3, 4, 11, 12, 13, 14, 16, 18, 19, and 21 pertain to a specific scale of labor-related intimidation. Questions 2, 5, 6–10, 15, 17, 20, and 22 relate to a scale of labor-related intimidation regarding the worker's personality. Question 23 concerns how often the respondent considers that there is moral harassment in his/her work after being given the definition. The questions are rated from 1 to 5 (5 point Likert scale), with the scale corresponding to: 1 = never, 2 = rarely, 3 = once per month, 4 = once a week, 5 = every day. The above answers are added together and the total score results in values ranging from 23 (lower) to 115 (higher), and the higher the sum, the higher the mobbing phenomenon. Based on the weighting of the Greek population, the interpretation of the results is as follows: nonexistence of mobbing: 23–25 points; low levels of mobbing: 26–34 points; moderate levels: 35–44 points; high levels: 45–55 points; very high levels of mobbing—frequent and extreme aggressive behaviors: 56 points or more [7].

### 2.3 Statistical analysis

Descriptive statistics were calculated for the study variables; continuous variables were summarized as mean (standard deviation, SD) and categorical ones as frequencies and percentages. Similarly, descriptive statistics were estimated for NAQ-22 items and overall score.

At the univariate analysis, the associations between NAQ-22 overall score with sociodemographic and work-related factors were evaluated with t-test and analysis of variance (ANOVA), as appropriate; the assumption of normality was verified with Shapiro-Wilk test.

At the multivariate approach, the independent associations between NAQ-22 score (treated as the dependent variable), sociodemographic and work-related factors (treated as independent variables) were evaluated by multivariate linear regression analysis. Model fit was evaluated with the examination of jackknifed residuals. The level of statistical significance was set at 0.05. Statistical analysis was performed with SPSS® version 16 statistical software (SPSS Inc, Chicago, IL, USA).

## 3. Results

### 3.1 Descriptive statistics

The sample of the present study consisted of 92 individuals, all medical residents in the UGHP. The demographic features of participants are shown in **Table 1**. Fifty-two percent (n = 48) were females. In terms of age, the majority (77.2%, n = 71) was 25–35 years old. With regard to sector-specialty, 41.3% (n = 38) of participants worked at the Internal Medicine, 31.5% (n = 29) Surgical, 21.7% (n = 20) Laboratory, 3.3% (n = 3) Psychiatric, and 2.2% (n = 2) at Clinical-laboratory Sector, respectively. Only 9.9% (n = 9) had an MSc and 7.7% (n = 7) a PhD degree. The majority of participants (59.8%, n = 55) worked overall as medical residents for 2–5 years and especially at UGHP for 0–2 years (51.1%, n = 47).

The questions that were related to possible negative issues at the workplace of participants have represented: Participants asserted that they had been "frequently" ordered to do work below their level of competence (M = 3.68), as well as having key areas of responsibility removed or replaced with more trivial or unpleasant tasks (M = 3.63). Also, participants' answers, regarding the statement "Being exposed to an unmanageable workload", were placed between the scale "sometimes" and "frequently" (M = 3.34). Furthermore, participants claimed that "sometimes" had been shouted at or being the target of spontaneous anger (M = 2.88) and under pressure not to claim something to which by right they were entitled (M = 2.83). Accordingly, "sometimes" someone withholds information which affects their performance (M = 2.79). Also, "sometimes" having been their opinions ignored (M = 2.75), were under persistent criticism of their errors or mistakes (M = 2.74), as well as "sometimes" there were spreading of gossip and rumors about them (M = 2.73) (**Table 2**).

Additionally, participants' answers were placed between the scale "rarely" and "sometimes" as for the statements "Repeated reminders of your errors or mistakes" (M = 2.62), "Being given tasks with an unreasonable deadline" (M = 2.55), and "Excessive monitoring of your work" (M = 2.38). Moreover, participants declared that "rarely" having been humiliated or ridiculed in connection with their work (M = 2.25),

| Variables | Categories | n (%) |
|---|---|---|
| Gender | Male | 44 (47.8) |
| | Female | 48 (52.2) |
| Age | 25–35 | 71 (77.2) |
| | 35–45 | 19 (20.7) |
| | 45–55 | 2 (2.2) |
| Sector-Specialty | Laboratory | 20 (21.7) |
| | Clinical-laboratory | 2 (2.2) |
| | Internal Medicine | 38 (41.3) |
| | Surgery | 29 (31.5) |
| | Psychiatric | 3 (3.3) |
| Level of education | PhD | 7 (7.7) |
| | MSc | 9 (9.9) |
| | Medical degree | 75 (82.4) |
| Total years of work as a medical resident | 0–2 | 27 (29.3) |
| | 2–5 | 55 (59.8) |
| | 6–10 | 10 (10.9) |
| Years of work as a medical resident especially at UGHP | 0–2 | 47 (51.1) |
| | 2–5 | 40 (43.5) |
| | 6–10 | 5 (5.4) |

*N: Frequency; f%: Valid Percent.*

**Table 1.**
*Sociodemographic and work-related parameters in the study sample (n = 92).*

ignored or facing a hostile reaction when they approach (M = 2.22), having allegations made against them (M = 2.16), having been ignored or excluded (M = 2.13), having insulting or offensive remarks made about their attitudes or private life (M = 2.10), having been a victim of mobbing in their work (M = 2.02) or the subject of excessive teasing and sarcasm (M = 2.00). Moreover, participants argued that there were "rarely" intimidating behaviors, (such as finger-pointing, invasion of personal space, shoving, blocking their way) (M = 1.78), hints or signals from others that made them quit their job (M = 1.68) or practical jokes, carried out by people they don't get along with (M = 1.68). In conclusion, participants' answers were placed between the scale "never" and "rarely", with regard to the statement "Threats of violence or physical abuse or actual abuse" (M = 1.36).

### 3.2 Associations between mobbing and potential correlates: results from univariate analysis

In this section, the main research aim will be examined which is to find possible dependencies between negative issues at work with demographic characteristics. Internal reliability was very satisfying as Cronbach Alpha value is 0.932 > 0.7.

| Questions | Mean | Std. deviation |
|---|---|---|
| **Labour-related intimidation** | | |
| Being ordered to do work below your level of competence | 3.68 | 1.30 |
| Being exposed to an unmanageable work load | 3.34 | 1.30 |
| Being shouted at or being the target of spontaneous anger | 2.88 | 1.20 |
| Being given tasks with unreasonable deadline | 2.55 | 1.30 |
| Excessive monitoring of your work | 2.38 | 1.10 |
| Being humiliated or ridiculed in connection with your work | 2.25 | 1.20 |
| Being ignored or facing a hostile reaction when you approach | 2.22 | 1.20 |
| Being ignored or excluded | 2.13 | 1.10 |
| Have you been victim of mobbing in your work? | 2.02 | 1.10 |
| Being the subject of excessive teasing and sarcasm | 2 | 1.10 |
| Hints or signals from others that you should quit your job | 1.68 | 1.04 |
| **Labour related intimidation regarding the workers' personality** | | |
| Having key areas of responsibility removed or replaced with more trivial or unpleasant tasks | 3.63 | 1.2 |
| Pressure not to claim something to which by right you are entitled (e.g. sick leave, holiday entitlement, travel expenses) | 2.83 | 1.3 |
| Someone withholding information which affects your performance | 2.79 | 1.2 |
| Having your opinions ignored | 2.75 | 1.1 |
| Persistent criticism of your errors or mistakes | 2.74 | 1.1 |
| Spreading of gossip and rumors about you | 2.73 | 1.3 |
| Repeated reminders of your errors or mistakes | 2.62 | 1.1 |
| Having allegations made against you | 2.16 | 1.0 |
| Having insulting or offensive remarks made about your person, attitudes or your private life | 2.1 | 1.2 |
| Intimidating behaviors such as finger-pointing, invasion of personal space, shoving, blocking your way | 1.78 | 1.1 |
| Practical jokes carried out by people you don't get along with | 1.68 | 1.0 |
| Threats of violence or physical abuse or actual abuse | 1.36 | 0.9 |

**Table 2.**
*Descriptive statistics for NAQ items.*

Due to high internal reliability, questions that referred to negative issues at work have been grouped in a new variable named "Score of negative issues at work" using the unbiased estimator of mean value. The mean value of "Score of negative issues at work" is 2.45 indicating that negative issues happen rarely to sometimes while standard deviation is 0.743.

**Table 3** indicates results of the univariate analysis regarding the associations between NAQ overall score, sociodemographic, and work-related features. **Table 3** indicates that mean value of variable "Score of negative issues at work" differs in different categories of demographic features "Age" ($p$-value = $0.0174 < 0.05$,

| Variable | Mean (SD) | p-value |
|---|---|---|
| Gender | | |
| Males | 53.6136 (17.8498) | 0.1473[t] |
| Females | 58.7917 (16.1324) | |
| Age | | |
| 25–35 | 58.4930 (16.3059) | **0.0174[A]** |
| 35–45 | 51.0000 (17.5816) | |
| 45–55 | 29.5000 (7.7782) | |
| Sector-specialty | | |
| Laboratory | 45.3500 (13.0274) | **0.0043[A]** |
| Clinical-laboratory | 40.5000 (4.9497) | |
| Internal Medicine | 57.6842 (17.0343) | |
| Surgery | 62.5517 (17.1435) | |
| Psychiatric | 62.3333 (7.7675) | |
| Years of work as a medical resident | | |
| 0–2 | 58.8889 (18.4835) | 0.4776[A] |
| 2–5 | 55.9636 (15.3067) | |
| 6–10 | 51.3000 (22.5490) | |
| Years of work as a medical resident at UGHP | | |
| 0–2 | 59.3830 (18.2525) | **0.0449[A]** |
| 2–5 | 54.6750 (15.3529) | |
| 6–10 | 40.60000 (7.8294) | |

*t: p-value derived from t-test; A: p-values derived from analysis of variance.*

**Table 3.**
*Univariate associations of NAQ overall score with demographic features. Bold cells denote statistically significant associations.*

ANOVA), "Sector-Specialty" (p-value = 0.0043 < 0.05, ANOVA) and "Years of work as a medical resident at UGHP" (p-value = 0.4776 < 0.05, ANOVA).

## 3.3 Associations between mobbing and potential correlates: results from multivariate regression analysis

Results of multiple regression model fit with dependent variable "Score of negative issues at work" and independent variables the demographic features. Null hypothesis that model does not fit and its data is rejected (p-value = 0.002 < 0.05). Level of adjustment is moderate as R2 = 0.212 < 0.4.

**Table 4** indicates coefficients of multiple regression model fit with dependent variable "Score of negative issues at work" and independent variables the demographic features. Null hypothesis is that coefficients are zero and the alternative is that they are statistically significant. Statistical significant are considered the coefficients of variables "Age" (p-value = 0.035 < 0.05), "Sector-Specialty" (p-value = 0.001 < 0.05). Linear model is described by the following mathematical formula:

| Independent variables | B | BETA | p-value |
|---|---|---|---|
| Gender | 0.1 | 0.06 | 0.539 |
| Age | −0.4 | −0.2 | **0.035** |
| Sector-specialty | 0.2 | 0.3 | **0.001** |
| Level of education | −0.04 | −0.03 | 0.722 |
| Years of work as a medical resident | 0.1 | 0.1 | 0.404 |
| Years of work as a medical resident at UGHP | −0.08 | −0.07 | 0.620 |
| *Dependent Variable: Score of negative issues at work.* | | | |

**Table 4.**
*Results of the multivariate regression analysis examining the associations between NAQ (dependent variable), sociodemographic and work-related parameters.*

$$\text{"Score of negative issues at work"} = 0.001 - 0.365 \times \text{Age} + 0.222 \times \text{Sector} - \text{Specialty}. \quad (1)$$

Results of independent variables affection in dependent variable "Score of negative issues at work" using BETA coefficients were as follows: Variable "Age" affects negatively (BETA = −0.238) dependent variable of model, while "Sector-Specialty" positively (BETA = 0.349). BETA coefficients have values in the interval [−1.1]. Values close to 1 indicate maximum positive affection while values close to −1 maximum negative. Values close to 0 indicate no affection.

The sample of medical residents in this study shows an average score of 56.32 ± 17.080 for NAQ-22, which means on average that there were very high levels of mobbing- frequent and extreme aggressive behaviors in the medical residents of UGHP. No statistically significant difference occurred in NAQ-22 relative to sex (p = 0.14), training (p = 0.735), the specialty years (p = 0.478), or years of work as a trainee in UGHP (p = 0.052). On the other hand, statistically significant difference (p = 0.0174) occurs with respect to: (a) age, where at the age group 25–35 the highest value is observed (mean = 58.5) in relation to ages groups 35–35 (mean = 51.0) and 45–55 (mean = 29.50), and (b) Sector, (p = 0.0043) with higher score in the Division of Surgery (mean = 62.55), and lowest in the Laboratory sector (mean = 45.4).

### 3.4 Multivariate regression analysis for subscales of NAQ

**Table 5** indicates the results of Cronbach Alpha coefficient for subscales of NAQ. Reliability of "labor related intimidation" was a = 0.864 while "labur related intimidation regarding the worker's personality" 0.902. Reliability of the total scale was 0.932.

Using as dependent variable "Labor related intimidation", statistically significant are considered the coefficients of variables "**Age**" (p-value = 0.003 < 0.05), "**Sector-Specialty**" (p-value = 0.001 < 0.05) and the coefficient of constant (p-value < 0.001). Linear model is described by the following mathematical formula:

$$\begin{aligned}\text{Labor related intimidation} = {} & 2.987 + 0.087 \times \text{Gender}–0.544 \times \text{Age} + 0.237 \\ & \times \text{Sector} - \text{Specialty}–0.118 \times \text{Level of education}(\text{A}) \\ & + 0.112 \times \text{Years of work as a medical resident}(\text{A})–0.098 \\ & \times \text{Years of workas a medical resident at UGHP}(\text{A}). \quad (2)\end{aligned}$$

| Category | Questions | Cronbach Alpha |
|---|---|---|
| Labour related intimidation | 1, 3, 4, 11, 12, 13, 14, 16, 18, 19, 21 | 0.864 |
| Labour related intimidation regarding the worker's personality | 2, 5, 6, 7, 8, 9, 10, 15, 17, 20, 22 | 0.902 |
| Victim of mobbing in work | 23 | — |
| Score of negative issues at work | 1–23 | 0.932 |

**Table 5.**
*Reliability analysis for subscales of NAQ.*

Using as dependent variable "Labor related intimidation regarding the worker's personality", statistically significant is considered the coefficient of variable "Sector-Specialty" ($p\text{-value} = 0.006 < 0.05$). No appropriate model was formulated.

Using as dependent variable "Victim of mobbing in work", statistically significant is considered only the constant ($p\text{-value} = 0.034 < 0.05$). No appropriate model was formulated.

Using as dependent variable "Score of negative issues at work" statistically significant are considered the coefficients of variables "Age" ($p\text{-value} = 0.035 < 0.05$), "Sector-Specialty" ($p\text{-value} = 0.001 < 0.05$) and the coefficient of constant ($p\text{-value} = 0.0001 < 0.05$). Linear model is described by the following mathematical formula:

$$\begin{aligned}\text{Score of negative issues at work} &= 2.122 + 0.092 \times \text{Gender} - 0.365 \\ &\times \text{Age} + 0.222 \times \text{Sector} - \text{Specialty} - 0.044 \times \text{Level of education(D)} \\ &+ 0.132 \times \text{Years of work as a medical resident(D)} - 0.084 \\ &\times \text{Years of work as a medical resident at UGHP(D)}.\end{aligned} \quad (3)$$

## 4. Discussion

In our study, statistically significant differences occurred with respect to age and Sector. Regarding the age, medical residents of 25–35 years were subject to highest values of mobbing (mean = 58.5) in relation to ages groups 35–35 (mean = 51.0) and 45–55 (mean = 29.50). Regarding the Sector, the higher score was objected in the Surgery Sector (p = 0.0043), (mean = 62.55), and lowest in the Laboratory Sector (mean = 45.4).

The sample of the present study consisted of 92 individuals, all medical residents in the UGHP. Males and females were almost equal and regarding age most of the participants were 25–45 years old. As far as sector specialty was concerned, the majority of individuals worked at the Internal Medicine Sector, at the Surgical Sector, and at the Laboratory Sector. In respect of the level of education, most of the participants had a medical degree and worked as medical residents at UGHP for 0–5 years.

Generally, negative issues at work happened rarely to sometimes. Participants stated that they had been frequently ordered to do work below their level of competence as well as having key areas of responsibility removed or replaced with more trivial or unpleasant tasks. Negative incidents at work happened more frequently to young participants age 25–35 years old, individuals with specialty in Internal Medicine or Surgery, and those who worked 0–2 years as medical residents at UGHP.

Specifically, participants stated that labor-related intimidation happens sometimes while labor-related intimidation regarding the workers' personality or being a victim of mobbing in work rarely. Analyzing labor related intimidation, participants stated that they had been frequently ordered to do work below their level of competence as well as having key areas of responsibility removed or replaced with more trivial or unpleasant tasks.

In our study, very high levels of mobbing - very frequent and extreme aggressive behaviors emerged (score 56.32±17.080 for NAQ-22). Regarding the Greek hospitals, these findings are consistent with the study of Gavrielatos [18] that referred to a sample of medical residents using the same tool (NAQ scale) [18]. Data from a cross-sectional quantitative empirical study from University General Hospital from Heraklion, Crete, in Greece, revealed that among health care professionals 41.3% of the participants were subjects of serious mobbing and 31.3% of occasional mobbing, with doctors more vulnerable from nurses. Also the upper the more highly educated were victims of mobbing. This survey also used the Negative Acts Questionnaire-Revised [25]. In accordance with those results is a study conducted in Bosnia and Herzegovina; where over three-quarters of doctors declared they were exposed to moral harassment, and with surveys in Turkey and Portugal, where non-specialist doctors were exposed to moral harassment at a rate of 87.7% and 60% respectively [5, 21]. In a survey conducted among primary health care workers in Turkey, 31.1% of health workers declared having been victims of mobbing in the last one year with a frequency of 1–3 times per year [26]. Lower rates were observed in hospital doctors in the United Kingdom and Finland [5, 21]. With international evidence demonstrating that in the healthcare sector the phenomenon of moral harassment is reinforced, but on the other hand not properly evaluated by the victim due to the stress of survival amidst the economic crisis and daily exposure to illness and death, these percentages are particularly important [6, 21, 27, 28].

In another study from Turkey among healthcare professionals, half of the participants declared exposure to "mobbing behaviors for targeting reputation" and to "mobbing behaviors for targeting occupational status" [29]. A qualitative study from Greece among health professionals in a public hospital revealed that the mobbing phenomenon was tangible and the abuse was mainly verbal and behavioral [30].

As far as gender is concerned, findings in literature are controversial [6, 20, 26, 31, 32]. In the present study, there was no statistically significant difference in NAQ-22 related to gender. A statistically significant difference was observed only in questions referring to the individual's intimidation about his/her personality, such as question 2 (Being humiliated or ridiculed in connection with your work), question 5 (Spreading of gossip and rumors about you), question 7 (Having insulting or offensive remarks made about your person), and question 16 (Being given tasks with an unreasonable deadline). In the above-mentioned questions, women had a higher score than their male counterparts. Despite the fact that the present study does not present a statistically significant difference in the NAQ-22 between the two sexes, those responses of female medical residents should be taken under consideration and redefine the attitude towards female doctors. A survey conducted in Turkey also revealed high rates of mobbing in females doctors, participants with low income, and also workers from other provinces [33, 34]. On the other hand, a survey from Turkey in healthcare professionals from three different cities included workers from private hospitals, state hospitals, university hospitals, and other health centers revealed that the level of mobbing did not vary depending on gender, but on the marital status and age. Singles and younger employees were subjected to mobbing more than the married and older ones [35].

In the international literature, there is a controversy about the relationship between age and the occurrence of the phenomenon of mobbing [20, 36]. In Uruguay 40.4% of hospital employees reported being the victim of mobbing at least once a week, with the majority being older and more highly educated [37]. In the current study, there appeared to be a particularly higher NAQ score in the youngest doctors (25–35-year-old). This pattern is in line with the study by Gavrielatos for physicians [18]. Possible explanations may include that older medical residents have learned how to handle similar incidents from their job experience or they are perpetrators themselves [38].

Regarding previous education, there was no statistically significant difference between medical residents with a medical degree, MSc degree, or PhD in our survey. A statistically significant difference occurred only in question 15 "Practical jokes carried out by people you don't get along with", with the maximum occurring in the case of people with an MSc degree. This finding is in part consistent with Gavrielatos's study, where doctors with an MSc or PhD seemed to be subject to higher mobbing rates [18]. Other studies also demonstrated that the selected victims were often more qualified than others [2, 39]. In Turkey healthcare professionals with a doctoral education level were exposed more to mobbing than their colleagues with lower education [40, 41].

In accordance, there is also a study conducted in Uruguay among hospital employees. In this study, there was more prevalent mobbing among the employees who had higher education [37].

According to the results of the present study, the highest rates of mobbing were observed in the Surgical Sector (62.55), whereas in the Laboratory sector the lowest (45.35). Issues of increased workload in connection with a lack of division of duties and responsibilities in connection with management deficiencies of the Surgical Sector are a possible explanation of these results. A strict hierarchical structure in an organization, combined with the ambiguity of tasks and lack of distinct responsibilities, may intensify and fuel the phenomenon as tensions are favored. Another potentially important parameter is the non-recognition of the efforts made by the employees, resulting in frustration and loss of confidence [2, 6, 19, 38, 42–44].

There was no statistically significant difference with respect to years of being a medical resident in this study. A difference was noted only in question 2 "Being humiliated or ridiculed in connection with your work" where people with 2–5 years of service (mean = 2.49) appeared to be more harassed than people with years of service 0–2 (mean= 2.11) and 6–10 (mean = 1.30). This is in contradiction with the findings of Gavrielatos [18] and Katsilaki [20], where those who accept very low levels of mobbing have more years of experience [18, 20, 45]. A cross-sectional study in a Malaysian Public University Hospital, using the validated Malay version of the 23-item Negative Acts Questionnaire—revised, revealed that workers in less than ten years were the victims [46].

## 5. Conclusion: limitations

Given the devastating effects of mobbing on the individual and the organization, management should take preventive and countermeasure acts [5]. Keeping the medical residents and Heads of the Sectors informed about the mobbing phenomenon is a positive step to that direction along with recording the current situation. The phenomenon of moral harassment requires immediate confrontation as the very high levels of mobbing observed should sound the alarm. In health care working environment hierarchies, respect is often related to power and status [47]. On the other hand, respect should be related to "positive attitudes toward human worth" especially when vulnerable individuals are involved. As far as medical residents are concerned, their time, opinions and privacy should not be ignored [47]. Trust and job satisfaction should build respect and professionalism [47].

Regarding limitations, the low response rate of the doctors in the completion of the questionnaire, despite the assurances of the anonymity of the participants, has troubled the investigators of this survey. Despite necessary explanations to the participants and the preservation of anonymity, the low response rate may have signaled selection bias.

The interpretation of the results of relevant surveys should be based on the particular characteristics of the organization in which the study is conducted and the nature of the work being done [3]. Comparing data with other research papers on the same subject is difficult when there are not used the same measuring tools [7]. Finally, the present research has a cross-sectional character, which on the one hand facilitates sample selection from the general population, but on the other hand, it cannot give information about the sequence of time or search for the cause of facts.

## Acknowledgements

Part of this work was presented during the sessions of International Conference on Business & Economics, Athens, Greece, 2018, available at shttp://icbe-hou.eap.gr › public › program-en_US. Special thanks to Professors Theodoros N. Sergentanis and Maria Trigoni, Management of Health Care Services, Hellenic Open University, Patras, Greece, for guidance and inspiration. The author received no financial support for the research, authorship, and publication of this article.

## Conflict of interest

The author declares no conflict of interest

## Author details

Panagiota Xaplanteri
General Hospital of Eastern Achaia, Kalavrita, Greece

*Address all correspondence to: panagiota.xaplanteri@gmail.com

## References

[1] Duffy MK, Ganster D, Pagon M. Social undermining and social support in the workplace. Academy of Management Journal. 2002;**45**:331-351

[2] Demirag S, Ciftci S. Psychological intimidation at workplace (Mobbing). Journal of Psychology and Psychotherapy. 2017;7:305. DOI: 10.4172/2161-0487.1000305

[3] Einarsen S, Raknes BI, Matthiesen SM. Bullying and harassment at work and their relationships to work environment quality: An exploratory study. European Work and Organizational Psychologist. 1994;**4**(4):381-401. DOI: 10.1080/13594329408410497

[4] Einarsen S, Hoel H, Notelaers G. Measuring exposure to bulling and harassment at work: Validity, factor structure and psychometric properties of the Negative Acts Questionnaire-revised. Work & Stress. 2009;**23**(1):24-44

[5] Pranjić N, Maleš-Bilić L, Beganlić A, Mustajbegović J. Mobbing, stress, and work ability index among physicians in Bosnia and Herzegovina: Survey Study. Croatian Medical Journal. 2006;**47**: 750-758

[6] Koinis A, Saridi M. Mobbing in the workplace. Mobbing effects on health. Hellenic Journal of Nursing Science. 2013;**6**(1):36-48

[7] Kakoulakis C, Galanakis M, Bakoula-Tzoumaka C, Darvyri P, Chrousos PG, Darviri C. Validation of the negative acts questionnaire (NAQ) in a sample of Greek Teachers. Psychology. 2015;**6**: 63-74

[8] Dede I. The mobbing phenomenon; Work intimidation]. 2017. Available from: https://www.inegsee.gr/wp-content/uploads/2017/.../NOEMBRIOS_DEKEMBRIOS.pdf. Article in Greek

[9] Papalexandri N, Galanaki E. Workplace bullying: It frightens workers and blocks the good climate even in Greek businesses. HR Focus. 2011;**42**: 24-27

[10] Makrakis C. Moral harassment in the workplace: Examining the example of a private and public sector hospital in Chania [diploma thesis]. Greece: Technological Educational Institute of Crete; 2009. Available from: lib.teicrete.gr/browse/seyp/ker/.../MakrakisCharalambos/.../Makrakis2009.pdf

[11] Keashly L. Emotional abuse in the workplace: Conceptual and empirical issues. Journal of Emotional Abuse. 1997; **1**:85-117. DOI: 10.1300/J135v01n01_05

[12] Vartia M. The sources of bullying: Psychological work environment and organizational climate. European Journal of Work and Organizational Psychology. 1996;**5**(2):203-214

[13] Zapf D, Gross C. Conflict escalation and coping with workplace bullying: A replication and extension. European Journal of Work and Organizational Psychology. 2001;**10**(4):497-522. DOI: 10.1080/13594320143000834

[14] Konstantinidis M. Work harassment: A proposal for research and intervention. Elinyae. 2011;**47**:4-11

[15] Lianos T. Brain drain and brain loss: Immigrants to Greece. Journal of Ethnic and Migration Studies. 2007;**33**(1): 129-140

[16] Okeke EN. Brain drain: Do economic conditions push doctors out of

developing countries? Social Science & Medicine. 2013;**98**:169-178

[17] Ferrinho P, Biscaia A, Fronteira I, Craveiro I, Antunes AR, et al. Patterns of perceptions of workplace violence in the Portuguese health care sector. Human Resources Health. 2003;**1**:11

[18] Gavrielatos G. The Mobbing syndrome among medical residents and the role of emotional intelligence in coping with it [Postgraduate thesis]. Hellenic Open University; 2015. Available from: https://apothesis.eap.gr/handle/repo/33752. Article in Greek

[19] Gök S. Prevalence and types of mobbing behavior: A research on banking employees. International Journal of Human Sciences. 2011;**8**(1): 318-334

[20] Katsilaki EC. Investigation of the mobbing syndrome among healthcare professionals (Doctors and Nurses) at a public sector hospital and the Role of Communication [Postgraduate thesis]. Hellenic Open University; 2017. Available from: https://apothesis.eap.gr/handle/repo/35048. Article in Greek

[21] Kivimäki M, Elovainio M, Vahtera J. Workplace bullying and sickness absence in hospital staff. Occupational Environmental Medicine. 2000;**57**: 656-660

[22] Ozdemir S, Tosun B, Bebis H, Yava A. Mobbing from nurse pencil: Psychological Harassment at Workplac. TAF. Preventive Medicine Bulletin. 2013;**12**(2):183-192

[23] Sahin B, Cetin M, Cimen M, Yildiran N. Assessment of Turkish junior male physicians' exposure to mobbing behavior. Croatian Medical Journal. 2012;**53**(4):357-366

[24] http://www.pgnp.gr/?section=2376&language=el_GR

[25] Katsounaki N, Kiaourtzi E, Manousaki E. Exploring the phenomenon of mobbing in health professionals at the university general hospital of Heraklion. Hellenic Journal of Nursing Science. Available at: http://journal-ene.gr/exploring-the-phenomenon-of-mobbing-in-health-professionals-at-the-university-general-hospital-of-heraklion/?lang=en

[26] Pinar T, Acikel C, Pinar G, Karabulut E, Saygun M, Bariskin E, et al. Workplace violence in the health sector in Turkey: A National Study. Journal of Interpersonal Violence. 2017;**32**(15): 2345-2365

[27] Hutchinson M, Vickers M, Jackson D, Wilkes L. Workplace bullying in nursing: Towards a more critical organizational perspective. Nursing Inquiry. 2006;**13**(2):118-126

[28] Trépanier SG, Fernet C, Austin S. Workplace psychological harassment in Canadian nurses: A descriptive study. Journal of Health Psychology. 2013; **18**(3):383-396. DOI: 10.1177/1359105312443401

[29] Sahin B, Dundar T. Examining factors that affect meeting levels of healthcare professionals who are exposed to mobbing: The example of Bolu Province. TİSK Academy. 2011;**11**:88-117

[30] Koinis A, Velonakis E, Kalafati M, Tziaferi S. Mobbing in a Greek Public Hospital and the views experiences and beliefs among Health Professionals: A Qualitative Study. International Journal of Quantitative and Qualitative Research Methods. 2019;**7**(4):11-25

[31] Ariza-Montes A, Muniz N, Montero-Simo M, Araquel-Padila A. Workplace

bullying among healthcare workers. Research and Public Health. 2013;**10**(8): 3121-3139

[32] Information and Consultation of Employees|Guide CIPD. Available from: https://www.cipd.co.uk ›

[33] Erdogan V, Yildirim A. Healthcare professionals' exposure to mobbing behaviors and relation of mobbing with job satisfaction and organizational commitment. Procedia Computer Science. 2017;**120**:931-938

[34] Kılıç T, Çiftçi F, Şener S. Journal of Health and Nursing Management. 2016; **2**:3. DOI: 10.5222/SHYD.2016.065

[35] Türkan AH, Kılıç I. Journal of Business Resaerch Turk. 2015;**7**(3):7-21

[36] Einarsen S, Skogstad A. Bullying at work: Epidemiological findings in public and private organizations. European Journal of Work and Organisational Psychology. 1996;**5**:185-201

[37] Buunk AP, Franco S, Dijkstra P, Zurriaga R. Mobbing in Schools and Hospitals in Uruguay: Prevalence and relation to loss of status. Journal of Interpersonal Violence. 2017;**32**(5): 623-634. DOI: 10.1177/ 0886260515625903

[38] Stephens T, Hallas J. Bullying and Sexual Harassment A practical handbook. Oxford, England: Chandos Publishing; 2006

[39] Khoo SB. Academic mobbing: Hidden Health hazard at workplace. Malaysian Family Physician. 2010;**5**(2): 61-67

[40] Karcioglu F, Akbas S. The relationship between psychological violence in workplace and job satisfaction. The Journal of Economic and Administrative Sciences. 2010; **24**(3):139-161

[41] Turkmen SN, Ustun C, Ozdemir C, Akyol T, Cokmus FP. Health professionals exposure to mobbing in a medical school hospital. Journal of Turgut Ozal Medical Center. 2017;**24**(4): 437-442. DOI: 10.5455/jtomc.2017. 05.072

[42] Dewe PJ. Identifying the courses of nurse stress: A survey of New Zealand Nurses. Work & Stress. 1987;**1**(1):15-24

[43] Jimmieson NL. Employee reactions to behavioral control under conditions of stress: The moderating role of self-efficacy. Work & Stress. 2000;**14**(3): 262-280

[44] Shallcross L, Sheehan M, Ramsay S. Workplace mobbing: Experiences in the public sector. International Journal of Organisational Behaviour. 2008;**13**(2): 56-70

[45] Hillard J. Workplace mobbing: Are they really out to get your patient? Current Psychiatry. 2009;**8**(4):45-51

[46] Awai NS, Ganasegeran K, Abdul Manaf MR. Prevalence of workplace bullying and its associated factors among workers in a Malaysian Public University Hospital: A Cross-Sectional Study. Risk Management and Healthcare Policy. 2021;**8**(14):75-85. DOI: 10.2147/RMHP. S280954

[47] Karnieli-Miller O, Taylor AC, Cottingham AH, Inui TS, Vu TR, Frankel RM. Exploring the meaning of respect in medical student education: an analysis of student narratives. Journal of General Internal Medicine. 2010;**25**(12):1309-1314. DOI: 10.1007/s11606-010-1471-1

Section 4

# New Diagnostic and Treatment Approaches

Chapter 8

# New Diagnosis and Treatment Approaches to Post-Traumatic Stress Disorder

*Nevzat Tarhan, Muhsin Konuk, Mesut Karahan, Öznur Özge Özcan, Sibel Öztürk Ayvaz, Gökben Hızlı Sayar, Nurper Ülküer, Hazal Ayas and Feride Zeynep Güder*

## Abstract

Post-traumatic stress disorder (PTSD) is a mental health condition and disorder causing psychological deterioration triggered by terrifying events or traumatic experiences either by experiencing or by witnessing it. Though many people have common feelings, PTSD symptoms vary from one person to another. So it is strongly recommended to focus on new diagnostic and therapeutic methods relying and structured on a neurobiological dimension by collecting and processing neuroimaging data. It is crucial to make a profound analysis of PTSD in terms of its ontological, biological, developmental, psychological, and sociological aspects. Both with the new treatment opportunities and involvement of in silico-based artificial intelligence applications, new psychotherapy techniques and new discourses in digital media will be possible. Within the scope of the study, ontological discussions are followed and juxtaposed by Neuro-Biological Perspectives on Genomics and Epigenomics as well as the clinical and neuro-imaginative perspectives and clinical overviews of PTSD. Besides, the neuro-developmental views in the context of children along with adverse childhood experiences (ACE) and their relation to PTSD are analyzed by emphasizing the significance of brain development. Sociological aspects of PTSD in the digital habitus are collocated to develop unique therapy approaches that embrace sociological perspectives of Information Society.

**Keywords:** PTSD, ontology, neurobiology, genomics, epigenomics, neuro-imaginations, ACE, toxic stress, cyber violence and traumas

## 1. Introduction

Tsunami-like digital revolutions cause a sharp transformation of the world from modern society to Information society that eventually changed the scientific paradigms and approaches. Therefore, there appear several problems related to major clinical problems. Similarly, there emerge gaps between the cathartic effect of clinical interviews and therapeutic alliance. This gap also exists in the deeper understanding of the real experiences of the client and the help of the therapist. This chapter discusses the new diagnosis and treatment opportunities of post-traumatic stress disorder (PTSD) that appeared in stunning psychotherapy techniques and approaches and the changing role of psychiatrists. Since the shift in society and technological advancements doubles the burden of psychiatrists to a large extent, conventional diagnoses and therapies for PTSD do not work properly. It seems inevitable that recent developments and challenges surpass conventional approaches to PTSD that can easily miss embracing the overwhelming realities that those people experience.

This study, therefore, aims to explore and exemplify new diagnostic and therapeutic approaches to PTSD cases by embracing the digital revolutions of society with their novel implications and insights. To search for new working diagnoses and treatment opportunities, PTSD issues are analyzed by different angles and multi perspectives developed by certain disciplines. For Tarhan, the algorithm for the diagnosis and treatment process of PTSD has three main dynamics—ontological, sociological, and clinical (see **Figure 1**). These three dynamics are expanded by two more additional dynamics. Recent research on genomics and epigenomics in neuro-biological perspectives along with clinical and neuro-imaging perspectives are presented that they conglomerate new insights and implications for PTSD. They are explained in detail in the second and third parts of the chapter, respectively.

The underlying reason for designing this chapter in five subsequent parts comes from the need to shed some new light on PTSD from different angles. The latest technological innovations in genomics, epigenomics in neuro-biological perspectives, and clinical and neuro-imaging perspectives challenge the psychiatrists' role as they are expected to update their reference frames related to PTSD for diagnosis and

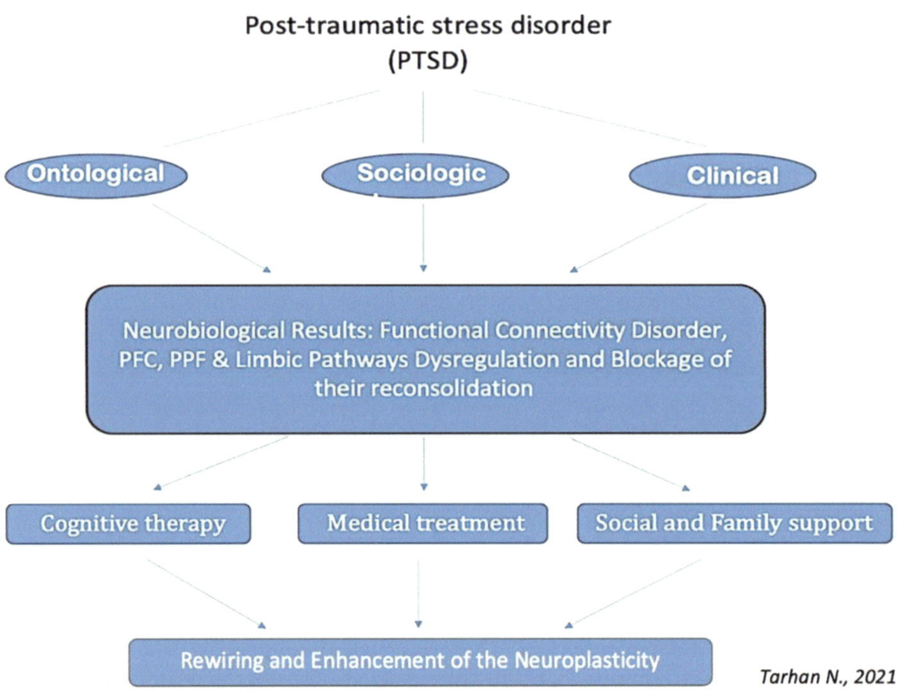


**Figure 1.**
*The algorithm for the diagnosis and treatment process of PTSD.*

treatment alternatives. Therefore, the study presents five interdisciplinary domains that are correlated with each other thematically as they particularly aimed to answer the question of what possible new approaches we have in terms of PTSD.

To pursue the goals mentioned above, the first part of the chapter starts with an ontological discussion that analyzes PTSD in terms of epidemiology and existential questions. In addition to those dimensions, the heavy impact of Coronavirus Disease (COVID-19) on PTSD cases and its sociopolitical consequences are portrayed in detail. This first part also throws a question as to whether post-traumatic growth is possible or not. It underlines that ontological well-being should not be ignored as healthy mindsets that eventually produce a healthy society. Ontological well-being and positive psychology are given as the ultimate aims of the science that would work for the benefit of the whole society counting PTSD patients. However, it is a challenging standpoint to offer a therapy that can work for the whole society. In the PTSD context, if social psychiatry utilizes cutting-edge approaches by wisely utilizing the technological advances of the cyber era, the mental and social well-being of society can be reached.

The second part follows the ontological discussions with Neuro-Biological Perspectives on Genomics and Epigenomics in PTSD. This part also discusses current Genome-Wide Association Studies and current Epigenome-Wide Association Studies. PTSD can occur at the organic, cellular, and molecular level due to the effect of an external event such as psychological trauma, as well as inherited from generation to generation. In PTSD, genetic and epigenetic studies are prioritized based on biological research because they are promising in elucidating molecular functioning and finding biomarkers. The goal of these studies is to lay the groundwork for new and preventive treatments to ameliorate the symptoms and the disease. In this context, there is current evidence for the potential of current genetic and epigenetic studies from the biological risk factors of PTSD.

In a similar vein, the third part of the chapter portrays the clinical and neuroimaging perspectives and clinical overviews of PTSD. This part argues the practical psychological treatments, such as neuromodulatory and neurobiological treatments. This part presents the Post-Traumatic Stress Disorder Checklist for DSM-5 as a self-report measure to evaluate the presence and severity of PTSD symptoms.

The fourth part expands the topic by adding the neuro-developmental perspective of PTSD, particularly in the context of children. Here, PTSD is analyzed by emphasizing the significance of Brain Development. This part is followed by a detailed explanation of adverse childhood experiences (ACE) and their relation to PTSD.

The fifth and final part of the chapter reviews PTSD in its correlation to the new paradigms and changes in Information Society. This part brings forward those transformations of society and media that necessitate searching for new discourses and alternative digital therapies for PTSD. Here, within the context of Attachment Theory, this final part warns of the potential evil that is inherent in new media, particularly in Digital Habitus and Dark Web. It would be wise to be cautious toward the widespread acts of cyber violence. It highlights the significance of a new emotional repertoire that can be identified as new types of traumas seen in digital habitus. In conclusion, since new trauma types emerged on cyber platforms, the mission and goal of social psychiatry are recommended to adopt these changes. Therefore, keeping pace with these transformations is widening the job definition of contemporary psychiatrists. Searching for new ways and counter activities to prevent society from demonic sides of social media ultimately shaped the agenda of psychiatrists.

## 2. Ontological discussions

*Trauma* can be roughly defined as an event that threatens the physical and psychological integrity of the person. However, the traumatic effect changes from one person to another. While the death of a cat has a traumatic effect on some people, the most severe war conditions do not have a traumatic effect on others. In the first step, therefore, we need to find the underlying reasons for these discrepancies. Why do these individual differences arise? It is worth explaining that the meaning ascribed to the event or a philosophy of life that is not afraid of death has an anti-traumatic effect.

Some basic information regarding the understanding of PTSD can be summarized as follows—PTSD is one of the few disorders among the Diagnostic and Statistical Manual of Mental Disorders (DSM) diagnostic categories regarding the etiology. Therefore, it is relatively easy and unproblematic to diagnose a PTSD case. The trauma mentioned there may appear in different situations and features. They can be concrete, obvious, extreme, unusual, unexpected, unforeseen, etc. The fact that the event's cause is not obscure ensures that the discomfort it causes is both predictable and fully comprehensible.

In the shock of the event, we can interpret cognitive blockage in many people as the brain shutting itself off to mental stimuli due to excessive adrenocorticotropic hormone (ACTH) and cortisol release. Later on, in other words, over-aroused state, avoidance behavior related to the event, insomnia, re-experiencing (Flashback), having nightmares are common symptoms. Even when awake, the person remembers the traumatic event over and over. S/he continues to experience the event that happened 10 years ago as if it happened yesterday. Since s/he feels like s/he is reliving the event, s/he tries to avoid the reminders.

Another definition of PTSD in DSM appears as follows: "The main feature of post-traumatic stress disorder is to experience the event of actual or threatened death, serious injury, or a threat to the physical integrity of the person, or the death or threat of death of another person. Extremely traumatic experiences, such as witnessing an event that poses a threat to one's life, injury or physical integrity, or learning that a family member or other relative has unexpectedly died or has been killed by being exposed to violence, was seriously injured or is under threat of death or injury. The development of specific symptoms following a source of traumatic stress. The person's reactions to the event in question are extreme fear, helplessness, or horror" [1].

### 2.1 Epidemiology

Studies conducted with large populations affected by the devastating earthquake, wars, and involvement in concentration camps found PTSD development risk between 20 and 50%. In one study conducted, data were analyzed from 26 population surveys in the World Health Organization World Mental Health Surveys. A total of 71,083 respondents aged 18+ participated. The cross-national lifetime prevalence of PTSD was 3.9% in the total sample and 5.6% among the trauma-exposed [2].

The experience of trauma is by no means exceptional, with all of its disruptive, jarring, deeply traumatic, intolerable, and "extremely terrifying, helpless, or terrifying" qualities. Moreover, both the frequency of PTSD that develops after a traumatic event and the acute stress disorder that occurs immediately after the trauma is often closely related to the threat to the person's psychological integrity.

It does not seem possible to establish a relationship between the nature of the trauma and the developing pathological picture that would require us to refer to the importance and severity of the current trauma. Of course, we should also note that different psychopathological conditions, such as post-traumatic depression and substance abuse, can occur utterly independent of PTSD. So, when we consider all these, we need to argue that the non-traumatic factors that determine the emergence of PTSD are essential enough and need to be carefully investigated [3].

### 2.2 Existential dimension

It is the ontological and cultural dimension that does not attract much attention from non-traumatic factors. Believing in and taking shelter in an unseen reality that knows everything, controlling the existence of belief in God when they feel helpless, powerless, and weak increases resilience to trauma. The conception of guardian angels, the Holy Spirit, or absolute monotheism (Tawhid) can be mental-sheltering. This approach, which changes our perceptions toward resilience, is also used in third-wave psychotherapies (Mindfulness, Metacognitive therapies) [4].

When mainly dealing with why evil exists, the Theodicy discipline proposes that it is significant to attribute more positive meanings to evil instead of ascribing it as a punishment. For the Positive Psychology approach, perceptions can change in the direction of endurance. Philosophers develop more or less similar ideas. Epicurus alleges that the Gods do not interfere with the earth, so evil belongs to the Gods. The motivation to enjoy is a sufficient measure for man. Giving the example of his famous cave allegory, Plato declares that God is absolute good and this world is not real life. While Kant says that evil has nothing to do with God, Leibniz claims that evil is for the benefit of good. For Comte, if he cannot prevent evil, God is helpless.

Unlike all these thinkers mentioned above, existential philosophy accelerated ferocious competition with the proposition that "God does not exist or cannot be proven, man's purpose is to seek self-interest and freedom in the world, and he must be selfish." As a result, many scholars, such as Nietzsche, Sartre, Kierkegaard, and Dostoevsky, changed the purpose, meaning, and values of life formed by human values in the name of hedonism and freedom. They even found Hegel and Kant to be prescriptive. On the other hand, Karl Popper said that if there is no evidence in epistemology, falsification is required. That is, it cannot be proven that God does not exist. Analytical philosopher Alvin Plantinga, on the other hand, argued that evils are necessary not because God does not exist but because God gives free will.

Heidegger, in 1966, accepted "time" as the most fundamental ontological category in the philosophical field. Today, people emotionally become vulnerable to traumatic experiences when existentialist philosophers Camus and Sartre defend absurdism by saying there is no meaning in life. Positive psychology, for this reason, has tried to fill the gap of this meaninglessness and meet the need to search for meaning. Today, when metacognitive genes related to the search for the meaning of life are mentioned, evidence has been sought against the approach of absurdism that reduces resilience to trauma. Psychological well-being is discussed in subjective, relational, semantic and temporal, and existential dimensions. The positive psychology literature confirms the importance of psychological well-being for resilience, so ontological well-being should not be ignored [5].

Ontological well-being, apart from subjective well-being, is the evaluation of life. Here, one's own life as a project should be examined together within the contexts of "past," "future," and "present." The meaningful combination of past, present, and future is the main focus of the evaluation of life [6].

People feel the need for a solid belief. The statement, "I believe, therefore I am," has been an area in which neuroscientists present their evidence [7, 8]. Being able to connect to that feeling in situations that one cannot control and cannot afford is considered in trauma therapies. For this reason, knowing the ontological dimension in the protection and prevention of PTSD and providing resilience training are recommended by Seligman under the name of the PERMA model.

### 2.3 COVID-19 impact

According to the March 2021 news in New York Times, the increase of existential questioning with the effect of social trauma globally draw our attention, particularly to the establishment of "Ministries of Loneliness" in England and Japan and on the search for solutions to suicide epidemics. The Ministry of Loneliness has an important mission as the existential needs of individual members of society have to be truly met by the systems. They can open new ways for the people who face trauma and allow them truly benefit from the effects of new diagnostic and therapeutic approaches. The existence of the ministry is highly significant, particularly in the case of the suicide epidemic. It can prevent suicidal people's feeling isolated and self-destructive action.

For this reason, studies on reorganizing the meaning of life and lifestyle have increased with the effect of social trauma. In a similar vein, Üsküdar University Senate reflected their studies and published a manifesto on Earth Day on April 22, 2021, to increase the resistance of world societies to trauma after the Pandemic and lead life toward the better tried to announce it globally. Üsküdar University here aims to help people who had a traumatic experience on a wider scale.

### 2.4 Can trauma have sociopolitical consequences?

After the cold war, the world became unipolar. As a result, global trends toward social justice have declined. Therefore, it is necessary to avoid the emergence of a new wealth hostility and to minimize opportunity and income inequality. For this reason, it is the right place to commemorate Marx and Engels together and talk about that extraordinary passage from the Communist Manifesto:

"Wherever the bourgeoisie has taken over, it has put an end to all feudal, patriarchal, rural relations. It has ruthlessly cut off the tangled feudal ties that bind man to his 'natural superiors,' leaving no other bond between man and man than pure self-interest, solid 'cash payment.' It has drowned the divine ecstasy of religious bigotry, the chivalric spirit, and petty-bourgeois sentimentality in the icy waters of selfish calculation. He has transformed personal dignity into exchange value and has replaced the innumerable freedoms so hard-won with that single, ruthless freedom, the freedom to trade. In short, it has replaced the exploitation of hidden religious and political illusions with open, indecent, direct, and brutal exploitation."

What will close that trauma bracket is obvious—the struggle of the poor/oppressed for liberation, equality, and freedom. Since the oppressed/poor are naked, all organizations and ties have collapsed, they are alone and helpless; since there is no light left for their hope, all ears to hear their voices are deaf [3].

### 2.5 Is post-traumatic growth possible?

As the sociopolitical consequence of the trauma, the global justice movement for worldwide peace must be initiated. We conducted a study in our field to turn trauma into an opportunity and presented it to the scientific world as evidence. In April 2020, 6318 cases were screened in all provinces of Turkey on Pandemic Fears, Anxiety, and Maturation, and there was a significant increase in six questions in the post-traumatic growth scale [9]. The primary aim of this investigation was to understand whether these findings are permanent after the Pandemic is over. These six questions are as follows:

1. The priority of the things I care about in life has changed, 59%
2. My interest in spiritual issues increased, 49%
3. I realized that I could handle the weaknesses, 56%
4. I can accept the events as they are, 56%
5. I started to give more importance to my social relations, 48%
6. I understand the value of the things I have, 74%

As a result, the causality relationship between Existence and Trauma draws attention. In addition, although 2 years have passed since COVID-19, it continues to force societies as a global social trauma. There are precursors to social crises that may occur. Such as migration and increase in mental disorders as post-pandemic. The rise of individual armament globally is worrying. We must find solutions so that there is no new break and disappointment in humanity. In conclusion, within the scope of this study, it is decided to present the aforementioned global well-being manifesto that will contribute to humanity's search for meaning and solution. In addition to this, it is lucid that the role of social scientists here plays a crucial role. For a better world, media, social and political scientists and leaders take several factors into consideration. Their function to lead to global peace and mental health is explained further in part six.

## 3. Neuro-biological perspective

### 3.1 Focus on genomics and Epigenomics in post-traumatic stress disorder

Post-traumatic stress disorder (PTSD) is a multifactorial disease characterized by structural, metabolic, and molecular changes in various brain regions and neural circuits, such as the limbic system, hippocampal region, and prefrontal cortex (in **Figure 2**), which regulate neurobehavioral functions [10]. Epigenetic and genetic current studies are included in this section. PTSD can occur at the organic, cellular, and molecular level due to the effect of an external event such as psychological trauma, as

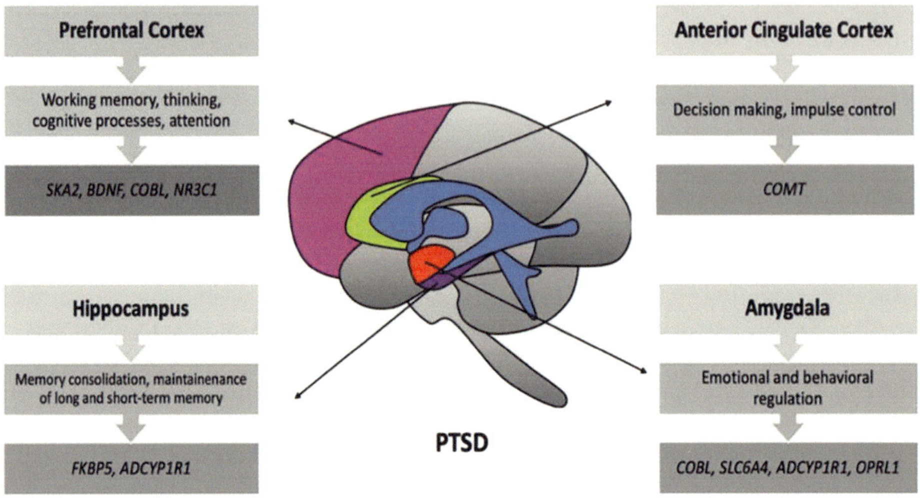


**Figure 2.**
*Current candidate genes associated with different brain regions and neuro-behaviors in PTSD [10]. Abbreviations: post-traumatic stress disorder (PTSD), catechol-O-methyltransferase (COMT), Cordon-Bleu WH2 Repeat Protein (COBL), Solute Carrier Family 6 Member 4 (SLC6A4), pituitary adenylate cyclase-activating polypeptide 1 receptor (ADCYP1R1), Opioid-Related Nociceptin Receptor 1 (OPRL1), FK506 binding proteins (FKBPS), Spindle And Kinetochore Associated Complex Subunit 2 (SKA2), Brain-Derived Neurotrophic Factor (BDNF), Nuclear Receptor Subfamily 3 Group C Member 1 (NR3C1).*

well as being inherited from generation to generation. In PTSD, genetic and epigenetic studies are prioritized based on biological research because they are promising in elucidating molecular functioning and finding biomarkers. The goal of these studies is to lay the groundwork for new and preventive treatments to ameliorate the symptoms that cause the disease. In this context, there is the current evidence for the potential of current genetic and epigenetic studies from the biological risk factors of PTSD.

Thousands or even hundreds of thousands of single nucleotide polymorphisms (SNPs) with a polygenic background are the genetic basis of PTSD according to Genome-wide association study (GWAS) summary statistic [11]. Considering the studies on twins with a traumatic history for hereditary dimensions, PTSD is inherited from 30% males and 70% females, SNPs play a major role in this hereditary process from women [12]. The heritability of PTSD following trauma has been demonstrated, but biological variations have not yet been fully defined. Elucidating the biological mechanisms underlying PTSD may contribute to a more accurate diagnosis and development of swelling-specific treatment interventions. Among the biological processes involved in PTSD and related conditions, this section focuses on epigenetic and genetic mechanisms. Genomic and epigenomic studies in large groups are valuable. Loci most recently examined in large-scale GWAS and Epigenome-wide association studies (EWAS) became candidate biological markers for PTSD.

### *3.1.1 Current genome-wide association studies*

Specific PTSD genetic variants that contribute to genetic studies have been most extensively researched and are currently known in the monoaminergic neurotransmission and hypothalamic-pituitary-adrenal (HPA) axis [13, 14]. The most frequently studied serotonin transporter gene (SLC6A4) polymorphisms in the monoaminergic system were associated with PTSD and identified with a prevalence of 45% in Europeans is the S allele frequency of SLC6A4. Association studies of 5-hydroxytryptamine 5-HT (5HTTLPR) and PTSD have been inconclusive, and a recent meta-analysis of 12 studies found no evidence of association overall, but the S allele was associated with PTSD in samples classified as having high trauma exposure [15]. Nominally significant associations between PTSD symptoms and many neurotransmitter-related genes, including 5-hydroxytryptamine (serotonin) 2A receptor gene (HRT2A), Solute Carrier Family 6 Member 3 (SLC6A3), Dopamine Receptor D3 (DRD3), Neuropeptide Y (NPY) Cannabinoid Receptor 1 (CNR1), and Regulator of G Protein Signaling 2 (RGS2) have been investigated [16–18].

One of the largest polymorphism studies of the Nurse's Health Study II, which included 845 PTSD cases and 1693 trauma-exposed controls, examined 3742 single nucleotide polymorphisms (SNPs) spanning more than 300 genes, but no gene was of clinical significance [19]. Meta-analysis and GWAS studies take an agnostic approach to the discovery of risk loci by comparing the frequencies of hundreds of thousands of SNPs and other genetic markers from the whole genome with those of controls, at least an update five gene markers are promising, including Zinc Finger DHHC-Type Palmitoyltransferase 14 (ZDHHC14), Parkinson Protein 2 E3 Ubiquitin Protein Ligase (PARK2), Kazrin, Periplakin Interacting Protein (KAZN), TMEM51 antisense RNA 1 (TMEM51-AS1), and Zinc Finger Protein 813 (ZNF813) [20–22]. The latest Military cohort study (29,539 PTSD cases and 166,145 controls) reported that Zinc Finger Protein 140 (ZNF140) is upregulated in blood, and Small Nuclear Ribonucleoprotein U11/U12 Subunit 35 (SNRNP35) is downregulated in the dorsolateral prefrontal cortex in Military PTSD [23]. Duncan et al. investigated strong evidence of overlapping SNPs and multi-loci risk between PTSD and schizophrenia (from 20,730 individuals) via 11 genome-wide case–control molecular genetic studies [24]. Chen et al. found two loci including chr10_6953246_D and rs2311207 that were associated with the severity of PTSD symptoms [25]. Other genome-wide significant loci were Ankyrin Repeat Domain 55 (ANKRD55) (rs1595))2 and Zinc Finger Protein 626 (ZNF626) on chromosome 19, moreover, the ANKRD55 gene was also related to rheumatoid arthritis and psoriasis that are additionally seen in patients with PTSD [26]. Maihofer et al. also found loci on four genes: Gamma-Aminobutyric Acid Type B Receptor Subunit 1 (GABBR1), Forkhead box protein P2 (FOXP2), Family with Sequence Similarity 120A (FAM120A), and ADP Ribosylation Factor Guanine Nucleotide Exchange Factor 2 (ARFGEF2) which had genome-wide significant ($p < 5 \times 10^{-8}$) from African American ancestry and the external Million Veteran's PTSD [27]. Pooler also discovered two SNPs; rs13160949 on chromosome 5 ($p = 7.33 \times 10^{-9}$) and SNP rs2283877 on chromosome 22 ($p = 2.55 \times 10^{-8}$) which have been firstly investigated in PTSD [28]. SNP rs267943 is located on chromosome 5 in the intron of the death-associated protein 1 (DAP1) gene had the strongest association from 396 chronic PTSD patients (Thai Tsunami survivors) and 457 controls [29]. Large-scale genome studies have identified heterogeneous and numerous SNPs and genes at multiple loci. Successful polygenic prediction models can be discovered in the future by increasing the number of current and large-scale studies. Current candidate genes associated with different brain regions and neuro-behaviors in PTSD are given in **Figure 2**.

### 3.2 Current epigenome-wide association studies

To better observe the Gene-Trauma Correlations in PTSD, epigenetic studies are also important to investigate the effects of environmental factors. Epigenome-wide association studies (EWAS) have identified epigenetic mechanisms for PTSD due to alteration of gene expression modifications without changing the genetic code. Epigenetic studies are carried out due to traumatic memory in the hippocampal region, frontal cortex associations, and extreme fear in the limbic system. An important regulation of gene function and phenotypic expression occurring in the understanding of PTSD occurs at the level of epigenetic regulation. Epigenetic changes include DNA methylation, histone modifications, and non-coding RNAs.

Animal research generally suggests that stress-induced epigenetic modification following environmental stress may affect stress-response functions as mediated by gene expression, HPA axis. Epigenetic factors, such as DNA methylation, have been shown to modulate the influence of the environment on gene expression [30]. McNerney et al. showed that the hippocampal volume/glucocorticoid receptor (GR) gene methylation interaction is an indicator of PTSD symptoms in 67 Veteran Patients [31]. Although animal and small sample epigenetic studies give clues about multiple genes and analysis, a major challenge for these studies is controlling the wide variety of stress factors that subjects are exposed to throughout their lives, and also they must be significant in EWAS measures. Hjort et al. reported that offspring of 72% of 117 mothers with PTSD had higher cortisol levels and differential methylation in candidate genes [NR3C1, 5-Hydroxytryptamine Receptor 3A (HTR3A), and BNDF] but the level of methylation differences did not reach epigenome-wide corrected significance levels [32]. Recent Epigenome-wide meta-analysis of military and civilian PTSD reported low DNA methylation in the four CpG regions of the Aryl-hydrocarbon repressor (AHRR) from blood DNA samples of 1896 PTSD patients [33]. Epigenetic meta-analysis of civilian PTSD (545 study participants) also found differential methylations in two CpG sites including NRG1 (cg23637605) and HGS (cg19577098) [34]. Interestingly, Yang et al. conducted two new different epigenetic biotypes for PTSD (G1 and G2). The G2 biotype has been associated with an increased risk of PTSD. The G1 biotype had higher polygenic risk scores and higher DNA methylation [35]. Logue et al. reported an epigenome-wide significant association with cg19534438 in the gene G0S2 (G0/G1 switch 2) and replicated it in other military cohorts. Although cg04130728 in Carbohydrate Sulfotransferase 11 (CHST11) had no genome-wide association, was significantly associated with PTSD in brain tissue (mostly prefrontal cortex) [36]. A longitudinal epigenome-wide association study identified three epigenome-wide significant CpGs, the intergenic CpG cg05656210 and Mitotic Arrest Deficient 1 Like 1 (MAD1L1) (cg12169700) and HEXDC (cg20756026).

Interestingly, cg12169700 was located within the same linkage disequilibrium block as a recently identified PTSD-associated (rs11761270) SNP in MAD1L1 [37]. In a meta-analytical review by Wolf et al., sex and immunity were strongly associated with the age of DNA methylation. However, they noted the lack of research into the underlying biological mechanisms [38]. In a multi-ethnic meta-analysis study (30,000 PTSD cases and 170,000 controls), non-coding RNAs such as Long Intergenic Non-Protein Coding RNA 2335 (LINC02335), microRNA 5007 (MIR5007), transcribed ultra-conserved region 338 (TUC338), (Long Intergenic Non-Protein Coding RNA 2571) (LINC02571), Long Intergenic Non-Protein Coding RNA 458 (LINC00458), microRNA 1297 (MIR1297) and Long Intergenic Non-Protein Coding RNA 558 (LINC00558) and PARK2 gene are involved in dopamine regulation, is associated with PTSD [20].

These studies support epigenetic differences in those with PTSD but it is also difficult to understand how persistent epigenomic changes affect a person's response to a traumatic event, and specifically to the molecular landscape of the brain. For this reason, it is inevitable to encounter multiple epigenetic effects in many parts of the brain and that these have not yet found their place in translational medicine. Current epigenetic studies are focused on research on blood DNA, and analysis of postmortem data from different brain regions can be used to understand how epigenetic regulation works in PTSD at a circuit, brain region, or whole-brain level [10]. Consequently, since the biological studies of PTSD are heterogeneous, it has not yet taken its place in translational medicine for a definitive diagnosis. More research with larger sample groups is needed in the biological diagnosis and treatment of PTSD.

## 3.3 Neuro-biological perspective

### *3.3.1 Fear and stress network in animal models*

The paucity of human studies investigating the neurobiological mechanisms of PTSD mirrored the understanding of this disease in animal models. Dysregulations of fear and stress-focused inflammatory responses detected in various brain regions have emphasized the importance of central nervous system centers that regulate fear memories (i.e., amygdala) and in response to acute or chronic stress response (i.e., the hypothalamus) since it began to be detected in PTSD patients. While animal studies continue to investigate fear-related processes for the amygdala, the medial prefrontal cortex (mPFC) and the hippocampus, interactions of the lateral (LA) (acquisition of fear and extinction concerning learning) and central nuclei (CeA) (behavioral expression of conditional fear) of the amygdala's nuclei regulating the inhibitory and excitatory effects of fear have been identified [39]. Connections between the hippocampus and the amygdala, particularly the LA, appear to be essential for the acquisition and reinforcement of contextual fear. At this point, it is thought that the somatosensorial projection of the hippocampus to the amygdala triggers contextual fear memory and may trigger fear-related learning through the LA nucleus. In addition, other evidence suggests that projections from the hippocampus to the mPFC can innervate neurons in the prelimbic (PL) and infralimbic (IL) regions that are active during fear and stress in animal models. PL and IL regions were important by creating neuronal potentials after the mPFC learned stress and conditioned fear on rodents, especially PL activity is responsible for regulating fear while its expression [40]. For instance, Richter-Levin developed a PTSD model in which animals are conditioned to pair a water-associated zero maze (WAZM) with underwater trauma that might be related to Amygdala LA and CeA nuclei. The remainder of underwater trauma rather than swimming stress, additional evidence of increased ERK phosphorylation (pERK) in the ventral dentate gyrus and basolateral amygdala [41]. Considering animal models of electrocution, this model is used more in learning and memory mechanisms than in PTSD, although it is associated with contextual reminders of trauma (associative fear) and ambiguous stimuli in a new setting (non-associative fear). Likewise, single long-term stress patterns were associated with neuronal apoptosis and dysregulation of autophagy in the hippocampus, amygdala, and prefrontal cortex (PFC), consistent with the findings in PTSD patients in terms of neurobiological background [42]. The social and psychological stressors animal model was mostly used for the PTSD behavioral measurements. In contrast, the social defeat stress (SDS) model was associated with optogenetic modulation of neuron projections to/from the ventromedial prefrontal cortex, ventral tegmental area, nucleus accumbens, and dorsal raphe nucleus in parallel with the PTSD clinic. Interestingly, amygdala-mPFC neuroadaptation was discovered in resting-state functional magnetic resonance imaging (rsfMRI) findings from Long-Evans rats exposed to the cat collar in predator-associated animal models [43].

### 3.3.2 Neurochemical and synaptical background

Serotonin (5-HT) is an important neurotransmitter for PTSD, targeting GABAergic neurons in response to fear-related acute stress in the amygdala, hippocampus, and ventromedial prefrontal cortex (vmPFC) regions. Clinical and animal studies have shown that symptomatic reduction associated with the use of antidepressants and/or anxiolytics in the treatment of PTSD is associated with stimulation and interaction of 5-HT1A, 5-HT1B, and 5-HT2A or 5-HT2C receptors. Sullivan et al. demonstrated positron emission tomography (PET) results of PTSD-like animals found higher 5-HT1A neuronal binding in all brain regions except the hippocampus and higher serotonin concentration in raphe nuclei compared to the healthy group [44]. Murrough et al. showed low 5-HT1B receptor density in the amygdala and anterior cingulate cortex (ACC) in PTSD patients [45]. The majority of the overactive noradrenergic activity associated with PTSD is due to the interaction of peripheral catecholamine (epinephrine, norepinephrine, and dopamine), transporter and receptor systems. In an animal and replicated study in humans, the high synaptic activity of norepinephrine (NE) in PTSD patients was detected in PFC projection areas. NPY also inhibits NE release and is found in high concentrations in the hippocampal and amygdala regions, it is associated with the projection of emotional values to memory and plays a role in the neurobiology of PTSD. Although intranasal NPY treatment reduces symptoms in many animal models of PTSD, efforts to develop NPY receptor-related pharmacological agents have failed [46]. Glutamate is an integral part of the learning, memory, and plasticity process. The glutamatergic system is studied as ionotropic and metabotropic. The PFC is transferred from the other to the amygdala and the bases of the whole brain regions to the amygdala are transmitted by glutamatergic contents and abnormal glutamate levels in PFC and N-methyl-D-aspartate (NMDA) receptor density in the hippocampus that is associated with synaptic plasticity underlying learning and memory, also have been reported in acute stress animal models. Especially metabotropic glutamate receptors have related with PTSD symptoms, high glutamate levels in the lateral temporal cortex and lower levels in ACC have been demonstrated. Research is ongoing that injection of subanesthetic doses of ketamine into rat brains increases glutamatergic neuronal activity in the PFC, which NMDA antagonists trigger learning and fear-related plasticity when examining the link between the glutamate system and dissociative symptomatology. Animal studies have shown that ketamine administration increases glutamate neurotransmitter levels and thus stimulates BDNF signaling, neurogenesis, and synaptogenesis [47]. GABA plays an important role in spatial and long-term memory, and directly in fear memory, in relation to neurogenesis in the hippocampal region. Fang et al. reported increased dysregulation of anxiety and fear memory with increased active GABAergic neurons in the CeA region of the amygdala in the single prolonged stress (SPS) animal model [48]. Behind the neurobiological mechanisms of PTSD, neuronal cell membrane damage due to stress and fear has also been researched. This damage is usually caused by oxidative stress-related free radicals (reactive oxygen species, for example, nitric oxide, glutathione, and hydrogen peroxide) damage to the cell membrane. In a recent study, Michels et al. found high higher levels of γ-amino butyric acid GABA and glutathione in PTSD patients via single-voxel proton magnetic resonance spectroscopy (MRS) in the dorsolateral prefrontal cortex (DLPFC) and ACC [49].

PTSD is also related to abnormal activity of the dopaminergic system, which has a mesolimbic pathway that is related to fear conditions and high plasma dopamine concentration was reported in PTSD patients. However, the dopamine metabolism of PTSD is unclear, so the genetic background is more studied. Most of these neurobiological explanations are accompanied by synaptic losses underlying PTSD. The clinical behavioral reflections (i.e., social disinhibition, apathy, attention and memory disorders, etc.) of these synaptic losses in various parts of the brain are tried to be explained. As a result of stress, disruption of intracellular signaling may result in a decrease in glutamate receptors and shrinkage of dendrite horns in postsynaptic neurons. The synaptic degeneration hypothesis is the basis of many neurodegenerative psychiatric disorders. Results of a postmortem pilot study reported that PTSD patients were immature, as the dendrites evaluated in vmPFC tissues were smaller in their spines compared to the control group [50]. In addition, neuroimaging studies conducted in PTSD were associated with volumetric and neuronal connectivity deficiencies in cortical areas and their resulting loss of cognitive functions in PTSD clinics. In particular, losses in dendritic connections are predominantly in hippocampal regions associated with neuroplasticity, resulting in chronic or acute stress-related learning disabilities. In short, the perspective on neuroplasticity has been developed by investigating neurochemical and receptor interactions in various brain regions of PTSD. In this context, antidepressants used clinically for PTSD may contribute to clinical improvement by promoting synaptic plasticity with this neurobiological infrastructure. In addition, inferences about synaptic connectivity based on neuroimaging methods are still unclear but may reveal various risks. Due to the limited knowledge about the neurobiology of PTSD, the inadequacy of the findings from animal stress models for the pathophysiology prevents us from making definite conclusions about the clarity of the applications for the clinical treatment of this disease. As a result, PTSD has been scientifically investigated with behavioral consequences related to neurobiological, genetic, and epigenetic, literature discussions continue especially in terms of both neuroscientific and clinical aspects. The importance of neurochemical, biological, and brain-regional neurologic interactions in human and animal models remains a mystery, and further studies need to unlock this mystery.

## 4. Clinical overview of PTSD

A cluster of psychiatric symptoms that persist for more than 1 month following a trauma, causing distress or a decrease in functionality in social, occupational, or other important areas of life is called PTSD [51].

**Trauma content**: There is actual or intimidating death, serious injury, or sexual assault. The person may have experienced this event directly and witnessed it. It may be the death of a family member or friend or learning that he or she has experienced trauma with a high probability of death. Persistent encounter with the adverse consequences of traumatic events (occupational exposure).

**What happens?** Recurrent involuntary distressing memories of traumatic events and recurrent distressing dreams involving these memories. Feeling as if traumatic events are recurring, dissociative reactions. Experiencing excessive or extended distress or physiological responses at exposure to stimuli that symbolize or evoke traumatic events.

**What are the avoidance behaviors?** Efforts to avoid and avoid distressing memories, feelings, and thoughts associated with the traumatic event. Avoidance or efforts to avoid people, places, conversations, activities, objects, and situations that may evoke distressing memories, feelings, and thoughts associated with the traumatic event.

**What is observed in cognitions and mood following the trauma?** Inability to remember the trauma, Negative beliefs, and expectations about self, others, or the world; Blaming self or others about the cause and consequences of the traumatic event, Persistent negative emotional states (e.g., fear, horror, anger, guilt, and shame); Decreased interest and participation in important activities; Feelings of detachment or alienation from others; Inability to constantly experience positive emotions (such as happiness and love).

**What are the changes in arousal and the reactions?** Verbal or non-verbal aggressive, angry behavior toward people or objects, outbursts of anger; Acting without restraint or engaging in self-destructive behavior; being alert all the time; Exaggerated startle response: It occurs in 88% of patients. Increased heart rate, greater skin conductance responses, and slower skin conductance in response to startling stimuli are well-defined findings [51, 52]. Focusing difficulties: The reason for the decrease in attention resources is the basic loss of sensory mechanisms before attention [52]. The dissociative subtype emphasizes a closure or blunted response to traumatic stressors characterized by dissociation [51–53]. The person constantly or recurrently experiences one of the following symptoms in response to the triggering factor:

1. Self-alienation (depersonalization): persistent or recurrent experiences in which the person feels detached from his mental processes or body, looking at them as if he were an outside observer (e.g, the sensation that he is in a dream; the sensation that he or his body is unreal, or that time is running slowly).

2. Unreality (derealization): persistent or recurrent experiences of feeling that the world or environment around the person is unreal or somewhat distorted).

**What is Delayed Onset PTSD?** If the symptoms are not fully appeared at least 6 months after the traumatic event (even if some symptoms start in a short time), it is called delayed-onset PTSD.

### 4.1 Diagnosis

In the face of severe stress, information processing is impaired, and it is not possible to resolve the traumatic event. An unintegrated traumatic experience can be easily aroused and affect daily life. Painful experiences cannot be suppressed or excluded. In experiences recorded with anxiety/fear, stimuli that stimulate one of the emotion-thought elements activate all of them. This general arousal and the unorganized cognitive processing behind it are considered as the source of symptoms, such as arousal, memory disorders, and impulsivity in PTSD. The individual who encounters the trauma first experiences confusion. This unprepared/unconditioned situation changes in the next step. By using the lived experiences before the trauma, the trauma is perceived as if it had been encountered before. The same emotional and physical reactions are given in the previous cases. This is a highly learned behavior. However, since this behavior is not suitable for the new situation, it is not an appropriate response and the answers become complex. Increasing confusion also increases anxiety. To diagnose PTSD, valid, objective/empirical methods other than previous trauma have not been defined. The diagnosis depends on the clinical interview.

The use of check-lists without recourse to clinical interviews may lead to the loss of significant clinical information that may be essential in the holistic provision of therapy and clinical care. To be diagnosed with PTSD, an adult must have all of the following for at least 1 month after a traumatic event: At least one re-experiencing symptom, one avoidance symptom, two arousals, and reactivity symptoms, and two cognition and/or mood symptoms.

The Post-traumatic Stress Disorder Checklist for DSM-5 (PCL-5) is a self-report measure to evaluate the presence and severity of PTSD symptoms (**Table 1**).

### 4.2 Factors facilitating the occurrence and persistence of PTSD

Inability to explain and share the effects of trauma, severity, and frequency of dissociative reactions during or immediately after trauma, childhood physical abuse, genetic predisposition, family history of psychopathology and PTSD, being a woman, excess physiological response during the traumatic event, acute stress disorder and early PTSD symptoms, previous psychiatric disease history, low socioeconomic level, and low education level, temporal intensity, and duration of trauma, memory disorders, soft neurological signs, low IQ, childhood attention deficit hyperactivity disorder symptoms are the factors related with increased risk or chronicity of PTSD [52].

PTSD is associated with many comorbidities besides causing disability on its own. Major depressive disorder, generalized anxiety disorder, alcohol and substance use disorders can be listed as the main comorbid conditions. The high-stress level accompanying PTSD increases the risk for many systemic diseases, such as hypertension, diabetes, and asthma [55].

One of the important comorbidities of PTSD is a borderline personality disorder. Borderline personality disorder causes the person to become prone to experiencing traumatic events by distorting the perception of risk. On the other hand, PTSD symptoms deepen the loss of functionality associated with a personality disorder.

#### *4.2.1 Acute and chronic PTSD*

If PTSD symptoms are present within 3 months following the trauma, it is defined as acute PTSD; and if symptoms persist for more than 3 months, it is defined as chronic PTSD [55].

#### *4.2.2 Complex PTSD*

PTSD is single-event trauma from traumatic experiences, such as rape, physical assault, or war. However, the traumatic event might be prolonged chronic victimization, such as interpersonal violence. Over time, chronic traumatization, often of an interpersonal nature, such as multiple and/or long-term developmentally negative traumatic events, came to be used to describe the term "complex trauma" [56].

#### *4.2.3 Course and prognosis*

The clinical course and outcome of PTSD vary depending on the factors before, during, and after the trauma. The nature of the symptoms observed after trauma,

| In the past month, how much were you bothered by: | Not at all | A little bit | Moderately | Quite a bit | Extremely |
|---|---|---|---|---|---|
| 1. Repeated, disturbing, and unwanted memories of the stressful experience? | 0 | 1 | 2 | 3 | 4 |
| 2. Repeated, disturbing dreams of the stressful experience? | 0 | 1 | 2 | 3 | 4 |
| 3. Suddenly feeling or acting as if the stressful experience were actually happening again? | 0 | 1 | 2 | 3 | 4 |
| 4. Feeling very upset when something reminded you of the stressful experience? | 0 | 1 | 2 | 3 | 4 |
| 5. Having strong physical reactions when something reminded you of the stressful experience? | 0 | 1 | 2 | 3 | 4 |
| 6. Avoiding memories, thoughts, or feelings related to the stressful experience? | 0 | 1 | 2 | 3 | 4 |
| 7. Avoiding external reminders of the stressful experience? | 0 | 1 | 2 | 3 | 4 |
| 8. Trouble remembering important parts of the stressful experience? | 0 | 1 | 2 | 3 | 4 |
| 9. Having strong negative beliefs about yourself, other people, or the world? | 0 | 1 | 2 | 3 | 4 |
| 10. Blaming yourself or someone else for the stressful experience or what happened after it? | 0 | 1 | 2 | 3 | 4 |
| 11. Having strong negative feelings, such as fear, horror, anger, guilt, or shame? | 0 | 1 | 2 | 3 | 4 |
| 12. Loss of interest in activities that you used to enjoy? | 0 | 1 | 2 | 3 | 4 |
| 13. Feeling distant or cut off from other people? | 0 | 1 | 2 | 3 | 4 |
| 14. Trouble experiencing positive feelings | 0 | 1 | 2 | 3 | 4 |
| 15. Irritable behavior, angry outbursts, or acting aggressively? | 0 | 1 | 2 | 3 | 4 |
| 16. Taking too many risks or doing things that could cause you harm? | 0 | 1 | 2 | 3 | 4 |
| 17. Being "super alert" or watchful or on guard? | 0 | 1 | 2 | 3 | 4 |
| 18. Feeling jumpy or easily startled? | 0 | 1 | 2 | 3 | 4 |
| 19. Having difficulty concentrating? | 0 | 1 | 2 | 3 | 4 |
| 20. Trouble falling or staying asleep? | 0 | 1 | 2 | 3 | 4 |

*Criterion B (1–5)—at least one ≥2 Criterion C (6–7)—at least one ≥2 Criterion D (8–14)—at least one ≥2 Criterion E (15–20)—at least one ≥2.*
*Mild 0–20; Moderate 20–40; Severe 40–60; Extreme 60–80.*

**Table 1.**
*The PTSD Checklist for DSM-5 (PCL-5) [54].*

the prognosis of the disease, or the information obtained from follow-up studies conducted at different periods makes it difficult to define a specific clinical situation for the course of the disease. PTSD starts when trauma is encountered or within the next few years, symptoms increase in the next few years and continue by drawing a plateau. Symptoms may fluctuate over time and intensify during stressful periods. Approximately 30% of patients show complete improvement, 60% have mild to moderate symptoms, and 10% have symptoms that remain unchanged or worsen. It is common for those who benefit from treatment to reappear after years of being exposed to a serious stressor.

### 4.3 Neuroimagination studies

Several neuroimaging studies have been implemented to investigate the pathophysiology of PTSD. Some symptoms associated with PTSD are related to changes in brain structure and function [57]. Brain regions implicated in the development of PTSD include the hippocampus, amygdala, and medial prefrontal cortex [58].

Advanced neuroimaging techniques contributed to our understanding of the possible pathophysiology of PTSD. The results of neuroimaging studies point to the importance of the hippocampus in PTSD. Exposure to chronic stress results in disturbances in memory function and neural damage to the hippocampus. The HPA axis controls stress response in the body by producing cortisol. The neural damage might be related to high levels of glucocorticoids, changes in serotonergic function, inhibition of neurogenesis in the hippocampus, or inhibition of brain-derived neurotrophic factors [59].

The magnetic resonance imaging (MRI) studies in PTSD consistently revealed reduced hippocampal and inferior temporal cortex volumes. The decreased volume of the inferior temporal cortex was inversely correlated with anxiety levels in PTSD [60]. Other neural structures often implicated in the pathophysiology of PTSD include the amygdala and prefrontal cortex. Amygdala is the integrative center for emotions, emotional behavior, and motivation. Functional magnetic resonance imaging (fMRI) studies with PTSD patients present increased activity in the amygdala in response to threat stimuli compared [57]. However, investigation of a large sample of nearly a hundred PTSD patients was characterized by reduced amygdala volumes [61].

Several methods have been used to study the pathophysiology of PTSD. Many neural networks and pathways that play a role in PTSD have been revealed, and these pathways can be studied in-depth due to the advances in techniques for neuroimaging.

### 4.4 PTSD treatment strategies

PTSD is associated with functional impairment and comorbidity. Therefore, early diagnosis and appropriate treatment are essential in PTSD. Existing treatment guidelines for the treatment of PTSD disorder generally aim to—reduce PTSD symptoms or achieve remission, loss of diagnosis, treatment of comorbid medical and psychiatric diseases, improvement of quality of life, correction of impairment in functional areas, return to work or duties. Treatment guidelines include psychological, pharmacological, and neuro-modulatory treatments [55]. However, a major limitation must be recognized: the current therapies described for PTSD are based on western cultures and modern technologies, and many of these approaches do not easily apply to rural communities in low- and middle-income countries. Clinicians or psychotherapists should, therefore, adopt psychotherapeutic strategies that are appropriate to the cultures in which they work.

### 4.5 Pharmacological interventions

It includes the use of various psychotropic drugs to target the core symptoms of PTSD. Medications that target key symptoms of PTSD, including intrusions, avoidance, negative changes in cognition and mood, and changes in arousal and responsiveness, include selective serotonin reuptake inhibitors, serotonin and norepinephrine reuptake inhibitors, atypical antipsychotics, β-blockers, and sleep medications (e.g., α-blockers, nabilone, hypnotics). Pharmacological treatments include antidepressants (e.g., sertraline), antipsychotics (e.g., risperidone), anticonvulsants (e.g., topiramate), hypnotics (e.g., zopiclone), and mood stabilizers (e.g., lithium), mood stabilizers; adrenergic agents; benzodiazepines; and other pharmacological agents [55].

Selective serotonin reuptake inhibitor (SSRI) stands out among pharmacological treatments because it is effective in most PTSD symptoms, easy to use, and has low side-effect profiles. They are the most valid and widely used drugs for the treatment of re-experiencing, avoidance, emotional blunting, and hyperarousal symptoms. SSRIs have been found to be effective in PTSD in double-blind, placebo-controlled randomized trials.

Mood stabilizers have the effect of reducing the sensitization of the limbic system, which develops in the first weeks and months after the traumatic event. Lamotrigine was found to be effective in re-experiencing and avoiding symptoms of PTSD. Studies are reporting that lithium, valproic acid, carbamazepine, oxcarbazepine, and gabapentin are effective. It has been found that propranolol, a beta-blocker, has positive effects on nighttime nightmares, remembering repetitive anxiety-provoking situations, jumping, sleep disturbances, and self-esteem.

### 4.6 Psychological interventions

Psychological treatments for PTSD are mainly in the form of cognitive-behavioral therapy. Cognitive processing therapy, trauma-focused cognitive behavioral therapy, and long-term exposure are largely within the framework of cognitive and behavioral therapy. Among the Cognitive Behavioral Therapies, especially Exposure Therapy and Systematic Desensitization techniques are successful in trauma treatment. In both techniques, it is aimed to desensitize the person and gradually reduce the traumatic effects by enabling the person to face the images and situations related to the trauma in a systematic and controlled manner.

Interpersonal psychotherapy was also found to be promising in recent research. Interpersonal psychotherapy is a form of attachment-based therapy. The patient is shown his / her own needs, and the support he/she needs. The client is taught how to get the support he/she needs from those around him/her. Thus, he/she will be able to recognize the attachment needs that have become active due to the trauma and will be able to provide appropriate social support for himself/herself.

During the traumatic event, the individual is exposed to intense fear and anxiety. The traumatic event cannot be processed by the brain as it should. The traumatic memory, which cannot be processed adequately and appropriately, disturbs the individual over time. Eye Movement Desensitization and Reprocessing (EMDR), developed by Shapiro and used in the treatment of PTSD, activates both halves of the brain through two-way eye stimulation and ensures healthy processing of the traumatic memory. With the EMDR method, the traumatic memory with high emotional intensity for the individual loses its vitality and the individual's hypersensitivity disappears.

### 4.7 Neuromodulation interventions

Neuro-modulatory treatments are viable treatment options for many psychiatric disorders. After U.S. Food and Drug Administration (FDA) approval of transcranial magnetic stimulation (TMS) as an option for treating depression, researchers also tried to use repetitive transcranial magnetic stimulation (rTMS) for depressive symptoms of PTSD [62]. rTMS and transcranial direct current stimulation (tDCS) are frequently employed as adjunctive options to pharmacotherapy for the treatment of several psychiatric disorders including PTSD. Several studies also investigated the potential of rTMS and tDCS in the treatment of PTSD to decrease the overactivity of the amygdala. The results of the studies revealed that both high-frequency and low-frequency rTMS can significantly reduce PTSD symptoms. rTMS may, therefore, be an effective add-on treatment option for treatment-resistant PTSD [63].

Deep TMS is a drug-free and non-surgical intervention, it does not require anesthesia. During the application, the patient is awake and conscious. The target area in the brain is physically stimulated by sending magnetic pulses under the skull with a mechanism placed in the skull. Thus, neurons working with electrical activity are activated by magnetic stimulation. It has been reported that recalling traumatic memories with activation and talking about it in the presence of an expert significantly reduces the burden of trauma.

The treatment method, which is based on the electrical processing of the data of the brain and bodywork and presenting it as feedback to the person, is called neurobiofeedback training. Thus, the patient learns to consciously control his/her own brain activity and bodily functions, such as breathing, muscle tension, and heart rate. Promising results are obtained in PTSD with the use of neurobiofeedback together with pharmacotherapy and psychotherapies.

## 5. Neuro-developmental perspective of PTSD

Human development starts from conception and continues until the end of life. Along this developmental pathway, earlier years witness the highest speed and the most complex changes. Moreover, recent neurological research studies have concluded that the human brain is the fastest developing organ in the first years of life. Not only physically that the child's brain reaches its almost full size by age four, but also by making almost 700 million snaps connections every second completing at least 80% of its functioning capacity. This makes neurological development the most decisive developmental process in the early years [64]. It also points to the fact that ACE become the major cause of long-term emotional problems, including PTSD.

Worldwide, children are often exposed to serious traumatic events, such as war, displacement, famine, and violence, that all disrupt a child's secure family structure and lead to long-term stress. Mental health problems affect around 10–20% of the child population worldwide [65]. Trauma is common in children and adolescents and may lead to PTSD. PTSD refers to maladaptive responses to at least one severe, threatening event (serious injury, threatened death, or sexual violence) by DSM-5, and the stress response, emotion regulation problems, and threat learning are indicated as common diagnostic symptoms of PTSD are; intrusion, avoidance, negative alterations in cognition and mood and arousal [66]. These cognitive symptoms have led researchers to examine the neurodevelopmental dimension of PTSD in the light of neuroscience studies.

According to the recent neurodevelopmental research results psychological as well as physiological responses to traumatic events such as being unable to bond with primary caregiver might lead to trauma having a long-term neurological impact on a child's psycho-social development and neurological functions [67, 68]. Such psychological problems, referred to as PTSD, are often associated with multiple psychosocial problems ranging from delinquency, poor academic performance to, alcohol and substance abuse, and even to suicidal attempts. Moreover, children exposed to traumatic events will have emotional, social, and physical developmental problems later in life [69]. It was observed that children exposed to traumatic events performed lower performance on cognitive and intellectual abilities than the children without a diagnosis of PTSD [70]. Besides, according to research results verbal and nonverbal intellectual capacity, mean IQ scores, language delay, sensory processing, memory, aggressive behavior, visual processing, affect, and behavior problems can be seen in children [71].

Neuroimaging research with PTSD indicates both functional and structural abnormalities in the front limbic area responsible for emotion regulation and threat processing. Such as decreased gray matter volume in ventromedial prefrontal and dorsal anterior cingulate cortex seen in structural analyses and hyperactivation of the insula, amygdala, and mid anterior cingulate cortex, smaller frontal-occipital circumference seen in functional analyses [72, 73]. Both structural and functional differences are also observed in the prefrontal cortex and limbic system (hippocampus and amygdala). Therefore, memory, emotion and excite function problems may accord exposure to stress [74].

### 5.1 Brain development

Most recent scientific studies on brain development reveal the fact that early experiences shape the architecture of a child's brain having a long-term impact on a child's social and emotional well-being [1]. A child's social, cognitive, and emotional development is heavily dependent on the quality of interaction between child and "significant" adult (e.g., mother, father. Caregiver. whoever s/he is bonded with). Neurodevelopmental studies claim that bonding problems and parenting inconsistencies might cause long-term mental health problems [75]. Although, the first years are critical for life-long success and healthy physical and mental development for the rest of their life, having a baby makes a significant change in the lives of parents. Lower stress of families is associated with lower stress levels and normal brain development in children [76].

Neurological development of the brain does not take place in a vacuum nor by itself. It is highly dependent on external stimulations and interactions. In other words, a child's early experiences shape the brain architecture from the beginning [1] and leave footprints that last a lifetime. Brain developmental functions also have critical moments providing "windows of opportunities" or challenges for specific developmental pathways (**Figure 3**).

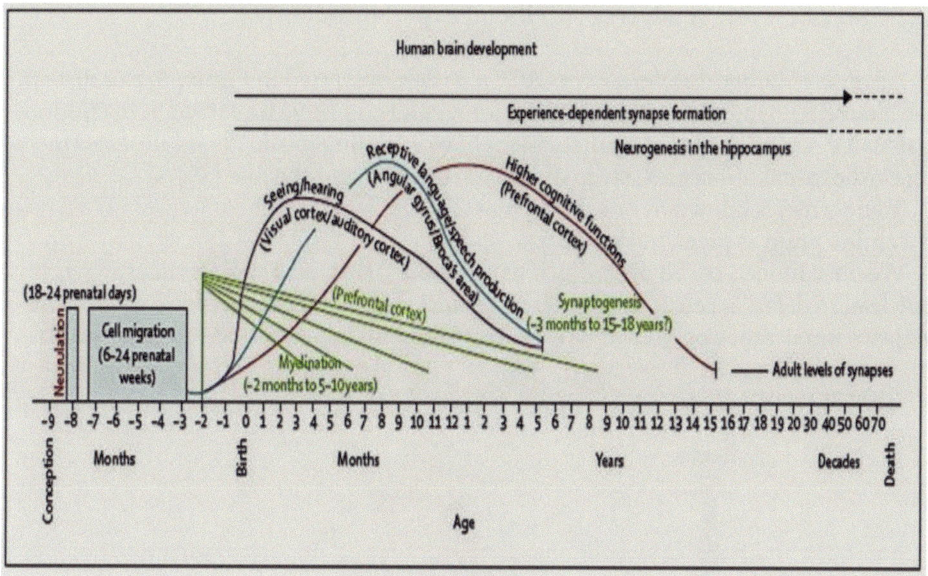


**Figure 3.**
*Human brain development [1].*

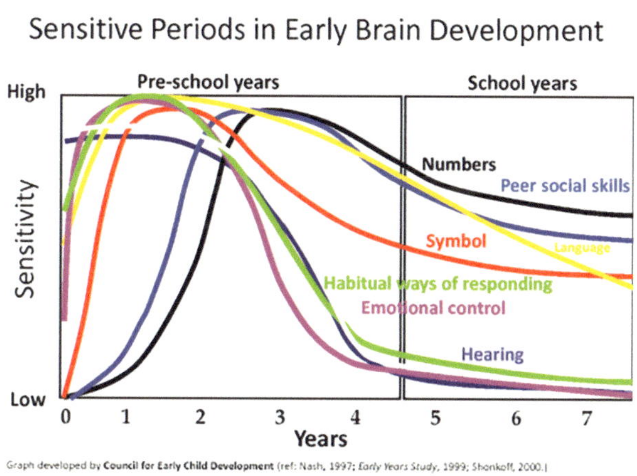


**Figure 4.**
*Sensitive periods in early brain development [77].*

Among all critical and sensitive periods, the first 3 years of life seem to be the most critical for emotional control responding to positive as well as adverse experiences as demonstrated in **Figure 4** [77].

Human brain development takes more years to reach maturity compared to other species. Although this long way to maturity is adaptive for the human species, the adolescent period is the second most important part of this journey of maturity because of its adaptive values of plasticity [78]. Therefore, the adolescent period is also sensitive and critical for stress factors. According to research about brain development, it claimed that exposure time to stress plays an important role in brain structure, the adolescent stage is more vulnerable to stress compared to the adulthood stage of development.

### 5.2 PTSD as a result of adverse childhood experiences (ACE)

Adverse childhood experiences (ACE), as demonstrated in **Figure 5**, can disrupt neurodevelopment causing social, emotional, and cognitive impairment in children that lead to the adoption of health-risk behavior leading to adulthood illnesses including cardiovascular diseases, sleep disorders, obesity, and the like [79].

Toxic stress is known as one of the most ACE in leaving almost irreversible damage in a child's brain as given in **Figure 6**.

Weems's model, based on evolutionary presentative, emphasizes that the stress may lead to delay, accelerate, or prolonged developmental process according to the adaptive importance of these changes. According to the model, the developmental

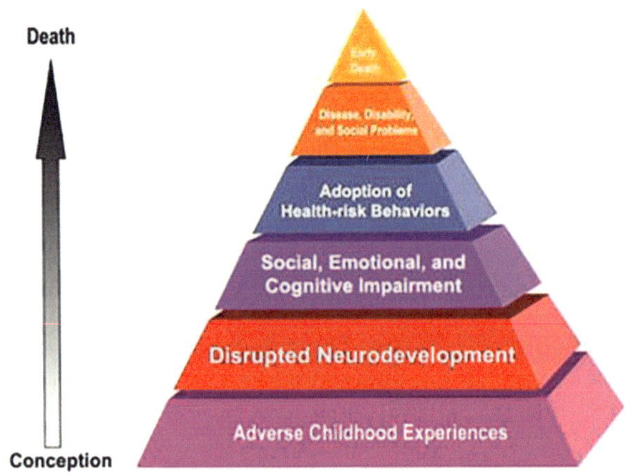


**Figure 5.**
*Mechanisms by which ACE influences health and well-being throughout the lifespan [79].*

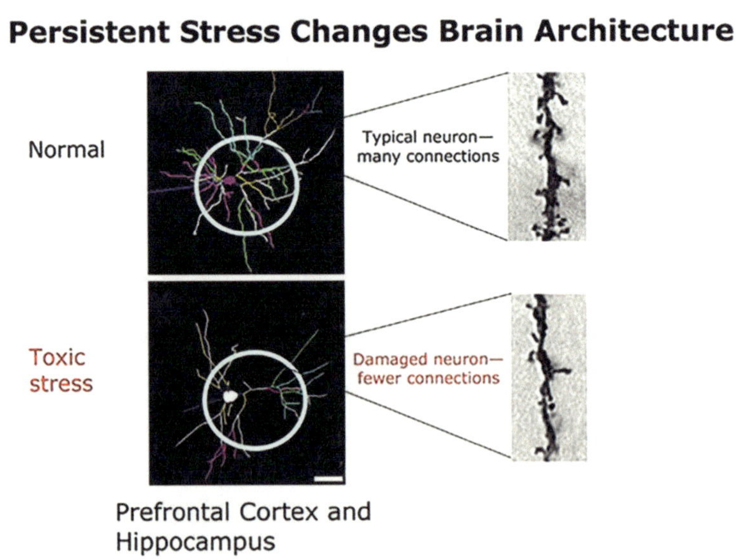


**Figure 6.**
*Persistent stress changes brain architecture [15].*

timing of stress exposure plays an important role in how the brain responds to the stressor, also they claimed that age and maturation are critical for amygdala volumes, which are responsible for emotion regulation [80]. Also, it is known that the prefrontal cortex and amygdala connection develop through childhood to adulthood and become stronger [79].

Coping with stress, if the stress is moderate level, is important for the healthy development of children and adolescents. In contrast, if the stress level is high, long term, and hard to cope with it, may cause damage to brain structural development, which is called toxic stress. Toxic stress defines as the activation of the human body's stress reaction system frequently and hardly reacting to long-term stressful stimuli or long-term activation of stress response to a stressful event with a failure of the human body. Toxic stress may cause prolonged physiologic and psychologic abnormalities, such as organ dysfunction or brain functional abnormalities. Abuse, violence, neglect, food scarcity are common types of toxic stress sources All these sources can also be considered as risk factors in the development of PTSD.

Toxic stress also negatively affects the neuroendocrine-immune system. Such abnormalities on cortisol levels might also be observed. Moreover, toxic stress preventing neural connections can have an adverse impact on brain architecture that impacts planning, reasoning, emotional and behavioral control areas. It is also claimed that these responses may play a role in psychopathological disorders including psychosis, depression, and PTSD [81].

Parenting style is considered as one of the major factors having an impact on the psycho-social development of young children as well as adolescents. It is known that parenting style plays an important role in the etiology of psychopathology in children and adolescents, both as a genetic factor and an environmental factor from a transgenerational perspective [82]. Parenting style can also be a protective factor when it has a positive role, whereas when it has a negative role, it is considered as a risk factor for the development of psychopathologies, such as depression, anxiety, obsessive-compulsive disorder, and schizophrenia. Also, according to evocative gene-environment correlations, symptoms of adolescent psychological disorders may affect parental psychological status [83]. Further, some studies have found that attachment styles are associated with both psychopathological and cognitive problems in adolescents, such as psychosomatic complaints, anxiety, verbal aggression, attention-seeking behavior, and thinking problems [84]. In conclusion, exposure to the traumatic event, negative parenting attitudes, or negative attachments may also have a negative effect on brain development.

All these developmental risk factors, evaluated from an evolutionary perspective, adaptational sensitivity in both young children and adolescents, from the perspective of toxic stress, exposure to toxic stress in the early developmental period, from the perspective of family attitudes, children growing up in an overprotective or authoritarian and inconsistent family structure, when faced with traumatic stress, are all considered risk factors for developing PTSD.

Developmental models of PTSD argue that an individual's biological, cognitive, and psycho-social characteristics are more decisive factors than the traumatic event itself in the emergence of PTSD. Such PTSD models, pointing to the importance of developmental processes of each individual argue that the brain will be affected by the traumatic event in a neurodevelopmental state. Likewise, it is thought that the neurodevelopmental state of the individual's brain is an important determinant in the development of PTSD reacting to the traumatic event.

According to neurodevelopmental research, the duration, intensity, timing of a traumatic event is important on how the brain and development will affect the event. Also, genetic vulnerabilities may affect the damage size, such as a genetically vulnerable child may develop psychopathology while a hardier child may not [73].

Preventing, early intervention and rehabilitation techniques are important for protecting the child from PTSD effects, especially neurodevelopmental damages. If possible, preventing children from possible traumatic experiences should be the first step. Later, for children who have been exposed to the traumatic event, early intervention and immediate action to remove the child from the traumatic environment should be the second step, finally, rehabilitation, such as psycho-social support mechanisms and programs, plays an important role in preventing neurodevelopmental damages. As a promising research Nelson et al. [85], studied with 136 abandoned children to examine their brain development, cognitive functioning, social and physical growth with 12 years' study. According to results, compared with children in foster care, the institutionalized children showed severe impairment in IQ and brain development, along with psychological disorders [85]. This study confirms that even if the child is exposed to a traumatic event, immediate action to remove the child from the traumatic environment afterward supports the reduction of traumatic effects and abnormal brain development.

## 6. New paradigms and changes in information society and PTSD

### 6.1 Transformations of society and media

The hegemony of the digital culture has changed and transformed the structure of society dramatically. The characteristics of those changes have a snowball effect on the layers of society. It is presumed that when people change, so are immediate consequences, and impacts are followed. The transformation of society ultimately dominates the way we think, feel, behave, and the way we use language. Nevertheless, the concepts, terminologies, and issues that are used in the present academia are now much more blurred compared to the clarity of the old modern days. Hence, creating a common and mutual language is plausible to comprehend the mental problems and the society with inclusive perspectives and views of digital habitus. Keeping all these digital reformations in mind, scholars try hard to keep pace with stunning developments. It seems inevitable that all academic references and mental archives should be re-read and digested accordingly.

For the well-being of public health, traumas should not be confined to individual levels. People in all walks of life are likely to suffer from PTSD. On a much broader scale, to help the victims of PTSD, diagnosis and therapy alternatives can be presented to society as a whole. If new diagnostic and therapeutic approaches regarding PTSD cases focus solely on personal levels, psychiatrists can easily fall into the trap by ignoring its widespread effect on society and on the culture of the individual that s/he lives. It is, therefore, significant to design unique therapy alternatives for PTSD patients by taking the cultural, social, and geographical facts into account. In addition to these alternatives, the experts should focus on cultural differences as well as individual differences. For example, the socio-cultural development in Turkey is in an eclectic form where the transition process from the traditional to the modern and postmodern period does not work in line. For this reason, the specific conditions of Turkish society and culture should be taken into account in social interpretations of individual problems.

Owing to the particular reasons mentioned above, social psychiatry should work for the benefit of the whole society counting PTSD patients. It is a challenging standpoint to offer a therapy that can work for the whole society. In the PTSD context, if social psychiatry utilizes cutting-edge approaches by wisely utilizing the technological advances of the cyber era, the mental and social well-being of society can be reached. It is, therefore, recommended to use new communication media, such as webinars, supervisions via the Internet, mental health apps, and developing "mind wares". These new discourses will automatically maximize the impact of social psychiatry particularly for PTSD cases [86].

### 6.2 Media and trauma

Media and television have a dangerous role as they can easily traumatize and continually retraumatize people with the vivid and graphic and horrifying pictures and videos that are broadcast on newscasts. They usually warn before they expose people pictures and videos full of violence. This is media violence. This warning cannot prevent people from trauma. So, they keep traumatizing people visually. Almost less than five decades before the digital reformation took place, George Gerbner, proposed in his Cultivation Theory that television negatively affect the mind of people [87]. TV news and programs usually exaggerate the violence of the outside world and depict the whole world as a bad, mad and cruel one. When particularly old people are exposed to media too long, they start to perceive the world as full of traumas, chaos, and tragedies. This is called Mean World Syndrome. As a result of that syndrome, three types of behavior or mood appeared: aggressive, depressive, and escaping. Unlike the world in which Gerbner lived, mass media today diversify with new technological opportunities within digital systems and affect the social sphere in a much shorter time and on a larger scale. While it is necessary to find an extra effort and time to encounter the mass media of the modern era, such as watching television, in the postmodern era, digital forms of communication tools have infiltrated the fabric of daily life. Now, without a special time requirement, individuals encounter multi-media messages in any part of daily life.

This infiltration of media in postmodern culture leaves us nowhere to escape. The risks of trauma are now scattered everywhere. Simmel associates the identity and mental problems of modern society with the over stimulus in the city life in his article Metropolis and Mental Life [88]. Whereas, in the postmodern age, we face a shift of paradigms as the rules of the game had changed. In the postindustrial society, identity and mental problems have different characteristics. Bernard Stiegler has correlated emotional problems with the digital revolution, as an inundation that carries with traumas, or at the very least the tensions.

The tsunami-like transformation of the communication landscape caused the sharp transformation from modern life to Information society that largely affected identity formation as the fragmented and episodic one [89]. People, for example, lost their feelings of belonging, and even their authentic ideology amidst uncertainty, which can be defined as social autism. The reasons highlighted here doubled the burden of psychiatrists in the post-capitalist/post-truth era. Conventional therapies, therefore, can miss embracing the overwhelming realities that those people experience.

### 6.3 Searching new discourses in digital therapies for PTSD

Digital media are now full of spiritual platforms providing solutions for people in trouble or suffering psychological disorders. There appeared new types of narration that quickly become popular in cyberspace. Some approaches like collective healing streams which offer to heal the past wounds of the society may have genuine reasons and philosophy behind them [90]. However, they are not free from problems. Disinformation is ubiquitous and misleading. Therapy-based applications and contents addressing PTSD are largely held in esoteric and unprofessional ways. Unfortunately, their popularity can be hazardous and confusing regarding a large number of PTSD cases.

When the whole world was haunted by the chaotic and sudden emergence of the COVID-19 pandemic, people were not ready to cope with this storm fully. This chaos and crisis have their unique problems. Many people suffer from that not only because they try to avoid being infected but also to escape from the harsh and odd situations that affected them mentally. It seems that it is hard to find isolation from this undefined fear atmosphere for everyone. People from all walks of life have suffered from the burden of digital works, ambiguity, and economic recession. As Chul Han discusses in *The Scent of Time*, the perception of time and its management worsened the situation [91]. While digital violence and crimes have been increasing, people have been pushed to live by the strict structures of discipline society and capitalism [92].

In these dark times, Turkish popular media resort to products that contain psychological consultancy contents. Here we come across a newly fledgling genre about digital media that works for Psychological Consultancy [93]. Some digital therapy contents, for example, act like postmodern witchcraft as they underestimate the real role of designing a therapy. These forms, which are grown in popular culture, also have an important function in maintaining the capitalist system. Expertise knowledge in the improvement of life created a new field outside of scientific knowledge and created a mystical field in postmodern culture. In places where modernization of society does not develop well, these forms of knowledge replace rational and scientific knowledge and present themselves in a form of reality.

Therefore, it takes professional psychiatrists to end this widespread cacophony and reverse the negative situation to positive ones [94]. If wisely used, digitalization gives several opportunities to implement new techniques regarding PTSD cases. Digital therapy sessions, awareness-raising activities can reach millions of people online. People can take online therapies or watch videos related to their problems. This is the natural outcome of the advent of the Internet and changing communication environments that widen the possibilities of civil protection services and emergencies [95].

As stated earlier in the study, changes in society challenge psychiatrists to diagnose and offer therapy by adding new perspectives to their conventional practices. Psychiatrists' role has changed as they now have to adapt these changes into their therapeutic diagnosis to follow the recent changes in society and find proper treatment. The pros of advanced technology should be used for the benefit of the people on the whole. It is true, digitalization challenges the psychiatrist to take PTSD cases by taking and addressing full sides of problems but digital narration opportunities allow them to lead fresh approaches in their discourse. Bennegadi, here, throws further questions: "Does the presence of a digital tool complicate the notion of empathy? Is confidentiality guaranteed? Is nonverbal language considered? And finally, how do we define the role of digital as a transitional element in the relationship?" [86]. The frame of these questions indicates that this is just the beginning of a new era. The methodology and their discourse that are shaped by the hegemony of the digital habitus must be arranged to offer the maximum of possibilities to the citizens in the art and the way of preserving their well-being.

### 6.4 Attachment theory and PTSD in digital habitus

Social media has been described as a double-edged sword. Beck's suggestions about The Risk Society have lost their validity. It is apparent that the types of risks that modern societies experience should be adapted to the de facto of the Information society. The risks are now scattered everywhere. There is no secure shelter in Information Age where people hide and protect themselves. The possibility of surviving without experiencing trauma is now a dream [96].

Bourdieu as the father of the term habitus declared that human beings are conditioned by their habitus [97]. Information society now created the term digital habitus where people now have to learn how to express constellations of new or previously unrecognized feelings, sensations, thoughts, and traumas to build an emotional repertoire, which assists them in emotional regulation. This is important because naming and expressing new experiences allows people to claim convenient agency in dealing with them.

To survive in the cyber world, we need to ensure that are we corresponding. Emotional and social attachments can create our little hells. Therefore, Attachment Theory can be reread to prevent dangerous attachments that can take place in digital areas. Attachment theory signifies the importance of our social interactions among trusted ones. In a similar vein, social baseline theory argues that social relationships play an important role in the well-being of society. Attachment theory argues that many people internalize attachment representations, such that mental representations of attachment figures acquire comparable soothing effects. So we humans learn from an early age to seek refuge in trusted others in times of need; caregivers provide us with food, nurture, and protection when we are vulnerable [98].

### 6.5 Cyber violence, dark web, and new emotional repertoire

Susan Sonntag underlines the importance of a basic human trait, such as empathy, in her book *On Regarding the Pain of Others*. Exposing visual violence in a voyeuristic gaze causes us to lose the feelings of empathy for others [99]. Unfortunately, indifference and showing no empathy toward the victims are now the new realities of society. The aestheticizing of the violence can decrease the real emotional reaction can cause paralysis of emotion. Here Baudrillard defines excessive and improper uses of violent images that cause "implosion of meaning." It is a kind of aphasia. This feeling of insensitivity, which is the general loss of meaning experienced in the social sphere, is read by Baudrillard as a feature of mass society. While the concept of the mass in the Frankfurt School was considered as a passive entity in communication studies, Baudrillard transformed the mass into an entity that could not be influenced by any information and on which no information could create effect [100].

While the general loss of meaning in the social field drags the mass into a sense of numbness, the tragedy, chaos, or violence experienced in the social field disappears without the slightest effect on the individual. This seemingly numbing state allows the legitimation and spread of violence as an impulse on every individual who constitutes the social sphere. In the social sphere, the individual gradually becomes the dynamo of a mechanism that produces or legitimizes violence, while the normative sphere of the society recedes. Reading, interpreting, and using technical tools from a critical perspective without being fetishized in the digital society will protect individuals from the possible negative effects of these tools.

When the September 11, 2001 attacks happened in New York, the collapse of the buildings and their visuals shocked the whole world. People who watched the planes plunging into the towers witnessed the commencement of a new era. This new era showed the vulnerability of the security of systems. Here, as explained above by Baudrillard's terminology implosion of meaning, people who watched the shootings of collapsing and jumping people from the towers are appalled by the heaviness of the tragedy. They were emotionally paralyzed. Feeling acedia or aphasia are two similar traumatic outcomes when exposed to violent visuals. As we can see, continual exposure to a persisting stress source or income has created new types of patients who have PTSD. To put in other words, PTSD in the postmodern society is the outcome of the post-modern city life we all witnessed.

To make things worse, capitalism eliminates the possibility of building a healthy community to get rid of the troubles. The fact that postmodern urban life forms are generally shaped in the axis of the dynamics of the capitalist system. As a result, elements such as competition, individualism, and hedonism become more visible in the cultural field. In this spatial practice, where the social collectivity is replaced by the hedonistic tendencies of the consumption culture, interpersonal communication forms are gradually falling apart [101]. In addition to the aforementioned paralysis of emotions caused by postmodern cultural, social, and economic problems, the COVID-19 pandemic time has appeared as a chaotic example for the present situation. People have begun to struggle with so many things with many new unknown emotions and trauma types that emerged on social media platforms. These unknown terminologies now become a big part of our emotional repertoire. They are multifarious such as thumbnailing, trolling, body shaming, gaslighting, cancel culture or de-platforming, #metoo campaign, toxic masculinity, stress to feed on social media, hashtagging posts, feeling acedia, losing the spatial sense in virtual and augmented reality, being immersed in the metaverse, having been cringed on social media. The list can be endless when it comes to the new phobia types of which may not be classified under the DSM-5 criteria yet to be accepted as legitimate trauma types [102]. Digital habitus is considered as the underlying reason of the problem cause or triggers many new phobias, such as netless phobia, fear of missing out (FOMO), nomophobia, or the feeling of being stalked by unknown gazes due to synoptic surveillance. The dark side of the digital world as we can see here turn many ordinary people's life into hell. Cyber violence is reinforced by professional criminals who used random pictures of people in deep fake porno. It takes a second to be the victim of deep fake porno. Hence, so-called naïve nudity trend-sending naked pictures to your beloved can be a real trauma for many young people. Similarly, some rather new terminologies, such as crowdsourcing or hive mind activities, can serve just for big data and nobody can guess the real outcome of those digital practices.

It follows that toward a more peaceful and healthy society, we need people who are emotionally healthy as well as mature. For many PTSD patients, time freezes. The past events occasionally haunt them. A similar haunting process can be seen in the Virtual Reality universe. The artistic use of visuals and space in VR technologies can cause new trauma in which time has been expanded as if it is a "duree" experience [103]. Aestheticizing the violence in those arts can trigger fears and worsen the situation. So all these new encounters have brought a new level of violence types in the new media. As it has been presented, each new media and innovation comes with its drawbacks.

Reversing this more positively, media content and AI should collaborate. Psychiatrists, therefore, here must carefully read the signs of digital habitus problems to address the issue by implementing new technologies wisely. One must be aware of the fact that not every innovation has positive effects on society. Reading, interpreting, and using technical tools adopting a critical perspective and without fetishizing things in the digital society will protect individuals from the possible negative effects of these tools.

### 6.6 Counter activities to prevent society from cyber violence

Prevention of PTSD should start by preventing and monitoring the activities of people on Digital Media. What we need is counter activities to stop the evil deeds and narrations all over the world. A narcissist can disguise himself/herself in social media groups with a hidden agenda camouflaging in amicable chats, can easily take advantage of PTSD people's vulnerability. They can easily hunt a new dependent person as his/her victim. A cyber sadist invites his/her victim in his digital tower-like Marquis de Sade captured and imprisoned his victims in his tower. Similarly, illegal groups can find their supporters from this digital bowl. Tracking the digital activities of potential criminals, sadists or schizophrenics can save many people's life. However, all these counter activities are hot topics and controversial as they are against the freedom of communication and privacy. These surveillance and counter-violence discussions are beyond the scope of this study. Pursuing digital technologies to find new ways to reach PTSD can be incomplete if people are not warned against the demonic uses of social media. As explained above, some narcissist people can find their victims via social media platforms. New media here not only digitalize the mindset of people but also offer new facets of crime, violence, and even terrorism. Now cybercrimes, digital violence, data mining, fake accounts, identity stealing, illicit money flows, the resonance of terrorists can cause new traumas in the cyber world. Counter activities to raise awareness of the malicious use of social media is surpassing the job description of social psychiatrists. To fight the root of the problems sometimes can minimize the number of people who would be traumatized in the cyber world. To create a peaceful society, one has a peaceful mindset that is free from restlessness, such as exaggerated startle responses, flashbacks, nightmares, and hypervigilance. Genuine and meaningful communication to lead a meaningful life should not be taken for granted. To provide sensitivity, it is necessary to construct a collective language in the social field by professionals working in the field of communication science and experts in the field of psychology. They should work together to build a new language that prevents social polarization. In addition to the polarized ideologies, digital media have also problematic discourse and contents. Aggressive language in social media is contagious. People who are traumatized, victimized, killed, raped, exiled had not escaped the same pattern of violent discourse. The wild and violent human nature has necessitated certain psychological support systems to cure the victims of tragic events. It is assumed that no society is immune from traumas, and postmodern societies are no exception. Depression, unhappiness, and the symptoms of burnout are highly correlated with the traumatic issues within the scope of postmodern society [91].

## 7. Conclusion

As stated above, this study brings Information Age traumas and psychological disorders to the forefront. First trying to find an answer to the questions that why and what types of traumas happen in the Information Age. And, secondly, what changes should be implemented in the discourse and the methodology of the psychiatrists. Trying to answer these questions can provide us a chance not only to define the problem accurately but also to seek valid discourses for the psychiatrists to be used in PTSD cases, particularly in postmodern society. Within the scope of the study, collecting and processing neuroimaging data or utilizing the latest AI techniques can be given as an example of designing new diagnostic and therapeutic methods that rely on neurobiological dimensions. In addition to these new approaches, sociological aspects of PTSD in the digital habitus can be added to develop unique therapy approaches that embrace sociological perspectives of Information Society with a full trajectory of healing practices and a chance of addressing PTSD in its full spectrum.

In conclusion, postmodern city life has worsened the situation of the Information Age regarding PTSD. It affects not only daily life, work-life, education, and academic life, but also affects the total health of society. A person who suffers from PTSD has a lot of issues to cope with. Since the main foci of this study are to explore and exemplify new diagnostic and therapeutic approaches to PTSD cases, a profound analysis of PTSD in terms of its biological, sociological, developmental, psychological, and even ontological aspects are provided by embracing the digital revolutions of the society with its novel implications and insights. To address the issue with its full sides and angles, new treatment opportunities are portrayed as a sine qua non for contemporary psychiatrists.

## Conflict of interest

The authors declare no conflict of interest.

## Author details

Nevzat Tarhan*, Muhsin Konuk, Mesut Karahan, Öznur Özge Özcan, Sibel Öztürk Ayvaz, Gökben Hızlı Sayar, Nurper Ülküer, Hazal Ayas and Feride Zeynep Güder
Uskudar University, Istanbul, Turkey

*Address all correspondence to: nevzat.tarhan@uskudar.edu.tr

## References

[1] American Psychiatric Association. The Diagnostic and Statistical Manual of Mental Disorders. 5th ed. Washington: American Psychiatric Association Publishing; 2013

[2] Koenen KC, Ratanatharathorn A, Ng L, McLaughlin KA, Bromet EJ, Stein DJ, et al. Posttraumatic stress disorder in the world mental health surveys. Psychological Medicine. 2017;**47**(13):2260-2274

[3] Özmen E. Bir İktidar Pratiği Olarak Psikiyatri ve Psikoloji: Travma Örneği [Internet]. 2013. Available from: https://birikimdergisi.com/guncel/715/bir-iktidar-pratigi-olarak-psikiyatri-ve-psikoloji-travma-ornegi [Accessed: September 19, 2021]

[4] Tarhan N. Çağın Vicdanı Bediüzzaman. Istanbul: Nesil Publishing; 2012

[5] Tarhan N. In: Tatlı A, Görmez İ, editors. Hakkın Dilinden Ontoloji. İstanbul: Üsküdar University Publishing; 2020

[6] Şimşek ÖF. Happiness revisited: Ontological well-being as a theory-based construct of subjective well-being. Journal of Happiness Studies. 2009;**10**:505-522

[7] Tanrıdağ O, İnanıyorum O. Halde Varım. İstanbul: Üsküdar University Publishing; 2017

[8] Tarhan N. Travmayı Anlamak. In: Travma Psikoloji Kongresi; Istanbul. 7-8 March 2020; İstanbul. Available from: https://www.nevzattarhan.com/travmayi-anlamak.html

[9] Hızlı Sayar G, Ünübol H, Tarhan N. Fears, concerns and maturation during the Covid-19 Pandemia (in Turkish). İstanbul: Üsküdar University Publications; 2020

[10] Nisar S, Bhat AA, Hashem S, Syed N, Yadav SK, Uddin S, et al. Genetic and neuroimaging approaches to understanding post-traumatic stress disorder. International Journal of Molecular Sciences. 2020;**21**(12):4503. DOI: 10.3390/ijms21124503

[11] Misganaw B, Guffanti G, Lori A, Abu-Amara D, Flory DJ, SBPBC, et al. Polygenic risk associated with post-traumatic stress disorder onset and severity. Translational Psychiatry. 2019;**9**:165. DOI: 10.1038/s41398-019-0497-3

[12] True WR, Rice J, Eisen SA, Heath AC, Goldberg J, Lyons MJ, et al. A twin study of genetic and environmental contributions to liability for posttraumatic stress symptoms. Archives of General Psychiatry. 1993;**50**(4):257-264. DOI: 10.1001/archpsyc.1993.01820160019002

[13] Dunlop BW, Wong A. The hypothalamic-pituitary-adrenal axis in PTSD: Pathophysiology and treatment interventions. Progress in Neuro-Psychopharmacology & Biological Psychiatry. 2019;**89**:361-379. DOI: 10.1016/j.pnpbp.2018.10.010

[14] Aliev G, Beeraka NM, Nikolenko VN, Svistunov AA, Rozhnova T, Kostyuk S, et al. Neurophysiology and psychopathology underlying PTSD and recent insights into the PTSD therapies—A comprehensive review. Journal of Clinical Medicine. 2020;**9**(9):2951. DOI: 10.3390/jcm9092951

[15] Gressier F, Calati R, Balestri M, Marsano A, Alberti S, Antypa N, et al. The 5-HTTLPR polymorphism and

posttraumatic stress disorder: A meta-analysis. Journal of Traumatic Stress. 2013;**26**(6):645-653. DOI: 10.1002/jts.21855

[16] Amstadter AB, Koenen KC, Ruggiero KJ, Acierno R, Galea S, Kilpatrick DG, et al. Variant in RGS2 moderates posttraumatic stress symptoms following potentially traumatic event exposure. Journal of Anxiety Disorders. 2009;**23**(3):369-373. DOI: 10.1016/j.janxdis.2008.12.005

[17] Beins EC, Beiert T, Jenniches I, Hansen JN, Leidmaa E, Schrickel JW, et al. Cannabinoid receptor 1 signaling modulates stress susceptibility and microglial responses to chronic social defeat stress. Translational Psychiatry. 2021;**11**(1):164. DOI: 10.1038/s41398-021-01283-0

[18] Wolf EJ, Mitchell KS, Logue MW, Baldwin CT, Reardon AF, Aiello A, et al. The dopamine D3 receptor gene and posttraumatic stress disorder. Journal of Traumatic Stress. 2014;**27**(4):379-387. DOI: 10.1002/jts.21937

[19] Solovieff N, Roberts AL, Ratanatharathorn A, Haloosim M, De Vivo I, King AP, et al. Genetic association analysis of 300 genes identifies a risk haplotype in SLC18A2 for post-traumatic stress disorder in two independent samples. Neuropsychopharmacology. 2014;**39**(8):1872-1879. DOI: 10.1038/npp.2014.34

[20] Nievergelt CM, Maihofer AX, Klengel T, Atkinson EG, Chen C-Y, Choi KW, et al. International meta-analysis of PTSD genome-wide association studies identifies sex- and ancestry-specific genetic risk loci. Nature Communications. 2019;**10**(1):4558. DOI: 10.1038/s41467-019-12576-w

[21] Sheerin CM, Lind MJ, Bountress K, Nugent NR, Amstadter AB. The genetics and epigenetics of PTSD: Overview, recent advances, and future directions. Current Opinion in Psychology. 2017;**14**:5-11. DOI: 10.1016/j.copsyc.2016.09.003

[22] Wilker S, Schneider A, Conrad D, Pfeiffer A, Boeck C, Lingenfelder B, et al. Genetic variation is associated with PTSD risk and aversive memory: Evidence from two trauma-exposed African samples and one healthy European sample. Translational Psychiatry. 2018;**8**:251. DOI: 10.1038/s41398-018-0297-1

[23] Huckins LM, Chatzinakos C, Breen MS, Hartmann J, Klengel T, da Silva Almeida AC, et al. Analysis of genetically regulated gene expression identifies a prefrontal PTSD gene, SNRNP35, specific to military cohorts. Cell Reports. 2020;**31**(9):107716. DOI: 10.1016/j.celrep.2020.107716

[24] Duncan LE, Ratanatharathorn A, Aiello AE, Almli LM, Amstadter AB, Ashley-Koch AE, et al. Largest GWAS of PTSD (N=20 070) yields genetic overlap with schizophrenia and sex differences inheritability. Molecular Psychiatry. 2018;**23**(3):666-673. DOI: 10.1038/mp.2017.77

[25] Chen C-Y, Stein M, Ursano R, Cai T, Gelernter J, Heeringa S, et al. Genome-wide association study of posttraumatic stress disorder symptoms in two cohorts of United States Army soldiers. European Neuropsychopharmacology. 2017;**27**:S472. DOI: 10.1016/j.euroneuro.2016.09.552

[26] Stein MB, Chen CY, Ursano RJ, Cai T, Gelernter J, Heeringa SG, et al. Genome-wide association studies of posttraumatic stress disorder in 2 cohorts of US army soldiers. JAMA Psychiatry. 2016;**73**(7):695-704. DOI: 10.1001/jamapsychiatry.2016.0350

[27] Maihofer A, Strom N, Mattheisen M, Torres K, Stein M, Ressler K, et al. Refined PTSD phenotyping identifies additional GWAS risk variants and broader domains underlying risk to psychopathology. Biological Psychiatry. 2020;**87**(9):S51-S52. DOI: 10.1016/j.biopsych.2020.02

[28] Pooler T. Genome-wide association study on the sleep symptom of post-traumatic stress disorder [thesis]. Minneapolis: Walden University; 2015

[29] Thavichachart N, Mushiroda T, Thavichachart T, Charoensook O, Prasansuklab A, Rutchatajumroon P, et al. Genome-wide association study in Thai tsunami survivors identified risk alleles for posttraumatic stress disorder. Open Journal of Genetics. 2015;**5**:43-57. DOI: 10.4236/ojgen.2015.52004

[30] Lee RS, Sawa A. Environmental stressors and epigenetic control of the hypothalamic-pituitary-adrenal axis. Neuroendocrinology. 2014;**100**(4):278-287. DOI: 10.1159/000369585

[31] McNerney MW, Sheng T, Nechvatal JM, Lee AG, Lyons DM, Soman S, et al. Integration of neural and epigenetic contributions to posttraumatic stress symptoms: The role of hippocampal volume and glucocorticoid receptor gene methylation. PLoS One. 2018;**13**(2):e0192222. DOI: 10.1371/journal.pone.01922

[32] Hjort L, Rushiti F, Wang SJ, Fransquet P, Krasniqi SP, Çarkaxhiu SI, et al. Intergenerational effects of maternal post-traumatic stress disorder on offspring epigenetic patterns and cortisol levels. Epigenomics. 2021;**13**(12):967-980. DOI: 10.2217/epi-2021-0015

[33] Smith AK, Ratanatharathorn A, Maihofer AX, Naviaux RK, Aiello AE, Amstadter AB, et al. Epigenome-wide meta-analysis of PTSD across 10 military and civilian cohorts identifies methylation changes in AHRR. Nature Communications. 2020;**11**(1):5965. DOI: 10.1038/s41467-020-19615-x

[34] Uddin M, Ratanatharathorn A, Armstrong D, Kuan PF, Aiello AE, Bromet EJ, et al. Epigenetic meta-analysis across three civilian cohorts identifies NRG1 and HGS as blood-based biomarkers for post-traumatic stress disorder. Epigenomics. 2018;**10**(12):1585-1601. DOI: 10.2217/epi-2018-0049

[35] Yang R, Gautam A, Getnet D, Daigle BJ, Miller S, Jett M. Epigenetic biotypes of post-traumatic stress disorder in war-zone exposed veteran and active duty males. Molecular Psychiatry. 2020;**26**:4300-4314. DOI: 10.1038/s41380-020-00966-2

[36] Logue MW, Miller MW, Wolf EJ, Huber BR, Morrison FG, Zhou Z, et al. An epigenome-wide association study of posttraumatic stress disorder in US veterans implicates several new DNA methylation loci. Clinical Epigenetics. 2020;**12**(1):46. DOI: 10.1186/s13148-020-0820-0

[37] Snijders C, Maihofer AX, Ratanatharathorn A, Baker DG, Boks MP, Geuze E, et al. Longitudinal epigenome-wide association studies of three male military cohorts reveal multiple CpG sites associated with post-traumatic stress disorder. Clinical Epigenetics. 2020;**12**:11. DOI: 10.1186/s13148-019-0798-7

[38] Wolf EJ, Maniates H, Nugent N, Maihofer AX, Armstrong D, Ratanatharathorn A, et al. Traumatic stress and accelerated DNA methylation age: A meta-analysis. Psychoneuroendocrinology. 2018;**92**:123-134. DOI: 10.1016/j.psyneuen.2017.12.007

[39] Quinones MM, Gallegos AM, Lin FV, Heffner K. Dysregulation of inflammation, neurobiology, and cognitive function In PTSD: An integrative review. CABN. 2020;**20**(3):455-480. DOI: 10.3758/s13415-020-00782-9

[40] Giustino T, Maren S. The role of the medial prefrontal cortex In the conditioning and extinction of fear. Frontiers in Behavioral Neuroscience. 2015;**9**:298. DOI: 10.3389/fnbeh.2015.00298

[41] Maren S, Phan KL, Liberzon I. The contextual brain: Implications for fear conditioning, extinction and psychopathology. Nature Reviews. Neuroscience. 2013;**14**:417-428. DOI: 10.1038/nrn3492

[42] Zheng S, Han F, Shi Y, Wen L, Han D. Single-prolonged-stress induced changes in autophagy-related proteins beclin-1, LC3, and p62 in the medial prefrontal cortex of rats with post-traumatic stress disorder. Journal of Molecular Neuroscience. 2017;**62**:43-54. DOI: 10.1007/s12031-017-0909-x

[43] Liang Z, King J, Zhang N. Neuroplasticity to a single-episode traumatic stress revealed by resting-state fMRI in awake rats. NeuroImage. 2014;**103**:485-449. DOI: 10.1016/j.neuroimage.2014.08.050

[44] Sullivan GM, Ogden RT, Huang YY, Oquendo MA, Mann JJ, Parsey RV. Higher in vivo serotonin-1a binding in posttraumatic stress disorder: A PET study with [11C]WAY-100635. Depression and Anxiety. 2013;**30**(3):197-206. DOI: 10.1002/da.22019

[45] Murrough JW, Czermak C, Henry S, Nabulsi N, Gallezot JD, Gueorguieva R, et al. The effect of early trauma exposure on serotonin type 1B receptor expression revealed by reduced selective radioligand binding. Archives of General Psychiatry. 2011;**68**(9):892-900. DOI: 10.1007/10.1001/archgenpsychiatry.2011.91

[46] Sabban EL, Alaluf LG, Serova LI. Potential of neuropeptide Y for preventing or treating posttraumatic stress disorder. Neuropeptides. 2015;**56**:19-24. DOI: 10.1016/j.npep.2015.11.004

[47] Krystal JH, Abdallah CG, Averill LA, Kelmendi B, Harpaz-Rotem I, Sanacora G, et al. Synaptic loss and the pathophysiology of PTSD: Implications for ketamine as a prototype novel therapeutic. Current Psychiatry Reports. 2017;**19**(10):1-11. DOI: 10.1007/s11920-017-0829-z

[48] Fang Q, Li Z, Huang GD, Zhang HH, Chen YY, Zhang LB, et al. Traumatic stress produces distinct activations of GABAergic and glutamatergic neurons in amygdala. Frontiers in Neuroscience. 2018;**12**:1-13. DOI: 10.3389/fnins.2018.00387

[49] Michels L, Schulte-Vels T, Schick M, O'Gorman RL, Zeffiro T, Hasler G, et al. Prefrontal GABA and glutathione imbalance in posttraumatic stress disorder: Preliminary findings. Psychiatry Research: Neuroimaging. 2014;**224**(3):288-295. DOI: 10.1016/j.pscychresns.2014

[50] Young KA, Thompson PM, Cruz DA, Williamson DE, Selemon LD. BA11 FKBP5 expression levels correlate with dendritic spine density in postmortem PTSD and controls. Neurobiology of Stress. 2015;**2**:67-72. DOI: 10.1016/j.ynstr.2015.07.002

[51] American Psychiatric Association. The Diagnostic and Statistical Manual of Mental Disorders. 5th ed. Washington:

American Psychiatric Association Publishing; 2013. pp. 271-272

[52] Wisco BE, Pugach CP, Nomamiukor FO. Sadness and depression in PTSD. In: Tull M, Kimbrell N, editors. Emotion in Posttraumatic Stress Disorder: Etiology, Assessment, Neurobiology, and Treatment. 3rd ed. Academic Press; 2020. pp. 89-116. DOI: 10.1016/B978-0-12-816022-0.00004-1

[53] Courtois CA, Elhai JD, Ford JD, Grasso DJ. Posttraumatic Stress Disorder Scientific and Professional Dimensions. Elsevier Academic Press; 2009. DOI: 10.1016/C2013-0-19408-1

[54] Weathers FW, Litz BT, Keane TM, Palmieri PA, Marx BP, Schnurr PP. The PTSD Checklist for DSM-5 (PCL-5) [Internet]. Scale Available From: The National Center for PTSD; 2013. Available from: https://www.ptsd.va.gov/ [Accessed: September 15, 2021]

[55] Forman-Hoffman V, Cook Middleton J, Feltner C, Gaynes BN, Palmieri Weber R, Bann C, et al. Psychological and Pharmacological Treatments for Adults With Posttraumatic Stress Disorder: A Systematic Review Update. Rockville: Agency for Healthcare Research and Quality; 2018. DOI: 10.23970/AHRQEPCCER207

[56] O'Shea BG. Healing Complex Posttraumatic Stress Disorder: A Clinicians Guide. New York: Springer; 2021. DOI: 10.1007/978-3-030-61416-4

[57] Bremner JD. Neuroimaging in posttraumatic stress disorder and other stress-related disorders. Neuroimaging Clinics of North America. 2007;**17**:523-538

[58] Bremner JD. Functional neuroimaging in post-traumatic stress disorder. Expert Review of Neurotherapeutics. 2007;7:393-405

[59] Fennema-Notestine C, Stein MB, Kennedy CM, Archibald SL, Jernigan TL. Brain morphometry in female victims of intimate partner violence with and without posttraumatic stress disorder. Biological Psychiatry. 2002;**52**:1089-1101

[60] Kroes MC, Rugg MD, Whalley MG, Brewin CR. Structural brain abnormalities common to posttraumatic stress disorder and depression. Journal of Psychiatry & Neuroscience. 2011;**36**(4):256-265

[61] Karl A, Schaefer M, Malta LS, Dörfel D, Rohleder N, Werner A. A meta-analysis of structural brain abnormalities in PTSD. Neuroscience and Biobehavioral Reviews. 2006;**30**(7):1004-1031

[62] Liu JJW, Nazarov A, Easterbrook B, Plouffe RA, Le T, Forchuk C, et al. Four decades of military posttraumatic stress: Protocol for a meta-analysis and systematic review of treatment approaches and efficacy. JMIR Research Protocols. 2021;**10**:10. DOI: 10.2196/33151

[63] Kan RB, Zhang B, Zhang J, Kranz GS. Non-invasive brain stimulation for posttraumatic stress disorder: A systematic review and meta-analysis. Translational Psychiatry. 2020;**10**:168

[64] National Research Council (US) and Institute of Medicine (US) Committee on Integrating the Science of Early Childhood Development. In: Shonkoff JP, Phillips DA, editors. From Neurons to Neighborhoods: The Science of Early Childhood Development. Washington: National Academies Press; 2000. DOI: 10.17226/9824

[65] Kieling C, Baker-Henningham H, Belfer M, Conti G, Ertem I, Ulkuer N, et al. Child, and adolescent mental health worldwide: Evidence for action.

Lancet. 2011;**22**:1515-1525. DOI: 10.1016/S0140-6736(11)60827-1

[66] American Psychiatric Association. Desk Reference to the Diagnostic Criteria from DSM-5. Arlington: American Psychiatric Association Publishing; 2013. DOI: 10.1176/appi.books.9780890425596

[67] Bremner JD. Does Stress Damage the Brain?: Understanding Trauma-Related Disorders from a Mind-Body Perspective. New York: W.W.Norton; 2005

[68] Creeden K. The neurodevelopmental impact of early trauma and insecure attachment: Re-thinking our understanding and treatment of sexual behavior problems. Sex Addict Compulsivity. 2004;**11**(4):223-247

[69] Putnam FW. The impact of trauma on child development. Juvenile & Family Court Journal. 2009;**57**(1):1-11. DOI: 10.1111/j.1755-6988.2006.tb00110.x

[70] Warshaw M, Fiermann E, Pratt L, Hunt M, Yonkers K, Massion AO, et al. Quality of life and dissociation in anxiety disorder patients with histories of trauma or PTSD. The American Journal of Psychiatry. 1993;**150**(10):1512-1516. DOI: 10.1176/ajp.150.10.1512

[71] Richardson M, Henry J, Black-Pond C, Sloanne M. Multiple types of maltreatment: Behavioral and developmental impact on children in the child welfare system. Journal of Child and Adolescent Trauma. 2008;**1**:317-330. DOI: 10.1080/19361520802505735

[72] Herring RJ. Trauma, PTSD, and the developing brain. Current Psychiatry Reports. 2017;**19**(10):69-78. DOI: 10.1007/s11920-017-0825-3

[73] Perry BD. Childhood experience and the expression of genetic potential: What childhood neglect tells us about nature and nurture. Brain and Mind. 2002;**3**: 7-100. DOI: 10.1023/A:1016557824657

[74] Weems CF, Russell JD, Neill EL, McCurdy BH. Annual research review: Pediatric posttraumatic stress disorder from a neurodevelopmental network perspective. Journal of Child Psychology and Psychiatry. 2019;**60**(4):395-408. DOI: 10.1111/jcpp.12996

[75] Winston R, Chicot R. The importance of early bonding on the long-term mental health and resilience of children. London Journal of Primary Care. 2016;**8**(1):12-14. DOI: 10.1080/17571472.2015.1133012

[76] Iruka IU, Sim J, Fort A. Black Parents and their Babies: Attending to the First 1,000 Days. Chapel Hill, NC: Equity Research Action Coalition at the UNC Frank Porter Graham Child Development Institute; 2021. Available from: https://fpg.unc.edu/publications/black-parents-and-their-babies-attending-first-1000-days

[77] National Scientific Council on the Developing Child. Excessive Stress Disrupts the Architecture of the Developing Brain: Working Paper 3. Updated Edition. 2005/2014. Available from: http://www.developingchild.harvard.edu [Accessed: November 15, 2021]

[78] Tottenham N, Galván A. Stress and the adolescent brain: Amygdala-prefrontal cortex circuitry and ventral striatum as developmental targets. Neuroscience and Biobehavioral Reviews. 2016;**70**:217-227. DOI: 1016/j.neubiorev.2016.07.030

[79] Kimberg L, Wheeler M. Trauma and trauma-informed care. In: Medical Management of Vulnerable and Underserved Patients: Principles,

Practice, and Populations. 2nd ed. New York: McGraw-Hill Medical Publishing Division; 2019. DOI: 10.1007/978-3-030-04342-1_2

[80] Weems CF. Severe stress and the development of the amygdala in youth: A theory and its statistical implications. Developmental Review. 2017;**46**(1):44-53. DOI: 10.1016/j.dr.2017.08.001

[81] Hillary AF. Toxic stress: Effects, prevention and treatment. Children. 2014;**1**(3):390-402. DOI: 10.3390/children1030390

[82] Raffagnato A, Angelico C, Fasolato R, Sale E, Gatta M, Miscioscia M. Parental bonding and children's psychopathology: A transgenerational view point. Children. 2021;**8**(11):1012. DOI: 10.3390/children8111012

[83] Avinun R, Knafo A. Parenting as a reaction evoked by children's genotype: A meta-analysis of children-as-twins studies. Personality and Social Psychology Review. 2014;**18**(1):87-102. DOI: 10.1177/1088868313498308

[84] Lacasa F, Ochoa S, Balluerka N, Mitjavila M. The relationship between attachment styles and internalizing or externalizing symptoms in clinical and nonclinical adolescents. Anales de Psicologia. 2015;**31**(2):422-432. DOI: 10.6018/analesps.31.2.169711

[85] Nelson C, Furtado E, Fox N, Zeanah C. The deprived human brain. American Scientist. 2009;**97**(3):222-229. DOI: 10.1511/2009.78.222

[86] Bennegadi R. Social psychiatry In the era of cyber age and globalization: Threatened, empowered, or both? World Social Psychiatry. 2019;**1**:62-66

[87] Shanahan J, Morgan M. Television and its Viewers Cultivation Theory and Research. Cambridge: Cambridge University Press; 2004

[88] Simmel G. The Metropolis and Mental Life. New York: Free Press; 1950. pp. 409-424

[89] Foshay R. The Digital Nexus: Identity, Agency, and Political Engagement. Athabasca: AU Press; 2016. DOI: 10.15215/aupress/9781771991292.01

[90] Hübl T, Avritt JJ. Healing Collective Trauma: A Process for Integrating our Intergenerational & Cultural Wounds. Colorado: Boulder; 2020

[91] Han B-C. The Scent of Time, a Philosophical Essay on the Art of Lingering. Cambridge: Polity Press; 2017

[92] Han B-C. The Burnout Society. Stanford: Stanford University Press; 2015

[93] Güder FZ. Psychological consultancy through digital media in times of Covid-19 pandemic: An analysis of the TV series "red room" and "apartments of innocents". In: IFIG 8th International Communication Days, Crisis Communication in the Digital Age Symposium; 26-28 May 2021; İstanbul

[94] Tarhan N. Toplum Psikolojisi ve Empati: Sosyal Şizofreniden Toplumsal Empatiye. İstanbul: Timaş Yayınları; 2016. pp. 82-83

[95] Öngün E. Renaming citizenship: An evolution from social citizenship to digital citizenship. In: Öngün E, Pembecioğlu N, Gündüz U, editors. Handbook of Research on Digital Citizenship and Management during Crises. USA: IGI Global; 2021. pp. 1-16. DOI: 10.4018/978-1-7998-8421-7

[96] Beck U. Pioneer in Cosmopolitan Sociology and Risk Society. Springer Briefs on Pioneers in Science

and Practice; 2014. p. 18. DOI: 10.1007/978-3-319-04990-8

[97] Costa C. Bourdieu, Habitus and Social Research the Art of Application. 1st ed. New York: Palgrave Macmillan; 2015

[98] Bryant RA. Social attachments and traumatic stress. European Journal of Psychotraumatology. 2016;7(1):29065. DOI: 10.3402/pt. v7.29065

[99] Sontag S. Regarding the Pain of Others. New York: Picador; 2003

[100] Baudrillard J. Simulacra and Simulation (the Body in Theory: Histories of Cultural Materialism). Michigan: University of Michigan Press; 1994

[101] Cem T. 6th International Communication Days Digital Transformation Symposium, Üsküdar University, Faculty of Communication; 02-03 May 2019; İstanbul, Turkey

[102] Zecher JL. Acedia: The Lost Name for the Emotion We're All Feeling Right Now [Internet]. 2020. Available from: https://theconversation.com/acedia-the-lost-name-for-the-emotion-were-all-feeling-right-now-144058. [Accessed: October 23, 2021]

[103] Restrepo JAF. Durée and temporality: A defense of Bergson's conception of time. Discusiones Filosoficas. 2015;**16**(27):49-61. DOI: 10.17151/difil.2015.16.27.4

Chapter 9

# Treating Trauma-related Disorders in Later Life: Moving Forward

*Jeannette C.G. Lely and Rolf J. Kleber*

## Abstract

Among stress-related disorders, post-traumatic stress disorder (PTSD) takes a central position. Although the percentage of older adults suffering from this condition appears to be lower than among younger adults, PTSD among them often presents a serious condition with high comorbidity rates. In this contribution, recent insights into post-traumatic stress disorder among older people as well as psychotherapeutic treatments are discussed. In particular, the results of recently completed investigations are discussed. In this research, treatment outcomes of two psychotherapeutic approaches considered suitable for older PTSD patients (Narrative Exposure Therapy or NET and Present Centered Therapy or PCT) were compared in terms of psychopathology and psychosocial adjustment. For older patients suffering from PTSD with varying backgrounds, both NET and PCT showed the potential for a significant reduction of symptoms (PTSD, depression and subjective distress). Moreover, it was found that older adults can change long-standing beliefs, even after long-past childhood trauma. In a patient's own words: "*I am still here, the past didn't bring me to my knees*". These findings disconfirm unfounded pessimism regarding psychotherapy in later life. Currently available treatment approaches in later life can be meaningful in improving the quality of life in older adults for years to come.

**Keywords:** older adults, PTSD, post-traumatic stress disorder, psychotherapy, quality of life

## 1. Introduction

Since the introduction of the latest version of the Diagnostic and Statistical Manual (DSM-5; [1]), Post-Traumatic Stress Disorder or PTSD takes a central position among stress-related disorders. This distressing and demoralizing disorder is triggered by exposure to a life-threatening or terrifying event, experienced in person or witnessed indirectly. The symptoms needed for a diagnosis are summarized as involuntary re-experiencing the adverse event(s), efforts to avoid such intrusive memories, negative cognitions or mood alterations, and increased arousal [1]. Although PTSD is precipitated by exposure to a severe life event, it is not clear why some people develop PTSD after potentially traumatic events (PTEs), while others do not. Several risk factors have been found, such as prior exposure to (and the number of types of) traumatic events [2], neuroticism, lack of social support or being female [3].

Although the percentage of older adults meeting full diagnostic criteria for this disorder appears to be lower than in younger adults [3, 4], PTSD among them often presents a serious condition [5] with high comorbidity rates [6] and showing a chronic, fluctuating course [7]. As older adults present the fastest-growing segment in the world population, evidence-based treatment approaches are required to address the needs of trauma-affected older populations. After all, PTE's can occur during all stages of life. Moreover, since populations of older adults not only grow in size, but also in life expectancy, trauma-related psychotherapy in later life can be followed by many more years to live.

In older adults, however, the symptoms are often misunderstood as depression, anxiety, somatic illness or memory problems due to aging. Consequently, PTSD has been described as a 'hidden variable' in the lives of older adults suffering from such a confusing array of symptoms [8]. Psychotherapy for older PTSD patients has been found to encounter several more barriers. To start with, long-standing stereotypes regarding older adults' capacity to change present a broadly generalized example of agism (age-related discrimination). Due to Freud's assumptions on psychoanalysis [9], advancing age was long considered a disadvantage in psychotherapy. Furthermore, low recognition of PTSD in primary care [5, 10], the reluctance of older adults to accept services of mental health professionals to deal with their problems [11] and insufficient empirical data [12] play a role. Taken together, in an age of a growing population of older adults, those suffering from PTSD risk receiving less-than-optimally efficacious treatment, which may be considered a research gap as well as a clinical problem challenging both researchers and clinicians.

Regarding trauma-related psychotherapy in later life, recent case studies reported encouraging results [13–15]. Trauma-focused exposure seemed to be well tolerated without adverse effects on comorbid cardiac conditions [16]. Some small controlled studies yielded preliminary positive treatment results for PTSD [17–19], although the small sample sizes did not allow for definitively bridging the research gaps. More robust studies [20, 21] suggested that (variants of) Trauma-Focused Cognitive Behavioral Therapy (TF CBT) can be safely and effectively used with older adult PTSD patients [22]. It must be realized, however, that the generalizability of those conclusions may be limited by the fact that most research has been conducted in Western countries, predominantly among Holocaust survivors or aging male military veterans. In addition, most studies are poorly reflective of the demographic context, as they do not include sufficient participants over the age of 74 [23].

To strengthen the existing evidence, a set of three studies (including a randomized controlled trial or RCT) was conducted, comparing treatment effects for PTSD of two psychotherapeutic interventions in treatment-seeking older adults with PTSD in the Netherlands [24], an exploratory analysis of self-reported symptoms and resilience measures in the same sample [25], and qualitative analysis of cognitions and emotions [26]. A global summary of these studies and their findings will allow for discussing current developments in the field of treating trauma-related disorders in later life.

## 2. Method

### 2.1 Participants

Participants enrolled in the RCT and the explorative analysis were recruited from two Dutch mental health centres (Centre'45/Arq and Sinai Centre), which specialized in treating trauma-related disturbances. To capture important age-related challenges and losses in terms of emotional attachment, physical independence and socio-economic setbacks [11], treatment-seeking, community-dwelling out-patients with PTSD aged 55 years and over were accepted for this trial. Participants were enrolled between April 2013 and April 2016. Exclusion criteria involved not meeting full PTSD-IV criteria, changes in psychotropic medication during the study, severe cognitive impairment, high suicide risk, psychosis or bipolar disorder, current substance use disorder and concurrent psychosocial treatment during the study. Half of the sample consisted of native Dutch participants, the other half of resettled refugees from various countries, mainly from the Middle-East. The 33 civilian trauma survivors reported traumatic events including persecution, political, domestic and sexual violence, including childhood abuse. These events took place throughout the life course. The participants' age ranged from 55 to 81 years; a mean age being 63.81 years, SD = 6.8 years; as for the gender distribution, 75% were men. All participants had encountered multiple adverse events. A total of 36.4% of the participants reported childhood trauma, implying Adverse Childhood Events (ACEs) between age 5 to 12; 30.3% reported sexual trauma. The majority (60.6%) of the participants suffered not only from PTSD (DSM-IV; 2000), but additionally from comorbid depression symptoms.

### 2.2 Interventions

In the first two studies, treatment effects from two well-known psychological interventions were compared: Narrative Exposure Therapy or NET [27] and Present-Centered Therapy or PCT [28].

In NET, TF CBT is embedded in an autobiography, offering a lifespan time-frame for imaginal exposure. Following the introductory session, the therapist and patient collaboratively create a timeline of the patient's life; subsequently elaborating this timeline in the next sessions. The final session allows the patient to receive the documented narration and focus on the future. This short-term treatment approach, which can be disseminated among local para-professional staff, is considered an innovative modification of TF CBT for vulnerable populations in low-resource regions. NET was extensively investigated in various populations of refugees and displaced persons in war- and disaster-affected areas, but also refugees and asylum seekers living in Western countries, demonstrating medium to large effect sizes and low dropout rates [29]. Some of those trials had investigated non-refugees, such as former political prisoners in Romania [17] or Chinese earthquake survivors [30, 31]. The lifespan perspective of NET suggests that this intervention shows high suitability for the population targeted in this trial.

As for PCT, in a trauma-informed context, the focus is explicitly *not* on traumatic content, but on problem-solving of current stressors or maladaptive interactions [28]. This equally innovative approach was developed as a control condition, contrasting the exposure-based technique in TF CBT. PCT, however, appeared to be an efficacious and acceptable stand-alone treatment for PTSD [9]. Just as NET, PCT showed low dropout rates [9]. Contrary to NET, PCT allows for systematically focusing on current problems associated with PTSD. Following the introductory session, psycho-education explaining the links between trauma and current distress is provided. The next sessions focus on relieving interpersonal and other current stressors. In homework assignments, patients select the relevant issues. Thus, a kind of self-help document is developed. The final session is dedicated to taking stock and looking forward.

### 2.3 Design, assessments and methods of analysis

The first two studies involved two conditions (NET vs. PCT) and three assessment timepoints (pre-treatment, post-treatment and at 4 months follow-up). Participants were randomly assigned to 11 sessions of NET or 11 sessions of PCT; each session covering 90 minutes.

In study 1 [24], the variables of interest were symptom severity and the symptom clusters (re-experience, avoidance and hyper-arousal) of PTSD (DSM-IV; [32]), using the well-validated Clinician-Administered PTSD Scale (CAPS; [33]). In addition to calculating group means, an individual clinically significant change [34] was rated.

In study 2, capturing the impact of PTSD in patients' daily life, exploratory analyses of self-reported symptoms and several measures of resilience were conducted [25]. This approach allowed patients to report self-reported distress from PTSD (using HTQ; [35]), depression symptoms (BDI-II; [36]), subjective general distress (BSI; [37]), self-efficacy [38], quality of life [39] and finally post-traumatic growth [40].

To enhance the external validity of this research project, inter-session intervals were adapted to patients' preferences and possibilities (weekly or once in 2 weeks). The resulting variation in treatment duration was addressed by advanced statistical analyses, using a (multilevel) piecewise mixed-effects growth model [41] to determine weekly change rates in the outcomes across time (therapy vs. follow-up) and conditions (NET- versus PCT-groups).

Finally, to explore post-traumatic cognitive processing during the treatment process, qualitative patient-reported outcomes were collected in study 3 [26]. This study consisted of the qualitative analysis of trauma narratives and individual interview responses in a subsample of four Dutch participants from the NET condition. All four participants reported multiple ACEs. Qualitative data analyses were conducted by using MAXQDA text software [42].

For all studies, methodological quality was addressed by trial registration, approval from the medical ethical committee (Leiden University), conducting a power analysis before starting the studies, randomization, blinding of assessors, protocol adherence, checks of treatment adherence and interrater reliability, and use of independent assessors.

## 3. Results

In study 1, both NET and PCT were found to be safe and efficacious psychological treatments for older adults suffering from PTSD. Both interventions demonstrated low dropout rates. Markedly, none of the participants in either condition left treatment prematurely because of intolerable stress increase. During treatment, PCT showed a steeper decline than NET for CAPS-scores (all PTSD symptom clusters). In the NET-group, a more gradual symptom decline was observed. This divergence resulted in a significant superiority at post-treatment (Cohen's $d = 0.44$), which was considered a medium effect [43]. At follow-up, however, the effects converged due to a partial symptom rebound in the PCT group and a persisting decline in the NET-group. The rebound in the PCT-group mainly involved the symptom clusters of re-experience and avoidance. **Figure 1** presents the outcomes for the PTSD total scale, centred around the post-treatment assessment timepoint.

The mean severity of PTSD symptoms in both groups decreased from severe at the mean timepoint pre-treatment to moderate at the mean follow-up. In addition to focusing on group means, an individual clinically significant change [34] was rated. On the individual level, 71% of NET completers achieved a clinically significant improvement, compared to 50% of the PCT completers.

In study 2, regarding self-rated PTSD, depression symptoms and perceived general distress, both groups (NET and PCT) showed equal, medium to large, within-group effects as well [25]. Whereas resilience (defined in terms of self-efficacy, quality of life, and personal growth) did not significantly improve in either group, it was not compromised, thereby confirming the treatment effects of both interventions.

In study 3, the question was addressed how the benefits of treatment by NET can be understood from a patients' perspective. Posttraumatic changes in thoughts and meanings are supposed to play an important role in recovering from PTSD [44, 45]. To explore cognitive processing during treatment, qualitative patient-reported outcomes were collected by analyzing autobiographic documents and interview responses. Would a cognitive and developmental framework clarify those outcomes? Would aging adults be able to change long-standing posttraumatic feelings and cognitions during treatment? In a sub-sample of NET-participants, the latter question could be answered with a convincing "Yes". The participants involved reported gradual, meaningful changes in self-awareness and self-esteem [24]. "*At the time of the violence in our family, I felt weak, helpless and guilty. Being a child, I was not able to defend my mother! Now I realize that I stood up for her when I was strong enough. Until this day, there is strength and endurance in me.*" Initial self-blame, shame, social alienation and anger gradually gave way to the realization that somebody else had to be blamed, that shame was not appropriate, to new feelings of attachment and rightful anger. In a patient's own words: "*I am still here, the past didn't bring me to my knees*". And: "*With help of the document, I might tell more about myself to my children. Maybe we can have a better time together in the years ahead*". As for the developmental framework, negative cognitions were associated with

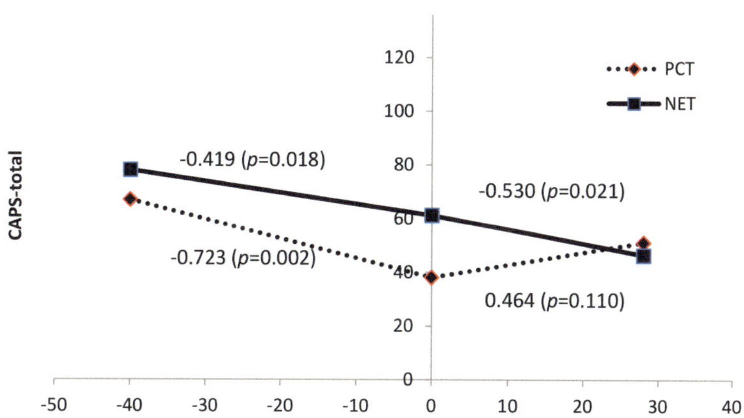


**Figure 1.**
*RCT outcomes of CAPS-total [24].*

traumatic episodes, retaining a strong centrality in emotional life. New contexts and relationships, however, offered opportunities for more self-asserting cognitions alongside the self-defeating ones. "*Learning the craft of cabinet-making helped me finding my own strengths and reconnecting to people*."

Pulling together the strings from the presented studies, the short-term treatment effects of the PCT-group exceeded those in the NET-group. Nevertheless, this superiority was lost at follow-up. The within-group treatment effects in the NET-group were found to extend beyond PTSD, drawing depression symptoms and general distress into the scope of recovering from PTSD. Resilience, quantitatively measured, did not show significant responses for either group. In other words, compared with NET, the PCT-group showed significantly stronger short-term reductions in PTSD pathology (study 1), whereas this group did not show significantly improved resilience, neither comparatively, nor longitudinally (Study 2). The qualitative analysis, however, showed gradual cognitive and emotional changes on a personal level, reflecting the processing of adverse events and regaining self-esteem and initiative.

## 4. Discussion

Taken together, the main findings of these studies suggest that both trauma exposure (NET) and a trauma-informed present-centred approach (PCT) are safe and effective interventions for older adults and that posttraumatic recovery in later life extends beyond clinician-rated PTSD symptoms, including mood and subjectively perceived distress as well. Moreover, older adults can change long-standing beliefs, even after long-past childhood trauma.

## 5. Strengths and limitations

To reflect the impact of PTSD symptoms on daily life, the presented studies were characterized by a broad approach to the subject of treating trauma-related disorders in later life. Consequently, PTSD, comorbid depression and several measures of resilience were included in the analyses. An additional strength is the multimethod approach of this research project. The studies used advanced and variable methods of analysis. A third strength is the controlled comparison of treatment response in two innovative psychotherapeutic interventions for PTSD in a sample of older adults. The interventions had contrasting treatment approaches: imaginal exposure (focusing on the past) versus a focus on problem-solving in the present. The resulting response patterns may provide a useful tool for clinicians to discuss treatment preferences with their patients. The equal efficacy at follow-up might be an important attribution to ongoing discussions concerning the necessity of exposure in trauma treatment [46]. The clinical meaningfulness of the results was increased by the inclusion of a heterogeneous sample of civilians, including both native Dutch civilians and refugees. In addition, the participants were allowed to determine session intervals in accordance with their preferences and possibilities. Advanced statistical analyses addressed the resulting variability of inter-assessment intervals. Within a clinical environment, methodological rigor was addressed by randomization, protocol adherence, checks of treatment adherence and interrater reliability, and the use of independent assessors.

Some limitations merit attention as well. The participants' mean age does not allow for generalizing the research findings to old age (over age 74). By using the 55 years limit, however, clinically important transitions could be captured and enough participants could be recruited to reach a sufficiently powered sample for the RCT on PTSD. Nevertheless, the study sample was small and mainly representative for the so-called young-old (ages 55 to 75), as distinguished [47] from the old-old (75 and over). In addition, out of fear of high dropout and concurrent influences in the follow-up interval, a short follow-up interval was chosen. In future research, a longer follow-up interval is strongly advisable. Therefore, the research findings from these studies have to be interpreted with caution. They can contribute, however, to ongoing discussions in the field of treating trauma-related disorders in later life, focusing on current issues and controversies, lessons learnt and future research. These topics will receive more attention in the following paragraphs.

## 6. Issues and controversies

### 6.1 Does age matter?

Reflecting the heterogeneity and etiological complexity of mental health in old age [48], a broad range of measures and a multimethod approach was selected in the presented studies. About late adulthood and young-old age, several questions were addressed. To begin with: Would advancing age matter in terms of treatment response? Meta-analytic findings on NET [29] did not support this hypothesis. Furthermore, in a recent study including 2578 adults – aged from 18 to 80 years [49], the single factor limiting treatment response in all outcomes was found to be the number of traumatic events, confirming the established dose-response correlation of higher trauma exposure and elevated PTSD symptom severity [2, 50]. Taken together, advancing age does not matter in terms of treatment response. In terms of etiological complexity and of biographical and historical context, however, age is highly influential, requiring historical sensitivity and detailed curiosity from therapists.

### 6.2 Past or present?

Like all exposure-based treatments, NET addresses the way patients cognitively cope with past events. The treatment strategies of NET have been described as re-organizing memories and restoring narrative continuity and coherence [27]. In the RCT comparing NET and PCT, present-centred therapy (PCT) served as an active comparator. PCT focuses on the present: coping with concurrent stressors, maladaptive interaction patterns and learning solution-focused techniques [9]. In addition to this contrast, there are similarities as well. Both 'dealing with the past' and 'coping with present stressors' refer to (cognitive and emotional) coping with either distressing memories and meanings or maladaptive behavior patterns. Similar considerations might be valid regarding other comparisons, such as Prolonged Exposure versus Relaxation training [51]. The conclusion might be that engaging in such a process in a therapeutic relationship allows for changing both kinds of coping. Patient-reported outcomes suggested a gradual shift in cognitions and emotions, not quite resulting in the complete extinction of old feelings, but expanding the patients' experiential repertory.

Since treatment changes in NET and PCT are found to be more similar than assumed, their direct comparison calls for close attention. The results of the RCT show that both approaches are safe and effective. Unexpectedly, at follow-up, NET and PCT show equal efficacy. Apparently, in this population dealing with the past and coping with the present show equal importance. Remarkably, change in terms of PTSD symptoms took place at a different pace per intervention. The gradual symptom decrease in the NET-group can be understood as an effect of the taxing exposure in NET. In contrast to the response pattern of PCT, the symptom decline in NET continued after treatment. This difference might be related to different learning strategies in both interventions. It could be suggested that increased coherence and habituation are more internalizing processes than problem-solving techniques, leading to more sustainable treatment results. The continuous symptom decrease in the NET-group tantalizingly suggests a further decline beyond the follow-up interval used and calls for a replication of the comparison with a longer follow-up interval. Meta-analytic findings regarding persisting within-treatment effects in NET justify such suggestions [29].

## 7. Clinical and research implications

Clinically, the importance of patient preferences for this population is illustrated. Some patients did not accept randomization, because they needed to tell their stories and did not accept any uncertainty about the possibility to do so. Following patient preferences can enhance treatment motivation, without, on the other hand, blindly following avoidance-based wishes. Regarding treatment outcome, in patients with chronic PTSD and comorbid depression, treatment matching was found to improve treatment response [52]. Careful information and preparation of treatment choices are necessary to reach shared decisions. Regarding further research, the findings of the RCT call for replication in a larger sample, including older age groups, and a longer follow-up interval.

## 8. Pathology and resilience

Both NET and PCT were found to be safe and efficacious treatments reducing PTSD symptoms in older adults suffering from PTSD. Compared with NET, the PCT-group showed significantly stronger short-term reductions in PTSD pathology, whereas this group did not show significantly improved resilience, neither comparatively, nor longitudinally. Nevertheless, the study findings suggest that posttraumatic recovery in later life extends beyond reductions in re-experiencing, avoiding and arousal symptoms, adding nuance to the current centrality of PTSD symptoms [53]. One might say that the current concept of PTSD in DSM-5 (including depression symptoms in the diagnostic criteria of PTSD), already reflects this nuance. These findings may inspire further research on resilience factors, both in individual and community contexts.

## 9. Lessons learnt

In addition to the described issues, several observations merit attention. Older adults suffering from PTSD report serious impairments in daily life. The presented studies show that patients who gain access to treatment can achieve a clinically significant treatment response. As for NET, the qualitative analysis showed that during and after treatment, renewed personal growth is found to be within reach for older adults, just as for younger patients. This renewed growth can be a sign of returning strength and vitality, notwithstanding residual symptoms. Even in later life, the taxing procedure of NET did not prevent significant symptom reductions, rendering credibility to interpreting treatment changes as results of cognitive and emotional reprocessing, without, however, ruling out the influence of the patient-therapist relationship.

Another observation refers to the age in terms of a remaining lifetime. Rapidly expanding life expectancies imply that improved quality of life after treatment offers new perspectives on potentially many more years of a satisfactory quality of life. This awareness may offset negative cognitions concerning the usefulness of treatment in later life. In these years, some patients hope for a new understanding between parents and children or grandchildren, potentially correcting existing intergenerational transmission of maladaptive interaction patterns [54]. In clinical practice, such intentions might call for careful preparation and timing, since self-disclosure of painful memories might evoke unexpected family dynamics. "*Wishing to be honest about my past experiences, I simultaneously fear the consequences. Will my children believe me? What will they think of me, and of my tormentor, who is one of their grandparents after all?*"

## 10. Treating trauma-related disorders in later life: moving forward

### 10.1 Treatment barriers

Psychological treatment for older adults has been characterized by several barriers: myths about older adults' incapacity to change, low recognition of PTSD in primary care, the reluctance of older adults to use the services of mental health services for solving their problems and a limited body of evidence concerning trauma-focused treatment for older adults [12, 17, 21, 46]. Without addressing these barriers, older adults with PTSD will not gain access to treatment. By showing the potential of psychotherapy with older adult PTSD patients to achieve clinically meaningful results (both with NET and PCT), without compromising resiliency, the presented studies addressed the latter barrier.

### 10.2 Adapting treatment formats

Previously, age-specific modifications for standard treatments were proposed, such as increasing the structure of treatment, utilizing memory aids and simplifying materials [55]. These modifications mainly refer to form: i.e., the way in which treatment and its environmental conditions are personalized in response to patients' individual needs. These adaptations do not appear to exceed adequate personalization of treatment in general. The present research does not call for conceptually changing current treatment protocols when treating older adults. Full information and careful psycho-education have been found to prepare senior participants sufficiently for their treatment, either including direct trauma exposure or focusing on current stressors. As for treatment duration, extension was not considered to be justified. In treatment modules of 11 sessions, at least half of the participants achieved clinically meaningful treatment changes for PTSD symptoms. When addressing specific symptoms, such as traumatic grief, trauma-related systemic problems or nightmares, alternative interventions may be considered, such as Brief Eclectic Psychotherapy for traumatic grief or BEP-TG [56], interpersonal therapy [52], or imaginary rehearsal therapy [57].

In case of persisting maladaptive cognitions, schema therapy – found to be safe and effective with older adults - might serve as a sequel treatment [58].

## 11. Future research

Future research calls for rigorous research methodology to be integrated in clinical-service provisions in ways that mutually improve both research and clinical practice [59]. Routinely assessing adverse childhood experiences by using the ACE (Adverse Childhood Events) Questionnaire (World Health Organization; WHO [60]) may support patients in better understanding their current health problems. Even if such experiences are initially denied, patients may hear the message that talking in therapy about such issues is acceptable. Since both age-related changes and PTSD symptoms can include attention and memory problems, cognitive functioning should be routinely assessed as well [61]. Extending routine assessments with cognitive and physiological measures (blood pressure or heart rate) could provide additional evidence on risks and outcomes of psychotherapy in older adults [22, 46]. Furthermore, directly comparing trauma-related psychotherapy with pharmacotherapy for older PTSD patients could improve treatment matching. Moreover, e-health applications for assessment and/or treatment (the timeline in NET or homework assignments in PCT) could bring interesting innovations and inspire yet further research. Summarizing, this field of research is still in its infancy and calls for expanding the scope of research. In particular, founding research sites outside Western countries and reaching new target populations will encourage researchers and clinicians in this fascinating field to move forward.

## 12. Treating trauma-related disorders in later life: in conclusion

For senior PTSD patients, both Narrative Exposure Therapy and Present Centered Therapy show the potential to significantly reduce symptoms of PTSD and related problems, whereas resilience factors are not compromised by either treatment procedure, Furthermore, gradual changes in posttraumatic feelings and cognitions mirror increasing self-esteem and initiative, implying that older adults can change long-standing self-related beliefs, even after long-past childhood trauma. These findings allow for three conclusions. First, whereas PTSD may be described as a hidden variable in the lives of older adults, their strength and flexibility are shown to be hidden factors in their recovery process. Second, psychological treatment in later life may be meaningful for years to come. Third, pessimism concerning the treatment of older adults with trauma-related psychopathology is unfounded. By overcoming these ungrounded convictions, treating trauma-related disorders in later life is coming of age.

## Author details

Jeannette C.G. Lely[1*] and Rolf J. Kleber[2,3]

1 ARQ Centrum'45, The Netherlands

2 Department of Clinical Psychology, Utrecht University, Utrecht, The Netherlands

3 ARQ National Psychotrauma Centre, Diemen, The Netherlands

*Address all correspondence to: j.lely@centrum45.nl

## References

[1] American Psychiatric Association. Diagnostic and Statistical Manual of Mental Disorders. Fifth ed. Washington, DC: APA; 2013

[2] Kolassa IT, Ertl V, Eckart V, Kolassa S, Onyut LP, Elbert T. Spontaneous remission from PTSD depends on the number of traumatic event types experienced. Psychological Trauma: Theory, Research, Practice and Policy. 2010;**2**:169-174

[3] Van Zelst WH, de Beurs E, Beekman ATF, Deeg DJH, van Dyck R. Prevalence and risk factors of posttraumatic stress disorder in older adults. Psychotherapy and Psychosomatics. 2003;**72**:333-342. DOI: 10.1159/000073030

[4] Reynolds K, Pietrzak RH, Mackenzie CS, Chou KL, Sareen J. Post-traumatic stress disorder across the adult lifespan: Findings from a nationally representative survey. The American Journal of Geriatric Psychiatry. 2016;**24**(1):81-93. DOI: 10.1016/j.jagp.2015.11.001

[5] Van Zelst WH, de Beurs E, Beekman ATF, van Dijck R, Deeg DJH. Well-being, physical functioning, and use of health services in the elderly with PTSD and subthreshold PTSD. International Journal of Geriatric Psychiatry. 2006;**21**:180-188. DOI: 10.1002/gps.1448

[6] Kang B, Xu H, McConnell ES. Neurocognitive and psychiatric comorbidities of posttraumatic stress disorder among older veterans: A systematic review. International Journal of Geriatric Psychiatry. 2019;*34*(4): 522-538. DOI: 10.1002/gps.5055

[7] Chopra MP, Zhang H, Pless Kaiser A, Moye JA, Llorente MD, Oslin DW, et al. PTSD is a chronic, fluctuating disorder affecting the mental quality of life in older adults. American Journal of Geriatric Psychiatry. 2014;*22*(1):86-97. DOI: 10.1016/j.jagp.2013.01.064

[8] Nichols BL, Czirr R. Post-traumatic stress disorder: Hidden Syndrome in Elders. Clinical Gerontologist: The Journal of Aging and Mental Health. 1986;**5**(3-4):417-433. DOI: 10.1300/J018v05n03_12

[9] Freud S. On Psychotherapy. London: Hogarth Press; 1905

[10] Ehlers A, Gene-Cos N, Perrin S. Low recognition of posttraumatic stress disorder in primary care. London Journal of Primary Care (Abingdon). 2009;**2**:36-42

[11] Laidlaw K, Thompson LW, Dick-Siskin L, Gallagher-Thompson D. Psychotherapy with older adults. In: Laidlaw K, Thompson LW, Dick-Siskin L, Gallagher-Thompson D, editors. Cognitive Behaviour with Older Adults. Chichester: Wiley; 2003

[12] Böttche M, Kuwert P, Knaevelsrud C. Posttraumatic stress disorder in older adults: An overview of characteristics and treatment approaches. International Journal of Geriatric Psychiatry. 2012;**27**:230-239. DOI: 10/1002/gps.2725

[13] Curran B, Collier E. Growing older with post-traumatic stress disorder. Journal of Psychiatric and Mental Health Nursing. 2016;**23**:236-242. DOI: 10.1111/jpm.12280

[14] Mørkved N, Thorp SR. The treatment of PTSD in an older adult Norwegian

woman using narrative exposure therapy: a case report. European Journal of Psychotraumatology. 2018;**9**(1):1414561. DOI: 10.1080/20008198.2017.1414561

[15] Reuman L, Davison E. Delivered as described: A successful case of Cognitive Processing Therapy with an older woman veteran with PTSD. Cognitive and Behavioral Practice, Advance Online Publication. 2021. DOI: 10.1016/j.cbpra.2021.06.004

[16] Chopra MP. PTSD in late life: Special issues. Psychiatric Times, Geriatric Psychiatry, part. 2018;**3**:1-10

[17] Bichescu D, Neuner F, Schauer M, Elbert T. Narrative exposure therapy of political imprisonment-related chronic posttraumatic stress disorder. Behaviour Research and Therapy. 2007;**45**(9):2212-2220. DOI: 10.1016/j.brat.2006.12.006

[18] Gamito P, Oliveira J, Rosa P, Morais D, Duarte N, Oliveira S, et al. PTSD Elderly War Veterans: A Clinical Controlled Pilot Study. Cyberpsychology, Behavior and Social Networking. 2010;**13**(1):43-48. DOI: 10.1089/cyber.2009.0237

[19] Ready DJ, Gerardi RJ, Backschneider AG, Mascaro N, Olasov Rothbaum B. Comparing Virtual Reality Exposure Therapy to Present-Centered Therapy with 11 U.S. Vietnam Veterans with PTSD. Cyberpsychology, Behavior and Social Networking. 2010;**13**:49-54. DOI: 10.1089=cyber.2009.0239

[20] Knaevelsrud C, Böttche M, Pietrzak RH, Freyberger HJ, Kuwert P. Efficacy and feasibility of a therapist-guided internet-based intervention for older persons with childhood traumatization: A randomized controlled trial. The American Journal of Geriatric Psychiatry. 2017;**25**(8):878-888. DOI: 10/1016/j.jagp.2017.02.024

[21] Thorp SR, Wells SY, Cook JM. Trauma-focused therapy for older adults. In: Gold SN, editor. APA Handbook of Trauma Psychology: Trauma Practice. Washington DC, USA: American Psychological Association; 2017. DOI: 10.1037/0000020-020

[22] Cook JM, McCarthy E, Thorp SR. Older adults with PTSD: Brief state of research and evidence-based psychotherapy case illustration. American Journal of Geriatric Psychiatry. 2017;**25**(5):522-530. DOI: 10.1016/j.jagp.2016.12.016

[23] Pless Kaiser A, Cook JM, Glick DM, Moye J. Posttraumatic stress disorder in older adults: A conceptual review. Clinical Gerontologist. 2019;**4**(42):359-376. DOI: 10.1080/07317115.2018.1539801

[24] Lely JCG, Knipscheer JW, Moerbeek M, ter Heide FJJ, van den Bout J, Kleber RJ. Randomised controlled trial comparing Narrative Exposure Therapy with Present-Centered Therapy for older Patients with post-traumatic stress disorder. British Journal of Psychiatry. 2019;**214**(6):369-377. DOI: 10.1192/bjp.2019.59

[25] Lely JCG, ter Heide FJJ, Moerbeek M, Knipscheer JW, Kleber RJ. Psychopathology and resilience in older adults with Posttraumatic Stress Disorder: A randomized controlled trial comparing. Narrative Exposure Therapy and Present-Centered Therapy. European Journal of Psychotraumatology. 2022;**13**(1). DOI: 10.1080/20008198.2021.2022277

[26] Lely JCG, de la Rie SM, Knipscheer JW, Kleber RJ. Stronger than my ghosts: A qualitative study on cognitive recovery in later life. Journal of Loss and Trauma. 2019;**24**(4):369-382. DOI: 10.1080/15325024.2019.1603008

[27] Schauer M, Neuner F, Elbert T. Narrative Exposure Therapy. A Short-term Intervention for Traumatic Stress Disorders after War, Terror or Torture. 2nd expanded ed. Göttingen: Hogrefe & Huber Publishers; 2011

[28] McDonagh A, Friedman M, McHugo G, Ford J, Sengupta A, Mueser K, et al. Randomised trial of cognitive behavioral therapy for chronic post-traumatic stress disorder in adult female survivors of childhood sexual abuse. Journal of Consulting and Clinical Psychology. 2005;**73**(3):515-0524. DOI: 10/1037/0022.006X.73.3.515

[29] Lely JCG, Smid GE, Jongedijk RA, Knipscheer JW, Kleber RJ. The effectiveness of narrative exposure therapy: a reviewmeta-analysis and meta-regression analysis. European Journal of Psychotraumatology. 2019;**10**(1):1550344. DOI: 10.1080/20008198.2018.1550344

[30] Zang Y, Hunt N, Cox T. A randomised controlled pilot study: The effectiveness of narrative exposure therapy with adult survivors of the Sichuan earthquake. BMC Psychiatry. 2013;**13**(41):1-11. DOI: 10.1186/1471-244X-13-41

[31] Zang Y, Hunt N, Cox T. Adapting narrative exposure therapy for Chinese earthquake survivors: A pilot randomised controlled feasibility study. BMC Psychiatry. 2014;**14**(262). DOI: 10.1186/s12888-014-0262-3

[32] American Psychiatric Association. Diagnostic and Statistical Manual of Mental Disorders, Fourth Edition (Text Revision). Washington, DC: APA; 2000

[33] Blake DD, Weathers FW, Nagy LM, Kaloupek DG, Gusman FD, Charney DS, et al. The development of a clinician-administered PTSD scale. Journal of Traumatic Stress. 1995;**8**(1):75-90

[34] Schnurr PP, Friedman MJ, Foy DW, Shea MT, Hsieh FY, Lavori PW, et al. Randomized trial of trauma-focused group therapy for posttraumatic stress disorder: results from a department of veterans affairs cooperative study. Archives of General Psychiatry. 2003;**60**:481-489. DOI: 10.1001/archpsyc.60.5.481

[35] Mollica RF, Caspi-Yavin Y, Lavelle J, Tor S, Yang T, Chan S, et al. The Harvard trauma questionnaire (HTQ): Manual; Cambodian, Laotian and Vietnamese versions. Torture. 1996;**6**:19-34

[36] Beck AT, Steer RA, Brown GK. Beck Depression Inventory: Second Edition Manual. San Antonio (TX): The Psychological Corporation; 1996

[37] Derogatis LR. The Brief Symptom Inventory. Baltimore: Clinical Psychometric Research; 1975

[38] Schwarzer R, Jerusalem M. Generalized self-efficacy scale. In: Weinman J, Wright S, Johnston M, editors. Measures in health psychology: A user's portfolio. Causal and control beliefs. Windsor, UK: NFER-NELSON; 1995. pp. 35-37

[39] WHOQOL Group. Development of the world health organization WHOQOL-BREF Quality of Life Assessment. Psychological Medicine. 1998;**28**(3):551-558

[40] Mooren TM, Kleber RJ. The Impact of War in Bosnia and Herzegovina: Devastated Trust. International Journal of Mental Health. 2001;**30**(2):6-21. DOI: 10.1080/00207411.2001.11449515

[41] Naumova EN, Must A, Laird NM. Tutorial in Biostatistics: Evaluating the

impact of critical periods in longitudinal studies of growth using piecewise mixed models. International Journal for Epidemiology. 2001;**30**:1332-1341

[42] VERBI. MAXQDA [Computer software]. Marburg, Germany: Author; 2007

[43] Cohen J. Quantitative methods in psychology. A power primer. Psychological Bulletin. 1992;**112**:155-159

[44] Foa EB, Ehlers A, Clark DM, Tolin DF, Orsillo SM. The Posttraumatic Cognitions Inventory (PTCI): Development and validation. Psychological Assessment. 1999;**11**(3):303-314. DOI: 10.1037/1040-3590.11.3.303

[45] Janoff-Bulman R. Shattered Assumptions: Towards a New Psychology of Trauma. New York: Free Press; 1992

[46] Dinnen S, Simiola V, Cook JM. Post-traumatic stress disorder in older adults: A systematic review of the psychotherapy treatment literature (Review). Aging and Mental Health. 2015;**19**:144-150. DOI: 10.1080/13607863.2014.920299

[47] Neugarten BL. Age groups in American society and the rise of the young-old. Political consequences of aging. Philadelphia: The Annals of the American Academy; 1974. pp. 187-198

[48] Kessler EM, Kruse A, Wahl HW. Clinical Geropsychology: A Lifespan Perspective. In: Pachana NA, Laidlaw K, editors. The Oxford Handbook of Clinical Geropsychology. Oxford: Oxford University Press; 2014. DOI: 10.1093/oxfordhb/9780199663170.01

[49] Sabey AK, Jensen J, Major S, Zinbarg R, Pinsof W. Are older adults unique? Examining presenting issues and changes in therapy across the life span. Journal of Applied Gerontology. 2018;**39**:1-18. DOI: 10/1177/0733464818818048

[50] Lonergan M. Cognitive Behavioral Therapy for PTSD: The Role of Complex PTSD on Treatment Outcome. Journal of Aggression Maltreatment & Trauma. 2014;**23**:494-512. DOI: 10.1080/10926771.2014.904467

[51] Thorp SR, Glassman LH, Wells SY, Walter KH, Gebhardt H, Twamley E, et al. A randomized controlled trial of prolonged exposure therapy versus relaxation training for older veterans with military-related PTSD. Journal of Anxiety Disorders. 2019;**64**:45-54. DOI: 10.1016/j.janxdis.2019.02.003

[52] Markowitz JC, Petkova E, Neria Y, Van Meter PE, Zhao Y, Hembree E, et al. Is Exposure Necessary? A Randomized Clinical Trial of Interpersonal Psychotherapy for PTSD. American Journal of Psychiatry. 2015;**172**(5):430-440. DOI: 10.1176/appi.ajp.2014.14070908

[53] Mooren GTM, Kleber RJ. The significance of experiences of war and migration in older age: Long-term consequences in child survivors from the Dutch East Indies. International Psychogeriatrics. 2013;**25**:1783-1791. DOI: 10.1017/s1014610213000987

[54] Danieli Y, Norris FH, Engdahl B. Multigenerational legacies of trauma: Modeling the what and how of transmission. American Journal of Orthopsychiatry. 2016;**86**(6):639-561. DOI: 10.1037/ort0000145

[55] Thorp SR, Glassman LH, Wells SY. PTSD and Trauma. In: Pachana N, editor. Encyclopedia of Gerontology. Singapore: Springer Science; 2015. pp. 1-8

[56] Smid GE, Kleber RJ, Rie SM de la, Bos JBA, Gersons BPR, & Boelen PA.

Brief eclectic therapy for traumatic grief (BEP-TG): Toward integrated treatment of symptoms related to traumatic loss. European Journal of Psychotraumatology. 2015;**6**:27324

[57] Van Schagen AM, Lancee J, De G, Spoormaker IW, VI & van den Bout, J. Imagery rehearsal therapy in addition to treatment as usual for patients with diverse psychiatric diagnoses suffering from nightmares: A randomized controlled trial. The Journal of Clinical Psychiatry. 2015;**76**(9):1105-1113. DOI: 10.4088/JCP.14m09216

[58] Videler AC, Rossi G, Schoevaars M, Van der Feltz-Cornelis CM, Van Alphen SPJ. Effects of schema group therapy in older outpatients: A proof of concept study. International Psychogeriatrics. 2014;**26**(10):1709-1717. DOI: 10.1017/S1041610214001264

[59] Carlsson J, Sonne C, Silove D. From pioneers to scientists. Challenges in establishing evidence-gathering models in torture and trauma mental health services for refugees. The Journal of Nervous and Mental Disease. 2014;**202**(9):630-637

[60] World Health Organization. Available from: http://www.who/Programmes/Violence [Accessed: 12 April 2018]

[61] O'Connor M, Elklit A. Treating PTSD symptoms in older adults. In: Schnyder U, Cloitre M, editors. Evidence Based Treatments for Trauma-Related Psychological Disorders: A Practical Guide for Clinicians. Springer International Publishing AG; 2015. pp. 381-397. DOI: 10.1007/978-3-319-07109-1_20

Chapter 10

# The COVID-19 Pandemic and Mental Health

*Swati Mittal, Smriti Sinha and Shilpi Bhat*


## Abstract

The COVID-19 crept in silently and subsequently spread at a rapid pace ultimately progressing into a pandemic with a high rate of morbidity, mortality, loss of income and sustained social isolation for billions of people. This sudden human tragedy required heavy adjustment and was difficult to adapt quickly as we humans are gregarious in nature and always need social connect in our lives especially during a crisis. History has shown that mental health impact of pandemics outlasts the physical impact. In general, mental health and related issues are not recognized in public and with global pandemic these silent and insidious issues can be either misdiagnosed or go unnoticed completely.


**Keywords:** coronavirus, COVID-19, psychological effects, mental health

> *"World leaders must move fast and decisively to invest more in life-saving mental health programmes–during the pandemic and beyond."*
>
> *- Dr. Tedros Adhanom Ghebreyesus*

## 1. Introduction

The novel coronavirus disease (COVID-19) has become the fifth pandemic reported since 1918 Spanish flu pandemic. COVID-19 first reported in December 2019, Wuhan, China and is caused by a virus called severe acute respiratory syndrome (SARS-CoV-2) It is an enveloped and spherical virus containing a positive-sense single-stranded RNA genome and belongs to the subfamily Coronavirinae. Like many other respiratory viruses, coronavirus is transmitted through droplets projected out during breath, cough or sneeze. The symptoms of respiratory tract infections vary from mild cold to severe acute respiratory distress [1]. It crept in silently and subsequently spread at a rapid pace progressing into a pandemic.

The Coronavirus Disease was unprecedented in recent history with a high rate of morbidity, mortality, loss of income and sustained social isolation for billions of people. Now it has been affecting the world at an alarming rate, unfolding a tsunami of changes and leaving it in shambles, at the same time triggering a global collaboration to disease containment. Being a novel disease, COVID-19 has presented itself as a mystery infection to the health and research field. SARS-CoV-2 has a tendency for genetic evolution resulting in quick mutation and multiple variants that may have different features compared to its ancestral strains. The coronavirus has created frequent challenges ranging from virus isolation, detection, prevention, vaccine development to clinical and mental health issues. Besides, the tremendous research and insights about nature of virus, the studies regarding short term and long-term consequences on mental and psychological health of the community need to be focused.

## 2. Effects of lockdown on the psyche of people

To restrict the rate of both infections and death of fellow-citizens from COVID-19 and meanwhile also to prepare ourselves for the pandemic of such a magnitude, inter-individual physical contacts were restricted in the form of social lockdown. Under this situation, minimal and only emergency movement of general public was allowed. The central objective was to forbid people from two different families or nearby inhabitants to come in close contact with each other and thus break the cycle of infection [2]. Following this there was a significant reduction in the growth rate and increase in doubling time of cases [3]. But this swift change in people's daily life in the form of loss of freedom and dissociation from family members led to dramatic consequences. Confinement of physical space, lack of mobility, fear of contraction, loss of income, hopelessness and growing ambiguity along with uncertainty and unpredictability over the disease were some of the observed collective experiences affecting the wellbeing during lockdown [4]. COVID-19 led to roughly 5–20% contraction of global economy which could result in an increased poverty rate for the first time since 1990 with Asia, Africa and Latin America enduring the hardest blow [5]. Factories and industries were shut down forcing thousands of informal workers to return back to their native villages in absence of any form of conveyance. A survey conducted by International Labor Organization in April 2020 estimated roughly 2.5 crores job loss in 2020 alone worldwide due to the pandemic, predicting a deep economic crisis in coming days. The situation of Crises often reveals the structural inequalities present in the social and political dimensions (such as the unequal distribution of resources or the uneven delivery of healthcare). United States unemployment rates rose and the country neared a recession and as the pandemic progressed it created a situation of socioeconomic crisis which was reflected across the borders. Unemployment rate in urban India rose to 20.9% during the April–June quarter of 2020 pushing over 40 crores informal workers jobless [6]. Roughly 80 million children of under 1 year missed their routine vaccination while an estimated 38% increase in maternal mortality was registered due to health system disruption resulting from COVID [5]. This sudden human tragedy required heavy adjustment and was difficult to adapt quickly as we humans are gregarious in nature and always need social connect in our lives especially during a crisis [4]. This was the largest psychological experiment ever conducted as 1/3rd of the world's population was living under some kind of lockdown, dealing with an intense stressor called "loneliness" [7].

## 3. Loneliness and mental health

According to the World Health Organization (W.H.O)., mental health is a "state of wellbeing in which an individual realizes his or her own abilities, can cope with normal stressors of life, work positively and fruitfully and is able to make a contribution to his or her community" [8]. Keyes identified 3 components of mental health: emotional, psychological and social well-being and its definition is said to be influenced by the culture that defines it [9].

Psychological distress, a common mental health disorder is defined as a state of emotional suffering typically characterized by symptoms of depression and anxiety [10]. An important point to remember here is that, mental health can change over time, and depends heavily over the prevailing conditions. More so, when the demand exceeds the resource of coping abilities, it is heavily impacted. People became vulnerable to psychological impact of COVID-19 infection due to both the pandemic and its cascading consequences worldwide including lockdown and economic recession. It negatively affected people's mental health and created new barriers for ones already suffering from mental illness. A broad body of work links social isolation and loneliness to both poor mental and physical health. Loneliness and frustration seemed to originate from inhibition of daily activities, interruption of social necessities and inability to indulge in social networking, leading to psychological distress and progressing to unhealthy ways of coping in form of overeating and substance abuse [11]. This abrupt situation exposed that individuals were largely emotionally unprepared to the detrimental effects of biological disasters and everyone was feeling frail and helpless. It had a remarkable and variable psychological impact in various countries, depending on the phase of the pandemic. Also, certain features were distinct to psychological presentations of the catastrophe. First, the overlapping of psychological issues was very frequent i.e. anxious people may also have depression and smoke or drink alcohol to reduce the problem. Second, normal individuals presented with psychological problems were overwhelmed by an exceptional stressor. And thirdly, a huge number of people presenting with pandemic associated psychological disturbances got better naturally over time or with brief psychological support. As a consequence, these presentations did not necessarily lead to an overtly psychiatric diagnosis. A report published by W.H.O. following a survey conducted on 130 countries provides the first global data screening the devastating impact of COVID-19 in form of compromised access to mental health services, reduced compliance and poor supervision of patients leading to disruption of mental health services in nearly 93% of countries worldwide, while the demand kept on increasing, underscoring the urgent need for surge in funding [12]. Unfortunately, in a frantic search for biological cure and vaccines against the virus, these issues were all the more neglected, contributing to an increased public health burden. Forced into physical separateness we were united by a common trauma, a common fear as all of us were terrified for our own safety and that of our loved ones.

## 4. Preceding pandemics and mental health

Previous researches reveal profound and wide range of impact on mental health of individuals, communities and countries, during past outbreak of infectious diseases primarily on disease survivors (Ebola, SARS) [13]. Studies report adverse psychological symptoms in the form of mood alteration, insomnia, anger and emotional exhaustion. The psychological trauma of bereavement during Middle East Respiratory Syndrome (MERS) outbreak showed that surviving individuals were stigmatized, marginalized and socially isolated even after successful treatment [11]. Literature published during Severe Acute Respiratory Syndrome (SARS) outbreak a decade ago suggested 50% of health care workers (HCW) were at an increased risk of acute distress syndrome (ADS) during these periods [14]. Moreover, long term behavioral changes in the form of vigilant hand washing and avoidance of crowds many months even after quarantine have been reported, depicting that pandemic and isolation has a definite long-term impact on the mental health of humans [15].

## 5. COVID-19 and its symptoms of mental disruption

The emotional and psychological effects of COVID-19 outbreak ranged from biological factors like the neurotropic effects of SARS-CoV-2 (causative agent of COVID-19) and involvement of limbic system along with its psychological factors of fear, discomfort, uncertainty, anger, addiction, socioeconomic issues of isolation, xenophobia, stigma, domestic-violence, loss of livelihoods and constraint of open spaces. Global studies have established COVID-19 to be increasingly associated with neuropsychiatric manifestations such as delirium, anxiety, depressive disorders, insomnia and incidences of increased self-harm. Meanwhile, COVID-19 itself can progress to neurological and mental complications like delirium, stroke, cerebrovascular accidents, seizures and agitation that can have added psychiatric associations. Further on, those with pre-existing psychiatric conditions might be at increased risk of COVID infection due to lack of supervision and inadequate compliance to many precautionary measures [16]. The emotional outcome of subjects who were quarantined compared to those who were not, shows presence of acute stress disorder, anxiety, irritability, insomnia, boredom, poor concentration and performance, post-traumatic stress disorder (PTSD) and nervousness. Other psychological reactions reported during mass quarantine were generalized fear, collective hysteria and pervasive community anxiety. These symptoms are typically associated with disease outbreaks and escalation of new cases, together with inadequate anxiety provoking information provided by the media [15]. Reports of people emptying supermarkets and panic buying was indicative of their escalated levels of anxiety [4]. Anxiety may be related to sensorial deprivation and pervasive loneliness initially in the form of insomnia and later progressing to depression and PTSD. Moreover, other health measures get compromised in presence of abnormally elevated anxiety. The butterfly effect of increased anxiety and depression could also lead to a global increase in chronic illnesses including heart-disease-related deaths as people diagnosed with depression are up to five-times more likely to die within six months of having had a heart attack than those without depression [17]. Factors associated with a greater psychological vulnerability seem to be more important than factors associated with the risk of infection in predicting mental health consequences of the pandemic. Furthermore, symptoms of the infection, such as fever, myalgia, hypoxia and cough, as well as adverse effects of treatment, such as insomnia caused by corticosteroids, led to feelings of fear of contracting COVID-19 causing worsening of anxiety and mental distress. As mental and physical health are equally important and closely connected, a sound state of mental health plays a crucial role in people's ability to maintain good physical health. **Table 1** shows the various research conducted globally to study the impact of COVID -19 on mental health.

Zhao et al. highlighted that even close contacts of people with COVID-19 experienced distress and prolonged mental health consequences including severe depression and chronic fatigue in the post-COVID period in a study comprising 1169 close contacts. The study revealed that old age, heavy financial loss and perception of poor health were significantly associated with depression in them while the cause of fatigue reported

*DOI: http://dx.doi.org/10.5772/intechopen.102947*

| Sl. No. | Study | Sample characteristics | Research tool | Outcome |
|---|---|---|---|---|
| 1. | Varshney et al. [18] | Cross- sectional study of 1106 participants across India | IES(R) | One-third participants had psychological impact (mostly mild) which was higher in younger age group and female participants |
| 2. | Khanna et al. [19] | 2355 Ophthalmologists | Mean patient health questionnaire score | One-third participants had depressive symptoms (mostly mild). Predictor of depression being young age, gender, marital status and profession |
| 3. | Chandu et al. [20] | 307 participants | COVID-19 related Anxiety scale | Higher anxiety in lower educational qualification group |
| 4. | Narsimhan et al. [21] | Hospital based study with 96 alcoholic middle-aged males | Changepoint analysis | 95% participants reported alcohol withdrawal symptoms due to sudden cessation of alcohol during lockdown. |
| 5. | Roy et al. [22] | Cross- sectional study with 662 participants in Indian Population | Online Semi-Structured Questionnaire | 80% participants were preoccupied with thoughts of COVID-19. 72% reported overuse of gloves and sanitizer, 37.8% had paranoia about acquiring the infection, 36.4% had distress related to social media and 12.5% had sleep disturbances |
| 6. | Grover et al. [23] | Cross sectional study with 1685 participants | PHQ-9, GAD-7 Warwick Edinburgh mental well- being scale | 74.1% had moderate stress, 40.5% had either depression or anxiety, 38.2% had anxiety and 10.5% had depression |
| 7. | Chakarborty and Chatterjee [24] | Regional survey of 507 participants from West Bengal, India | Self-designed questionnaire | 71.8% and 24.7% showed increased worries and depressive symptoms during pandemic. 69.6% were worried about the financial loss, 30.8% perceived higher health anxiety and feared it to continue post lockdown |
| 8. | Chatterjee et al. [25] | Cross sectional study of 152 doctors | DASS-21 | 34.9%, 39.5% and 32.9% were depressed, anxious and stressed respectively. Stigma and discrimination against frontline workers were important factors contributing to stress. |
| 9. | Mohindra et al. [26] | 3083 HCWs across north India | Interview | 23.9% of HCWs reported anxiety disorder and 20% depression which was higher in females, aged and unmarried participants |
| 10. | Wang et al. [27] | 1210 participants across China | IES(R) and DASS-21 scales | 53.8% participants had a psychological impact (moderate or severe); 16.5%, 28.8% and 8.1% reported moderate to severe depression, anxiety and stress |

| Sl. No. | Study | Sample characteristics | Research tool | Outcome |
|---|---|---|---|---|
| 11. | Rehman et al. [28] | 403 participants | Family affluence scale, Response accuracy scale and DASS | Students and HCWs had higher depression, anxiety and stress, which was negatively correlated with family affluence. |
| 12 | Gao et al. [29] | Cross sectional study of 4827 participants China | GAD-7, WHO-5 | 22.6% had anxiety while 48.3% suffered from depression |
| 13 | Gonzalez Sanguino et al. [30] | Cross sectional study of 3480 participants across Spain | GAD-2, PCL-C-2, PHQ-2 | 21.6% had Anxiety, 18.7% had Depression while 15.8% had PTSD symptoms |
| 14 | Mazza et al. [31] | Cross-sectional study of 2766 participants conducted in Italy | DASS-21 | 18.7% suffered from anxiety, 32.7% Depression and 27.2% had stress |
| 15 | Sonderskov et al. [32] | Cross-sectional study of 2458 participants conducted in Denmark | WHO-5 | 25.4% suffered from Depression |

**Table 1.**
*Various studies conducted across globe depicting adverse impacts of COVID-19 on mental health.*

was frequent use of mass media [33]. Among the varied corollaries of the pandemic, one among them was diametrically opposite incidences of both alcohol abuse as well as alcohol withdrawal symptoms in different circumstances due to sudden lockdown. The migrant labourers who represent 4.7% of the global labour workforce along with refugees, having limited access to healthcare, living in overcrowded environments, working in marginalized sectors and lacking workplace and social protection were the worst sufferers of pandemic and economic shutdown [16]. Researches depict that people working on site, within lower income bracket, job loss and households with children under the age of 18 yrs. were more likely to report negative mental health outcome in form of anxiety, stress or depression [34]. Lack of authentic information, dissatisfaction with fulfillment of basic needs, poor sleep quality, ambiguity about SARS-CoV-2 and a relatively lower confidence in health care fraternity could be the stipulated reason for ongoing extreme stress.

## 6. Challenges faced with age, sex and profession

Even though the SARS-CoV-2 was considered a public health calamity, certain sections of the society were at clearly defined risk and the morbidity as well as mortality correlated well with age, sex, profession and socio-economic conditions. This exposed the existing socio-economic, gender, ethnic and health inequities present in the social determinants of health community and exacerbated it some extent [35].

### 6.1 Children

In March 2020, schools across India were shut down to curb the transmission of infection. But now, children have been at home for longer periods of time than ever before in recent memory. Closure of schools led to disruption of their daily routine along with lack of extracurricular and outdoor activities. This sudden unexpected

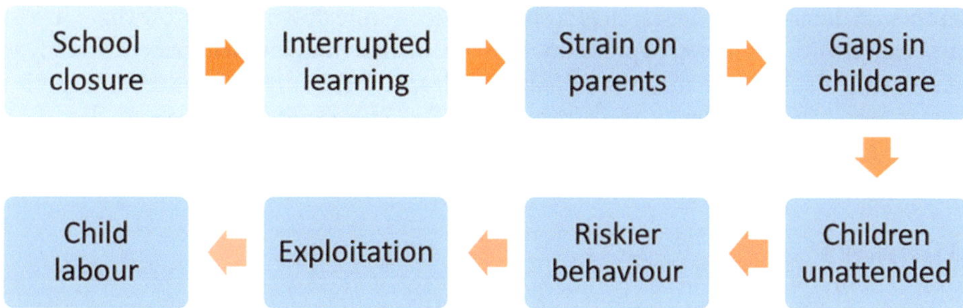


**Figure 1.**
*Depicting the domino effect of school closure on children.*

change caused altered eating and sleep habits, anguish, irritation and lack of peer time fostering monotony and diverse neuropsychiatric symptoms in them. Commonly reported psychological problems among them were inattention, clinginess, boredom, irritability, restlessness, nervousness, distraction and stress about the pandemic with the risk greatly increasing in those already suffering from some form of mental disorder. The domino effect of school closure on children is shown in **Figure 1**.

The social disruption which happened due to job loss, progressed to financial insecurity and threatened loss of loved ones impacting the quality of family relationship between parents and children causing a significant risk of adjustment to more than 370 million children in India, given their dependence on positive family processes for a host of developmental outcomes [30]. As COVID deaths among adults occurred within weeks, the families had little or no time to prepare for mental trauma and agony that a child underwent in a case of death of a parent or caregiver. An estimated 1.5 million children globally, experienced orphanhood either due to sudden death of their parents or death of their custodian grandparents or kin due to COVID-19. Such children usually face poverty, physical, emotional and sexual violence apart from depression, family separation and institutionalization in upcoming days [36]. Although home is the safest place for a child, physical, sexual and psychological abuse saw a significant rise in numbers and severity during the pandemic leading to heightened child abuse related hospitalizations. Child abuse leads to immediate emotional and psychological problems and an adverse childhood experience linked to possible mental illness, substance abuse and suicidal ideation later in life.

### 6.2 Adults

Young adults (<35 yrs.) experienced pandemic related consequences in form of closure of universities, uncertainty about future, financial crisis and space crunch that contributed to poor mental health. The stigmatizing psychological pressure of performance during the timespan when universities were shut led to aggravated feeling of guilt, shame, regret, sadness, self-pity, anger, internalized emotions, overwhelmed feelings, negative self-talk, unrealistic expectations and perceived sense of failure among the ones who could not perform due to various reasons [11]. Some of the reviewed studies have highlighted increased correlation of social media exposure with psychological issues like hampered social communication, sleep deprivation and increased gaming behavior, that was inversely related to physical activity in students and finally impairing their overall health [16]. Researches from prior economic downturns show that job loss is associated with increased depression, anxiety, distress and low self-esteem leading to higher rates of substance abuse and "deaths of despair". A study done on 1543 respondents to assess the prevalence of distress found 21–35 years old more prone to distress as compared to other age groups, maybe due to heavy pressure of managing finances along with reduced resilience and coping mechanisms [4, 33].

### 6.3 Geriatrics

Older adults were susceptible both to the virus and to its psychological impact as they have unique physical, psychosocial and environmental vulnerabilities owing to frailty [37]. Latest reports from Nature Medicine quoted those below 30 and above 59 years were 0.6 and 5.1 times more likely to die after developing symptoms respectively. According to the Centre for Disease Control and Prevention (CDC), people having chronic illness such as chronic lung diseases, asthma, serious heart conditions and diabetes are at an increased risk of COVID-19. Moreover, mental health disorders are a common comorbidity among older adults, which may get exacerbated by their fear and trepidation of being vulnerable to severe illness from COVID-19 [34]. This form of stress is associated with reduction in immunity compounding the already weakened physiological defense systems in an elderly. Recently, a study found that 18% individuals who received a COVID-19 diagnosis were later diagnosed with a mental health disorder such as anxiety or mood disorder and both was found to have a higher prevalence in the older age group as compared to middle aged and youngsters [38]. Neglected older people can even serve as vulnerable 'hidden pockets' of viral load that can contribute to increased infection spread due to under-reporting of the psychiatric symptoms in them. This leads to under-detection of symptoms, faulty treatment and increased prevalence of them being asymptomatic carriers. Higher viral load and virulence among geriatrics increases the fatality rate from 3.6% in 60–69 yrs. suddenly to 18% in more than 80 years [37]. Loneliness, especially when chronic and associated with lack of physical activity is a potent risk factor for depression and cognitive disorders. In 2018, an estimated 27% adults aged 65 and above were reportedly living alone [34]. In face of older elderlies not being well-versed with technology, their inability to conduct virtual meetings led to increase distancing during the pandemic. Finally, the social stigma of ageism magnified by COVID-19 outbreak led to marginalization, segregation, abuse, increased institutionalization and suicidal ideation among senior citizens. Banerjee et al. has shown increased depressive disorders, PTSD and adjustment reactions in geriatrics due to the pandemic [38]. On the other hand, poor perception of one's own health could lead to health-related anxiety which may further result in depression, headache, insomnia, and even suicidal tendency in the aged [33].

### 6.4 Females

Females reported elevated distress due to closure of schools and day care with increased household chores along with their regular professional work during times of crisis and quarantine. Apart from this, women also faced the brunt of domestic violence, which was reportedly at an all-time high since last 10 yrs. in India during COVID lockdown [30]. Generally, both prior to and during the pandemic, women have reported higher rates of anxiety and depression compared to men. Further, it was observed that the recovery rate of unemployment post-national lockdown in India was lower in case of females as compared to males and the gaps seems to have widened [6].

### 6.5 Health Care Workers

It appears that disaster management workforce was itself not immune to the psychological consequences of the pandemic. While others were under strict vigil of lockdown and quarantine, the local hospitals continued to receive suddenly thousands of critically ill COVID-19 patients and were forced to implement their emergency protocols [15]. With overwhelming hospitals and a rapidly increasing demand along with supply shortage, frontline HCW were put to immense stress. Previous studies on the infectious outbreaks of SARS, MERS and Ebola have revealed the severity of emotional distress among medical practitioners and law enforcing agents who faced PTSD, depression, anxiety, exhaustion and burnout at the onset, during and even after the outbreak of such epidemics [11]. A study conducted on 1563 health professionals found roughly half of them to suffer from depression, whereas 44.7% and 36.1% from anxiety and sleep disturbances. Higher depression, anxiety and acute overall psychological burden was reported particularly in those directly diagnosing and treating COVID cases [34]. Spoorthy et al. suggested that 68.7%–85.5% of medical staff comprises of females and were likely to be affected in the COVID-19 pandemic by elevated degrees of anxiety, distress and depression [39]. Psychological symptoms were frankly correlated with increased duty hours, lack of shift rotations, societal stigma, inadequate medical protective equipment, increased witness to death and dying, increased risk of exposure and self-blame, as well as the guilt and fear of spreading the infection to the family members [39, 40]. They suffered the worst sleep quality and sleep time. The discrimination, isolation, negative emotions of patients and lack of contact with own families for long led to frustration and hopelessness. Some studies have even depicted burnout of young nurses and found them to be more anxious and depressed when compared to doctors, which could be accounted due to low nurse to patient density (**Figure 2**) [39].

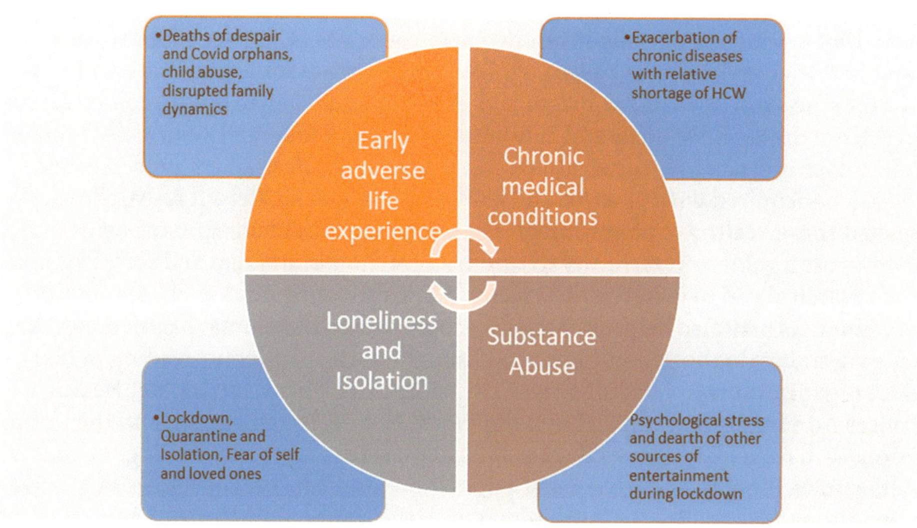


**Figure 2.**
*The text in the inner circle depicts the probable causes of mental health disorders while that in the boxes depict how those circumstances were created and got aggravated due to COVID-19.*

## 7. What can be done now?

Although government regulations were necessary to maintain social balance and guarantee the safety of individuals, a strategy to deal with psychosocial issues related to the crisis and its consequences in the community was relatively lacking [15].

History has shown that mental health impact of pandemics outlasts the physical impact, suggesting that today's elevated mental health need may continue well beyond the coronavirus outbreak itself and we may be heading towards an outbreak of a second pandemic, that of mental health crisis. As people faced the onslaught of pandemic related stressors, they wished and wanted to lean over, on each other for connection and coping strategies to ease the weight of public health crisis on their mental health, which was sadly cut down due to lockdown and isolation. Dissatisfaction with levels of social interaction led to negative affect which was further associated with a slowing of passage of time. The slower the passage of time, the higher was the negative emotions experienced escalating the feelings of helplessness and anxiety. A report highlights that the number of adults with anxiety or depression in U.S. increased four-hundred percent in the sixteen months following COVID-related lockdowns [11].

As rightly said by Dr. Tedros Adhanom, DG of W.H.O. "Good mental health is absolutely fundamental to overall health and wellbeing" [12]. During this public health emergency when the external environment is not in our control, it is imperative to focus on building and strengthening our mental immunity. People with strong psychological resilience and a healthy life appear to be less affected by COVID-19. This statement underpins that fear of pandemic disrupts people's psychology and the psychology of those who had an underlying illness before the pandemic or had family or friends who were infected or had died. Therefore, psychological resilience and being healthy are important individual characteristics that can be developed in facing the fear of COVID-19 and the psychological problems caused by this fear [41]. Other lessons learnt are that safety policies, accurate information dissemination about pandemic prevention and pandemic prevention impacts should be emphasized. There was a negative influence of attitudinal construct and mythical behavior on disease prevention practices especially in South-Asian countries [42]. Peer support, risk averse behavior and internet based cognitive behavior are some pragmatic implications for stress management at macro and micro level during an epidemiological level. Apart from these, individuals and communities could deliberately cultivate resilience, healthy coping strategies, mindfulness and well-being. These all are processes and they can be acquired with practice and learned dynamically. Recent researches have depicted those healthy coping strategies have helped individuals to stay positive, view lockdown as a golden opportunity to ruminate on their individual and social identity and to march ahead to enhance their skills [43]. Cultivating a sense of community belongingness may also help and prepare people to face the mental health issues that they may endure in the upcoming days. Throughout the pandemic, leading public health organizations — including the CDC, Substance Abuse and Mental Health Services Administration (SAMHSA), the World Health Organization, and the United Nations — have released general considerations and resources addressing the mental health and well-being of both general populations and specifically high-risk groups during the pandemic [34]. In India, along with the National Institute of Mental Health and Neurosciences (NIMHANS), the Indian Psychiatric Society also brought out a rulebook for effective mental health management titled "Mental Health Challenges during COVID-19 pandemic: Guidance for psychiatrists. It covers telepsychiatry, psychopharmacology, and brain stimulation practices during COVID-19, also catering to special populations like children and adolescents, older adults, perinatal groups and rehabilitation settings and can be referred.

In general, mental health and related issues are not recognized in public and with global pandemic these silent and insidious issues can be either misdiagnosed or go unnoticed completely. Thus, the role of mental health professional can be vital in this regard especially in educating, training, encouraging mental health-promoting behaviors, maintaining cross-specialty integration, facilitating problems solving approaches, empowering patients and allied professionals, and finally enabling self-care strategies for resilience [16]. Despite the common mental health problems and disorders among patients and HCW during the pandemic, most health professionals working in isolation units and hospitals did not receive any training in providing mental health care [13]. In this regard, mental health services, facilities and specialized psychiatric treatment teams including psychologists, psychiatrists and psychiatric nurses should be established to address psychological health concerns in the general public and we need to validate and value their immense selfless contribution. W.H.O. has previously highlighted the chronic underfunding of mental health prior to the pandemic, but the pandemic has suddenly increased its requirement, especially in the South Asian countries which suffer from an inadequate psychiatrist-patient ratio. Based on this, the Primary Care first and Collaborative Care model which has been suggested by Türközer and Öngür, teletherapy: Telemedicine and teletherapy should be established to provide psychological help which can be a boon during restrictive conditions of an infectious disease outbreak like COVID-19, but at the same time, limited accessibility and poor Internet connectivity in various areas are the existing challenges. Standardization of treatment, online surveys and local management of stable patients to reduce risk of infections can also be of help during this crisis [16]. It is suggested that public health machinery should conduct mental health audits during epidemiological emergencies which are critical for effective management of community mental health. Bouncing forwards for a new normal, we need to:

- Identify people at risk during clinical visit or teleconsultation, especially younger age, females and those having a preexisting mental health condition for which COVID-19 data disaggregated by characteristics such as age, gender, sex and race are needed to help tackle the health inequalities.

- Screen for psychiatric and psychosocial effects of social distancing of vulnerable population.

- Ask direct questions about wellbeing and safety at home.

- Specialized psychiatric treatments and appropriate mental health services for patients with comorbid mental disorders.

- Tremendous interconnectedness including cross country collaboration and research [4, 13, 16].

## 8. Prevention of future pandemics

Intergovernmental Platform on Biodiversity and Ecosystem Services (IPBES) hints at more severe and frequent pandemics in coming times. SARS, MERS, H1N1 to name a few along with COVID-19 testify to its damage [44]. With more than 2/3rd of the recently emerging diseases and almost all known pandemics being zoonotic diseases, following are some of the probable reasons of spill over of diseases from other organisms to humans, which needs to be addressed on a priority basis:

- **Deforestation:** With deforestation of over 25%, human and their livestock are likely to contact wildlife leading to vectors probably feeding near human settlements. Such contacts lead to and determine risk of novel human virus transmission.

- **Wildlife trade spill over:** Markets that sell wild animals have been the hotbeds of diseases. The US agency for international development (USAID) PREDICT project analyzed the spill over of viruses in people with high wildlife contact in as high as 31 countries.

The risk further increases with climate change, intensive farming and international travels enabling disease to spread across the world at an alarming rate. The estimated present cost of prevention of pandemics for 10 years is estimated to be only 2% of the cost incurred during the COVID-19 pandemic. A few stringent steps can go a long way in detection and managing them. Working on these lines, December 27th is proclaimed as the international day of Epidemic Preparedness – a day to embark on the importance of prevention of, preparedness for and partnership against epidemics like COVID-19. To prevent and be prepared for future pandemics, we need to invest in 4 core spheres i.e., surveillance, early detection and control, manufacturing and coordinated research and development.

- **Surveillance:** Effective surveillance for faster detection and control of diseases requires a multidisciplinary approach integrating meteorological, veterinary and medical surveillance with livestock farmers and local community playing a key role. It includes risk characterization and participatory surveillance of unusual events along with animal supply chains. Laws enforcing the ban of national and international trade in high-risk diseases reservoir species should be enforced to control zoonotic diseases. In this context, Regional Wildlife Enforcement Network (WEN's) and Convention on International Trade in Endangered Species of Fauna and Flora (CITES) should be strengthened which could form part of an effective response frontier. Building locally owned and internationally connected genomic surveillance network will also ensure that we can spot potential dangers and prevent future pandemics.

- **Early detection and Control**: SARS and COVID emerged as respiratory disease outbreaks in Guangdong and Wuhan respectively but the serological survey of people at Yunnan, a nearby province showed 3% had antibodies to similar virus species from their principal reservoir. This proves that there's substantial under-reporting of exposure to zoonotic diseases. Lags in detection and identification of diseases have decreased with time but still varies geographically, especially in economically weaker countries.

- **Manufacturing:** There is an urgent need to increase the regional manufacturing capacity for drugs and vaccines in low- and middle-income nations or regions, which go a long way to prevent and control future pandemics globally and ensuring that local needs are met. Kusuma et al. revealed that unavailability of protective gears including face masks and sanitisers adversely affected the COVID-19 prevention adoption in 4 south Asian countries including India.

- **Co-ordinated Research and Development**: Since the inception of pandemic, the world has seen an incremental investment in research, distribution and manufacturing of COVID-19 tests treatment and vaccines. Paradoxically the same increase in Research and Development for other infectious diseases of becoming pandemics of tomorrow is not witnessed. Given the cross-border nature of pandemics, international boards like world health organization (W.H.O.) or the Global fund should work through existing global health architecture [45].

And for such a rigorous pandemic preparedness, we need to have a sound financial footing and a collective investment globally, to support the key gaps in infrastructure. The emergence of SARS-CoV-2 showed the limits of current approach and the overall long reaction time of international reporting systems. The need of the hour is to improve global coordination and leadership while action is needed at local, national and regional levels. Establishing a trusted dialog between scientists, politicians and public could also be helpful if we want to act fast. The participation of community health workers who play a crucial role in covering the last mile in delivery of services also cannot go unacknowledged. International agencies like FAO, WHO need to endorse these decisions on a slow roll out plan when the prevalence of cases is low and show the advantages of long-term investment in proper system [46].

## 9. Conclusion and future directions

The infamous COVID-19, apart from being highly contagious, had severe physical, social and psychological manifestations in the form of isolation, quarantine and lockdown which hampered our social support system on a large scale. COVID-19 looks to be a lingering stressor and is bound to induce acute panic, anxiety, obsessive behavior, paranoia, depression and PTSD in long term even if the cases subside. The notable psychological consequences looming out of this disaster need to be addressed. Altered mental status and behavioral changes have been mentioned to be acute effects of the virus, and a putative link between those affected with COVID-19 and long-term psychiatric comorbidities might merit further research. So, all efforts should be directed towards minimizing the negative effects of this traumatic pandemic event on mankind including its mental health implications. Lessons learnt from this pandemic can help shape interventions and legislations in the near future. Therefore, either we identify the probable rising impact on mental health and work upon it or we will pay the price in the form of worsened quality of life in the post pandemic aftermath when we will need all the able bodies to help the world economy recover.

## Author details

Swati Mittal[1*], Smriti Sinha[2] and Shilpi Bhat[3]

1 Department of Physiology, All India Institute of Medical Sciences, Deoghar, Jharkhand, India

2 Department of Physiology, Apollo Institute of Medical Sciences and Research, Hyderabad, Telangana, India

3 Department of Physiology, School of Medical Sciences and Research, Greater Noida, Uttar Pradesh, India

*Address all correspondence to: drswatimittals@gmail.com

## References

[1] Umakanthan S, Sahu P, Ranade AV, Bukelo MM, Rao JS, Abrahao-Machado LF, et al. Origin, transmission, diagnosis and management of coronavirus disease 2019 (COVID-19). Postgraduate Medical Journal. 2020 Dec;**96**(1142):753-758. DOI: 10.1136/postgradmedj-2020-138234

[2] Paital B, Das K, Parida SK. Inter nation social lockdown versus medical care against COVID-19, a mild environmental insight with special reference to India. Science of the Total Environment. 2020;**728**:138914

[3] Lau H, Khosrawipour V, Kocbach P, Mikolajczyk A, Schubert J, Bania J, et al. The positive impact of lockdown in Wuhan on containing the COVID-19 outbreak in China. Journal of Travel Medicine. 2020 May 18;**27**(3):taaa037

[4] Anand V, Verma L, Aggarwal A, Nanjundappa P, Rai H. COVID-19 and psychological distress: Lessons for India. PLoS One. 2021;**16**(8):e0255683

[5] Tirivayi N et al. A rapid review of economic policy and social protection responses to health and economic crises and their effects on children. Innocenti Working Papers. No. 2020-02. Innocenti, Florence: UNICEF Office of Research; 2020

[6] Kumar O, Srivastava S. Impact of COVID-19 on employment in urban areas. 17 Sept 2021. Available from: https://prsindia.org/theprsblog/impact-of-covid-19-on-unemployment-in-urban-areas

[7] Kaplan J, Frias L, McFall-Johnsen M. A third of the global population is on coronavirus lockdown — Here's our constantly updated list of countries and restrictions. Morgan Mcfail: Juliana Kaplan, Lauren Frias; 2020. Retrieved from: https://www.businessinsider.com/countries-on-lockdown-coronavirus-italy-2020-3?IR=T

[8] World Health Organization. Promoting Mental Health: Concepts, Emerging Evidence, Practice (Summary Report). Geneva: World Health Organization; 2004

[9] Galderisi S, Heinz A, Kastrup M, Beezhold J, Sartorius N. Toward a new definition of mental health. World Psychiatry. 2015;**14**(2):231-233

[10] Schäfer SK, Sopp MR, Schanz CG, Staginnus M, Göritz AS, Michael T. Impact of COVID-19 on public mental health and the buffering effect of a sense of coherence. Psychotherapy and Psychosomatics. 2020;**89**(6):386-392

[11] Mukhtar S. Psychological health during the coronavirus disease 2019 pandemic outbreak. The International Journal of Social Psychiatry. 2020;**66**(5):512-516

[12] World Mental Health Day on 10 October to highlight urgent need to increase investment in chronically underfunded sector. 5 October 2020. Available from: https://www.who.int/news/item/05-10-2020-covid-19-disrupting-mental-health-services-in-most-countries-who-survey

[13] Xiang YT. Timely mental health care for the 2019 novel coronavirus outbreak is urgently needed. The Lancet Psychiatry. 2020;**7**:228-229

[14] Wu KK, Chan SK, Ma TM. Posttraumatic stress after SARS. Emerging Infectious Diseases. 2005;**11**:1297-1300

[15] Serafini G, Parmigiani B, Amerio A, AgugliaA, Sher L, Amore M. The psychological impact of COVID-19 on the mental health in the general population, QJM: An International Journal of Medicine. Aug 2020;**113**(8):531-537

[16] Banerjee D, Vaishnav M, Sathyanarayana Rao TS, Raju MS, Dalal PK, Javed A, et al. Impact of the COVID-19 pandemic on psychosocial health and well-being in south-Asian (world psychiatric association zone 16) countries: A systematic and advocacy review from the Indian psychiatric society. Indian Journal of Psychiatry. 2020;**62**(Suppl S3):343-353

[17] Khawaja IS, Westermeyer JJ, Gajwani P, Feinstein RE. Depression and coronary artery disease: The association, mechanisms, and therapeutic implications. Psychiatry (Edgmont). 2009;**6**(1):38-51

[18] Varshney M, Parel JT, Raizada N, Sarin SK. Initial psychological impact of COVID-19 and its correlates in Indian community: An online (FEEL-COVID) survey. PLoS One. 2020;**15**:e0233874

[19] Khanna RC, Honavar SG, Metla AL, Bhattacharya A, Maulik PK. Psychological impact of COVID-19 on ophthalmologists-in-training and practising ophthalmologists in India. Indian Journal of Ophthalmology. 2020;**68**:994-998

[20] Chandu VC, Pachava S, Vadapalli V, Marella Y. Development and initial validation of the COVID-19 anxiety scale. Indian Journal of Public Health. 2020;**64**:S201-S204

[21] Narasimha VL, Shukla L, Mukherjee D, Menon J, Huddar S, Panda UK, et al. Complicated alcohol withdrawal-an unintended consequence of COVID-19 lockdown. Alcohol and Alcoholism. 2020;**55**:350-353

[22] Roy D, Tripathy S, Kar SK, Sharma N, Verma SK, Kaushal V. Study of knowledge, attitude, anxiety perceived mental healthcare need in Indian population during COVID-19 pandemic. Asian Journal of Psychiatry. 2020;**51**:102083

[23] Grover S, Sahoo S, Mehra A, Avasthi A, Tripathi A, Subramanyan A, et al. Psychological impact of COVID19 lockdown: An online survey from India. Indian Journal of Psychiatry. 2020;**62**:354

[24] Chakraborty K, Chatterjee M. Psychological impact of COVID19 pandemic on general population in West Bengal: A cross-sectional study. Indian Journal of Psychiatry. 2020;**62**:266-272

[25] Chatterjee SS, Bhattacharyya R, Bhattacharyya S, Gupta S, Das S, Banerjee BB. Attitude, practice, behavior, and mental health impact of COVID-19 on doctors. Indian Journal of Psychiatry. 2020;**62**:257-265

[26] Mohindra RRR, Suri V, Bhalla A, Singh SM. Issues relevant to mental health promotion in frontline health care providers managing quarantined/isolated COVID19 patients. Asian Journal of Psychiatry. Jun 2020;**51**:102084. DOI: 10.1016/j.ajp.2020.102084. Epub 2020 Apr 7. PMID: 32289728; PMCID: PMC7138416

[27] Wang C, Pan R, Wan X, Tan Y, Xu L, Ho CS, et al. Immediate psychological responses and associated factors during the initial stage of the 2019 coronavirus disease (COVID-19) epidemic among the general population in China. International Journal of Environmental Research and Public Health. 2020;**17**:1729

[28] Rehman U, Shahnawaz MG, Khan NH, Kharshiing KD, Khursheed M,

Gupta K, et al. Depression, anxiety and stress among Indians in times of COVID-19 lockdown. Community Mental Health Journal. 2020;**57**:42-48

[29] Gao J, Zheng P, Jia Y, Chen H, Mao Y, Chen S, et al. Mental health problems and social media exposure during COVID-19 outbreak. PLoS One. 16 Apr 2020;**15**(4):e0231924. DOI: 10.1371/journal.pone.0231924. PMID: 32298385; PMCID: PMC7162477

[30] Parekh BJ, Dalwai SH. Psychosocial impact of COVID-19 pandemic on children in India. Indian Pediatrics. 15 Dec 2020;**57**(12):1107

[31] Mazza C, Ricci E, Biondi S, Colasanti M, Ferracuti S, Napoli C, et al. A nationwide survey of psychological distress among Italian people during the COVID-19 pandemic: Immediate psychological responses and associated factors. International Journal of Environmental Research and Public Health. 2020;**17**:3165

[32] Sønderskov KM, Dinesen PT, Santini ZI, Østergaard SD. The depressive state of Denmark during the COVID-19 pandemic. Acta Neuropsychiatrica. Aug 2020;**32**(4):226-228. DOI: 10.1017/neu.2020.15. Epub 2020 Apr 22. PMID: 32319879; PMCID: PMC7176490

[33] Zhao YJ, Zhang SF, Li W, et al. Mental health status and quality of life in close contacts of COVID-19 patients in the post-COVID-19 era: A comparative study. Translational Psychiatry. 2021;**11**:505

[34] Song L, Wang Y, Li Z, Yang Y, Li H. Mental health and work attitudes among people resuming work during the COVID-19 Pandemic: A Cross-Sectional Study in China. International Journal of Environmental Research and Public Health. 2020;**17**(14):5059 [Published: 2020 Jul 14]

[35] Mittal S, Sinha S. Impact of coronavirus disease-19 lockdown on psychological and mental health status among residents of Delhi-National Capital Region. National Journal of Physiology, Pharmacy and Pharmacology. 2021;**11**(9):964-970. [cited February 19, 2022] DOI: 10.5455/njppp.2021.11.02057202109042021

[36] Hillis SD, Unwin HJT, Chen Y, Cluver L, Sherr L, Goldman PS, et al. Global minimum estimates of children affected by COVID-19-associated orphanhood and deaths of caregivers: A modelling study. Lancet. 31 Jul 2021;**398**(10298):391-402. DOI: 10.1016/S0140-6736(21)01253-8

[37] Banerjee D. Age and ageism in COVID-19′: Elderly mental health-care vulnerabilities and needs. Asian Journal of Psychiatry. 2020;**51**:102154

[38] Panchal N, Kamal R, Cox C, Garfield R. The implications of COVID-19 for Mental Health and Substance Use. 10 Feb 2021. Available from: @cynthiaccox on Twitter

[39] Spoorthy MS, Pratapa SK, Mahant S. Mental health problems faced by healthcare workers due to the COVID-19 pandemic-a review. Asian Journal of Psychiatry. 2020;**51**:102119

[40] Kar SK, Yasir Arafat SM, Kabir R, Sharma P, Saxena SK. Coping with mental health challenges during COVID-19. Coronavirus Disease 2019 (COVID-19). Apr 2020;**30**:199-213. DOI: 10.1007/978-981-15-4814-7_16. PMCID: PMC7189395

[41] Koçak O, Koçak ÖE, Younis MZ. The psychological consequences of COVID-19 fear and the moderator effects of individuals' underlying illness and witnessing infected friends and family. International Journal of Environmental

Research and Public Health. 13 Feb 2021;**18**(4):1836. DOI: 10.3390/ijerph18041836. PMID: 33668655; PMCID: PMC7917729

[42] Ahmad M, Akhtar N, Jabeen G, Irfan M, Khalid Anser M, Wu H, et al. Intention-based critical factors affecting willingness to adopt novel coronavirus prevention in Pakistan: Implications for *Future Pande*mics. International Journal of Environmental Research and Public Health. 7 Jun 2021;**18**(11):6167. DOI: 10.3390/ijerph18116167. PMID: 34200335; PMCID: PMC8200947

[43] Sharma AJ, Subramanyam MA. Psychological Impact of Covid-19 Lockdown in India: Different Strokes for Different Folks. med Rxiv preprint. 2020

[44] IPBES workshop on biodiversity and pandemics executive summary. Intergovernmental Platform on Biodiversity and Ecosystem Services. Available from: https://ipbes.net/sites/default/files/2020-11/20201028%20IPBES%20Pandemics%20Workshop%20Exec%20Summ%20Laid%20Out%20Final.pdf

[45] Dobson AP, Pimm SL, Hannah L, Kaufman L, Ahumada JA, Ando AW, et al. Ecology and economics for pandemic prevention. Science. 24 Jul 2020;**369**(6502):379-381

[46] Conversation Media Group. In: Peyre M, Goutard FL, Roger F, Olive M-M, editors. 28 January 2021. Available from: https://www.preventionweb.net/news/keys-preventing-future-pandemics

Section 5

# Traumatic Stress and Suicide Behaviour

Chapter 11

# Lay Counselors' Mental Wellness in Suicide Prevention after Prolonged Mass Trauma: A Pre- and Post-Training Appraisal

*Emilio Ovuga, Henry Oboke, Anne Abio, Felix Kaducu Ocaka, Morten Sodemann and Ask Elklit*

## Abstract

Information on the mental wellness of lay counselors in Uganda is unavailable. Sixty representatives of three sub counties in Gulu District in Northern Uganda were equipped with counseling skills through 40 hours of training over 5 days. The trainees completed the 32-item Response Inventory for Stressful Life Events (RISLE) immediately before the commencement of the training and soon after the completion of the training. Pretest prevalence of suicide ideation was 9.3%, and posttest prevalence was 11.1%. Immediate post-training assessment showed better overall mental wellbeing as judged by overall RISLE scores, which were statistically significantly lower post-training than pre-training for gender ($P = 0.05$) and marital status ($P = 0.001$) on most RISLE scores. Qualitative assessment after 3 months of training showed that trainees were less suicidal, and they had improved psychosocial functioning. The current results point to the need to pay attention to the mental wellness of volunteer counselors and support them in their role in preventing suicide in areas of mass trauma. We recommend robust randomized community trials to determine the role of the mental wellbeing of volunteer lay counselors in the provision of psychological first aid to communities exposed to prolonged mass trauma.

**Keywords:** mass trauma, lay counselors, mental wellbeing, mental disorders, suicide ideation, suicidality, psychological first aid, northern Uganda

## 1. Introduction

Stress in the lives of humans under different names has attracted myriads of studies and publications since World War I (WW I). One of the most compelling books in the field is Herman's publication [1]. Protracted, catastrophic, and life-threatening events happen in daily life behind closed doors of families in the form of domestic violence, sexual abuse and defilement, political terror and wars, and natural disasters, and the diagnosis of terminal illness. Mental disorder in the form



IntechOpen

of post-traumatic stress disorder (PTSD) is so complex that misdiagnoses are common. Another influential book by Varmik Volkan [2] theorize that society accepts "*widespread violence,*" which begins with what Volkan has described "*chosen trauma.*" The defeat of one of the groups involved in intergroup conflict carries the painful memories of their humiliation for centuries as a result of historical details passed on from generation to generation in the hope that a future generation might be able to avenge them. Likewise, the victor in intergroup conflict keeps alive their chosen glory for as long as history can tell to ensure that their victory remains in memory. The stark implication of this is that traumatic stress remains in memory for the entire lives of affected people. According to Volkan, mass psychosis and suicide may follow organized ethnic or political violence. Several traumatic stress-related psychiatric disorders appear in the two main diagnostic systems, namely the Fifth Edition of the Diagnostic and Statistical Manual of Mental and Behavioral Disorders (DSM-V) of the American Psychiatric Association [3], and the eleventh edition of the International Classification of Diseases and Behavioral Disorders (ICD-11) of the World Health Organization [4].

Though not strictly a disorder, but rather, a consequence of other medical and psychiatric conditions, suicide has come to take a central position as one of the leading complications and comorbid health and social problems of stress disorders, occurring together with post-traumatic stress disorder (PTSD), depression, anxiety disorders, alcohol and substance use disorders, and general medical conditions. The risk of suicide is higher than in the general population as reported in anxiety disorders [5, 6], general physical conditions (Dome et al., 2019), and bipolar disorder [7]. In Uganda, a landlocked country in East Africa, a violent war took place between the Uganda government armed forces, the Uganda People's Defense Forces (UPDF), and a rebel army of the Lord's Resistance Army (LRA) in Northern Uganda from 1986 to 2006. Several publications have documented varying prevalence rates for depression, suicide, suicide ideation, and other consequences of the decade long civil war in Northern Uganda [8–10], Ovuga and Wasserman [11, 12].

As would be expected, one of the main goals of trauma therapy should aim to help trauma-affected persons to recover from trauma, minimize mental distress, improve community resilience and psychosocial functioning, and prevent suicide in the aftermath of mass trauma exposure. Unfortunately, little or no attempt aims to prevent suicide among trauma-exposed people. In situations of mass trauma, psychosocial support to trauma-exposed persons is limited to the provision of social amenities, the provision of protection and security guarantees, and other actions that aim to promote community cohesion and resilience. Suicide prevention work, which should be a key component of trauma therapy and psychosocial support, should include the creation of an awareness of potential self-destructive behavior occurring in communities affected by trauma. Following this step is the institution of measures to provide psychological services to trauma victims; and recognizing, assessing, and offering quality counseling services and specialist mental health care to people showing symptoms and signs of psychological distress or mental illness. An optimal outcome of such an intervention occurs when suicide prevention work takes place at community level close to where trauma victims live, and with the full participation of war-exposed communities. To do this, trained laypersons will deliver the suicide prevention therapy as an integral component of generic psychosocial support services [13]. A setback to this approach is the potential resistance of trauma-affected communities concerning the role of laypersons to deliver psychological first aid in their own areas of abode. In the words of one community member, "*What can our colleagues do that we do not know? We live with them, they know our problems, and we have suffered with them. How can they help us?*"

The present chapter describes the outcome of training laypersons to deliver psychological support for distressed war-affected individuals in Gulu District in Northern Uganda. In doing so, we hypothesized that vulnerable members of traumatized people would show evidence of psychological distress even though they seem to "*function normally.*" If this is the case, we expected that laypersons would offer psychological services to their colleagues more effectively if they themselves receive psychological care before they assume responsibility for the psychological wellness of their distressed colleagues. We therefore hypothesized that training distressed war-affected individuals would constitute the means to improve their mental health.

## 2. Materials and methods

### 2.1 Selection of 60 lay counselor recruits

Leaders of the host communities of the participating volunteer lay counselors, based on the predefined criteria and in consultation with communities, selected the 60 trainees. Each person should have shown that they were kind, friendly, and approachable to other persons in distress, be willing to help distressed individuals, be trusted, be of good social standing, be male or female, be a youth or of older age, and be willing to work on voluntary basis. Preparations and selection process followed several levels of discussions as depicted in **Figure 1**.

The research team held several consultative meetings with Gulu District Officials, which delegated the District Community Development Officer (DCDO), as the contact person to oversee the suicide prevention initiative. The DCDO accordingly appointed the various Assistant Community Development Officers (ACDOs) based in the Sub Counties of District. The ACDOs in term granted authority to the Parish Community Development Officers (PCDOs) of the participating parishes. Each PCDO selected lay community volunteers for the training. The goals of the consultative meetings, preparation, and processes were to gather information from the various stakeholders about suicidal behavior, introduce a self-help community response to the wave of self-destructive behavior at the time, explain the mental health philosophy behind the response, and align it with the prevailing traditional, cultural, and religious belief systems concerning suicidal behavior.

There were 20 participants at each of three Sub-County Headquarters. The trainers were a senior psychiatrist, a clinical psychologist who was a doctoral research student, two social workers, and a senior physician assistant in mental health. Training consisted of 8 hours of a review of the learning objectives of the previous day, a short introductory talk by one of the trainers on the areas to cover during the day, life problems that commonly cause psychological or social distress, plenary discussions, and examples of recent suicide or suicide attempt, or other life problems. The short introductory lecture on the very first day of training provided an overview of the entire 5-day training. The assessment of mental wellbeing followed the overview of the training after which the training progressed smoothly. In the course of the training, each trainee provided personal accounts of their own difficulties whenever they wished to. In this way, the trainers supported the

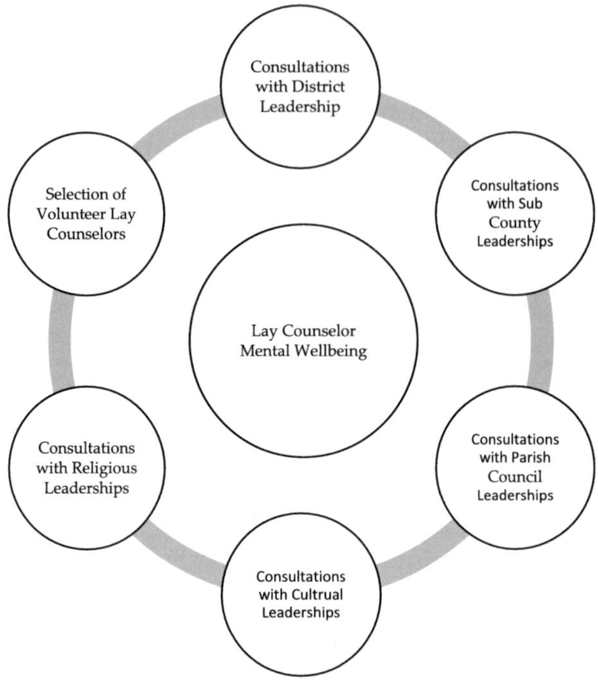


**Figure 1.**
*Preparation and process of selection of volunteer lay counselors.*

individual to tell their own lived story, and the rest of the trainees to listen without interruption or show of judgmental attitude. The training reference material was a standard mental health teaching methodology adopted in Uganda's health training institutions [13].

## 2.2 Self-assessment

Every selected layperson participated in two waves of self-assessment for the risk of suicide behavior; the first wave of self-assessment took place immediately prior to the start of training, and the second wave, at the close of the training. Participants used the revised 32-item Response Inventory for Stressful Life Events (RISLE) [12] to determine their suicidal behavior risk. The participating laypersons were members of the same communities that lived with the experience of distress in the forms of suicide, suicide attempts, suicide ideation, alcohol use disorders, and domestic violence. The underlying principles in suicide risk self-assessments were as follows:

a. Since the volunteer lay counselors experienced the decade long brutal war in Northern Uganda, as the rest of their community members, it would be expected that they too would show evidence of psychological distress;

b. It would be ethically prudent to offer psychological support to participants who screened positive for suicidal behavior; and

c. Because of training, laypersons who screened positive for psychological distress would benefit from the experience of training.

### 2.3 Instruments and screening for mental wellbeing

#### *2.3.1 Conceptual framework of the Response Inventory for Stressful Events (RISLE)*

**Figure 2** presents the conceptual framework of three factors that interact in dynamic ways to engender suicidal behavior. An interaction of two of these factors, depicted as *individual predisposition*, *stressful life events*, and *quality of social capital*, may lead to impulsive self-destructive act or deliberate self-harm, failed suicide act, completed suicide act, recurrent suicide ideation, or repeated suicide urge in response to the experience of difficulties in life. Individual predisposition may take the form of genetic predisposition, the existence of a major psychiatric disorder such as major depressive disorder, affective disorder, or schizophrenia; the diagnosis of a debilitating somatic illness or terminal illness such as malignancy, or an endocrine disorder such as diabetes mellitus. Examples of stressful life events are multiple, and these include unexpected business collapse, loss of employment, failed marriage or sudden end of a relationship, teenage pregnancy, domestic violence, and dropping out of school due to lack of school fees. Examples of quality of social capital include lack of social support to elderly parents who, as a result, may choose to end their lives. Constant harassment of a child or teen by stepmother, neglect of a child by a father, and child abuse or defilement are often potent risk factors for suicidal behavior.

The actual occurrence of a lethal suicidal act happens when all three factors (individual predisposition, a stressful life event, and lack of social capital) act in combination and create the environment for the affected person to view life as intolerable, hopeless, worthless, and meaningless.

#### *2.3.2 The RISLE and self-assessment*

**Table 1** presents the content of the Response Inventory for Stressful Life Events (RISLE). The instrument consists of five subscales that comprise of items, which describe situations relating to one or other of the three pillars of suicidal behavior.

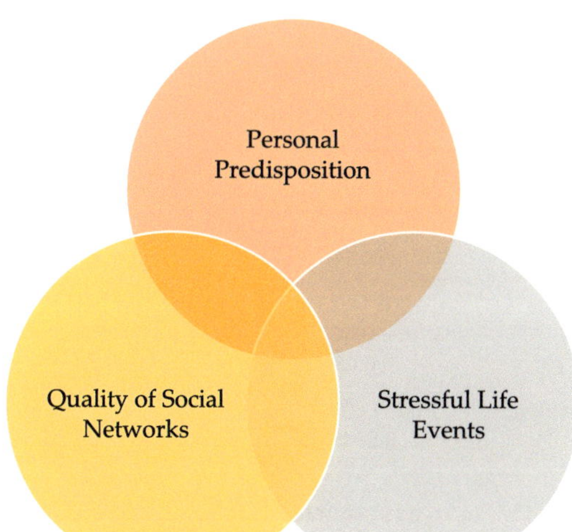


**Figure 2.**
*Three pillars of suicide behavior.*

| | Variable | Sex (females = 0, males = 1) (95% CI) | Marital status (other = 0, married = 1) (95% CI) | Age (34 and less = 0, 35 and above = 1) (95% CI) |
|---|---|---|---|---|
| 1. | Life is intolerable | −0.32 (−0.49 to – 0.15) P; 0.000*** | −0.13 (CI −0.28 to 0.01) P; 0.08 | 0.04 (CI −0.10 to 0.18) P; 0.54 |
| 2. | Life is hell on earth | −0.08 (−0.21 to 0.05) P; 0.25 | −0.10 (CI −0.22 to 0.01) P; 0.08 | −0.02 (CI −0.12 to 0.09) P; 0.74 |
| 3. | The world has nothing to offer | −0.02 (−0.15 to 0.11) P; 0.77 | −0.05 (CI -0.16 to 0.07) P; 0.43 | −0.08 (CI −0.19 to 0.03) P; 0.15 |
| 4. | Wish to be out of this world | −0.11 (−0.22 to – 0.01) P; 0.04* | −0.05 (CI −0.14 to 0.04) P; 0.28 | 0.001 (CI −0.09 to 0.09) P; 0.97 |
| 5. | Extent of pain | −0.064 (−0.24 to 0.11) P; 0.46 | −0.05 (CI −0.20 to 0.10) P; 0.50 | −0.07 (CI −0.21 to 0.07) P; 0.29 |
| 6. | Reaction to latest hardship | 0.06 (−0.36 to 0.02) P; 0.68 | −0.24 (CI −0.50 to 0.02) P; 0.08 | 0.06 (CI −0.19 to 0.30) P; 0.64 |
| 7. | Nervousness | −0.13 (−0.45 to 0.19) P; 0.42 | 0.002 (CI -0.29 to 0.28) P; 0.99 | 0.04 (CI −0.22 to 0.30) P; 0.77 |
| 8. | Confusion | −0.19 (−0.49 to 0.11) P; 0.22 | −0.31 (CI −0.58 to – 0.05) P; 0.02* | −0.71 (CI −0.20 to 0.29) P; 0.71 |
| 9. | Difficult times | −0.07 (−0.25 to 0.11) P; 0.44 | −0.17 (−0.32 to – 0.01) P; 0.04* | 0.03 (CI −0.11 to 0.18) P; 0.64 |
| 10. | Kill myself immediately | −0.09 (−0.29 to 0.04) P; 0.16 | −0.03 (CI −0.15 to 0.08) P; 0.57 | 0.04 (CI −0.07 to 0.15) P; 0.47 |
| 11. | Kill myself after business collapses | 0.04 (−0.07 to 0.15) P; 0.48 | 0.03 (CI −0.06 to 0.13) P; 0.50 | 0.08 (CI −0.01 to 0.17) P; 0.09 |
| 12. | Worry | −0.01 (−0.29 to 0.29) P; 0.94 | −0.003 (CI −0.24 to 0.24) P; 0.98 | −0.02 (CI −0.24 to 0.21) P; 0.89 |
| 13. | Kill myself before they do so | −0.17 (−0.34 to – 0.001) P; 0.05* | −0.21 (CI −0.36 to – 0.07) P; 0.005** | −0.02 (CI −0.16 to 0.11) P; 0.73 |
| 14. | Give myself one more chance | −0.17 (−0.35 to 0.004) P; 0.06 | −0.13 (CI −0.29 to 0.02) P; 0.08 | 0.02 (CI −0.12 to 0.16) P; 0.77 |
| 15. | No way out | −0.13 (−0.27 to 0.02) P; 0.09 | −0.13 (CI −0.26 to – 0.004) P; 0.04* | 0.02 (CI −0.10 to 0.13) P; 0.79 |

| | Variable | Sex (females = 0, males = 1) (95% CI) | Marital status (other = 0, married = 1) (95% CI) | Age (34 and less = 0, 35 and above = 1) (95% CI) |
|---|---|---|---|---|
| 16. | Relieve relatives of problems | −0.17 (−0.32 to − 0.01) P; 0.03* | −0.17 (CI −0.30 to − 0.04) P; 0.01* | 0.12 (CI −0.01 to 0.24) P; 0.06 |
| 17. | Remind relatives of responsibilities | −0.10 (−0.33 to 0.13) P; 0.38 | −0.18 (CI −0.38 to 0.02) P; 0.08 | 0.22 (CI 0.03 to 0.41) P; 0.02* |
| 18. | Punish my relatives | −0.14 (−0.25 to − 0.040 P; 0.01* | 0.03 (CI −0.07 to 0.12) P; 0.58 | −0.01 (CI −0.09 to 0.08) P; 0.87 |
| 19. | Teach my relatives a lesson | −0.09 (−0.32 to 0.14) P; 0.45 | −0.13 (CI −0.33 to 0.07) P; 0.21 | 0.05 (CI −0.14 to 0.24) P; 0.60 |
| 20. | Die to get away from problems | −0.01 (−0.14 to 0.13) P; 0.92 | −0.06 (C−I 0.17 to 0.06) P; 0.36 | −0.01(CI −0.12 to 0.10) P; 0.81 |
| 21. | Death solution to problems | −0.06 (−0.14 to 0.02) P; 0.12 | −0.02 (CI −0.09 to 0.05) P; 0.53 | −0.03 (CI −0.10 to 0.03) P; 0.31 |
| 22. | Go to another town | −0.27 (−0.56 to 0.01) P; 0.06 | −0.09 (CI −0.34 to 0.16) P; 0.49 | −0.19 (CI −0.42 to 0.04) P; 0.11 |
| 23. | Wish died with relatives | −0.08 (−0.27 to 0.12) P; 0.44 | −0.13 (CI −0.30 to 0.04) P; 0.13 | −0.06 (CI −0.22 to 0.10) 0.46 |
| 24. | Wish kill myself | −0.03 (−0.14 to 0.08) P; 0.59 | −0.07 (CI −0.17 to 0.02) P; 0.13 | −0.05 (CI −0.14 to 0.04) P; 0.28 |
| 25. | Kill myself to end suffering | −0.14 (−0.29 to 0.004) P; 0.06 | −0.12 (CI −0.25 to 0.004) P; 0.06 | −0.05 (CI −0.17 to 0.07) P; 0.39 |
| 26. | Kill myself before full features develop | −0.16 (−0.29 to − 0.04) P; 0.01* | −0.08 (CI −0.19 to 0.03) P; 0.15 | 0.04 (CI −0.07 to 0.14) P; 0.49 |
| 27. | Lost control | −0.07 (−0.25 to 0.11) P; 0.44 | −0.17 (CI −0.32 to − 0.01) P; 0.04* | 0.03 (CI −0.11 to 0.18) P; 0.64 |
| 28. | Wish to be dead than alive | −0.16 (−0.31 to − 0.01) P; 0.04* | −0.05 (CI −0.18 to 0.08) P; 0.41 | 0.01(CI −0.11 to 0.13) P; 0.91 |
| 29. | End life rather than live with problems | −0.09 (−0.22 to 0.04) P; 0.17 | −0.09 (CI −0.21 to 0.02) P; 0.10 | −0.09 (CI−0.19 to 0.02) P; 0.11 |
| 30. | No appreciation | 0.05 (−0.22 to 0.32) P; 0.70 | −0.07 (CI −0.30 to 0.17) P; 0.57 | 0.02 (CI−0.20 to 0.24) P; 0.88 |

| | Variable | Sex (females = 0, males = 1) (95% CI) | Marital status (other = 0, married = 1) (95% CI) | Age (34 and less = 0, 35 and above = 1) (95% CI) |
|---|---|---|---|---|
| 31. | Wonder why born | −0.18 (−0.42 to 0.08) P; 0.15 | −0.16 (CI −0.36 to 0.05) P; 0.14 | 0.01(CI−0.19 to 0.20) P; 0.94 |
| 32. | No practical assistance | −0.23 (−0.52 to 0.06) P; 0.11 | −0.01 (CI −0.26 to 0.24) P; 0.92 | −0.12 (CI −0.35 to 0.12) P; 0.32 |
| 33. | All variables | −2.11 (−4.21 to −0.02) P; 0.05* | −3.36 (−5.22 to −1.49) P; 0.001** | −0.08 (−1.78 to 1.63) P; 0.93 |

**Significant at P < 0.05.*
***Significant at P < 0.001.*
****Significant at P < 0.000.*

**Table 1.**
*RISLE regression analysis for the mean scores with sex, marital status, and age of participants as demographic characteristics post-training.*

The subscales are *Reaction to stressful events, Attitude to the social world, Attitude to life, Passive death wishes,* and *Active death wishes.* Suicidal persons have poor ability to adapt to and manage stressful events. The characteristic response to encounters with stressors, however minor, is bewilderment, confusion, and failure to be at ease. The overall pattern of behavior in the face of difficulties is maladaptive. Suicidal behavior in the Ugandan setting occurs in an environment of rich social networks. However, suicidal persons view their social networks as not being supportive; their attitude to their social networks is thus negative. In the face of life's difficulties, suicidal individuals view their life situation as intolerable, unbearable; they view themselves as having lost control over their personal and social lives. Passive death wishes refer to a constellation of thoughts, feelings, and urges reminiscent of suicide. Active death wishes, on the other hand, refer to thoughts, plans, and other activities that precede and culminate in a completed suicide. The score on the RISLE is the total of the scores on the five subscales. A high score indicates a high suicide risk. Details of how the score on the RISLE validation is described elsewhere.

In addition to the actual measures of responses to stressors, the RISLE has a section that captures sociodemographic characteristics of every respondent. The instrument is self-administered and asks the respondent to provide his or her response to the experience of each stressful event in the 2 weeks prior to the self-assessment. Respondents choose from one out of four possible responses to every stressful event. The four alternative responses grade the respondent's potential response from a positive and adaptive reaction to a negative maladaptive response depending on his or her life experiences. The content of the RISLE describes the presence of any chronic somatic illness such as HIV/AIDS, the respondent's adequacy of social support, type and level of stress tolerability such as in response to marital difficulty or business collapse, coping ability, and adaptive behavior in the face of difficulty such as impending natural death or execution for murder, etc. Trainee lay counselors completed the 32-item translated *Luo* version of the RISLE questionnaire [11, 12] on the first day of training and immediately after the end of training on the fifth day.

### 2.4 Statistical analyses

Multivariable logistic regression using STATA version 11.2 determined if there was a significant difference in mean RISLE scores between males and females, on the basis of marital status, and between respondents aged 35 years and older and those aged 34 years and younger (See **Table 1** above). The potential outcome of training on the mental wellness of trainee lay counselors. Three months post-training, three lay counselors who scored positive for suicidality and depression participated in in-depth interviews during support supervision by two of the trainers. The findings from in-depth interviews appear in the section of summaries in the following section. Uganda National Council for Science and Technology (UNCST, SS3678) and St. Mary's Hospital Lacor Ethics Review Committee (054/09/14) provided approval for the suicide prevention in the community.

## 3. Results

### 3.1 General characteristics

Seventy-eight percent of the respondents were male, and 100% were Christian. The mean ages of males and females were not statistically significantly different. Sixty trainees participated in the training, but only 48 had complete test scores for pretest and posttest scores. Of the 12 trainees that missed either pretest or posttest screens, 6 were absent at the time of the posttest assessment while 10 missed the pretest assessment. Of the 54 trainees who took the pretest assessment, 5 (9.3%) screened positive for medium to high suicide risk. At posttest assessment, 6 trainees out of 54 (11.1%) screened positive for suicidality. Part of the explanation for the higher proportion of trainees screening positive for medium to high suicide risk lies in the respective trainees having joined the training on the second or third day of training. Because of this, the trainees missed much of the information and discussion about psychosocial distress that results from exposure to traumatic stress.

### 3.2 Independent t-test (RISLE)

Immediate post-training assessment indicated statistically significant overall reductions in RISLE mean scores based on gender (−2.11, 95% CI -4.21 to −0.02, P = 0.05) and marital status (−3.36, 95% CI -5.22 to −1.49, P = 0.001). The reductions in test items based on gender levels occurred for *"life is intolerable"* P = 0.000), *"wish to be out of this world"* (P = 0.04), *and "kill myself before the authorities execute me for alleged murder"* (P = 0.05). Other statistically significant reductions occurred for *"relieve my relatives of my problems"* (P = 0.03), *"punish my relatives"* (P = 0.01), *"kill myself before the full features of HIV/AIDS show up"* (P = 0.01), and *"wish to be dead than alive"* (P = 0.04). Based on marital status, significant reductions in RISLE mean scores occurred for *"during difficult times"* (P = 0.04), *"kill myself before they do so for alleged murder"* (P = 0.005), "if there is no way out" (P = 0.01), *"relieve relatives of my problems"* (P = 0.01), and *"lost control"* (P = 0.04). However RISLE mean score increased significantly for respondents aged 35 years and older over those aged less than 35 years for the test item regarding social support from significant others *"remind relatives of their responsibilities"* (P = 0.02).

### 3.3 Findings on support supervision

Three months after training, a doctoral student and member of the trainers conducted support supervision. During the supervisions, three of the lay counselors who had high scores on the RISLE indicative of severe suicide risk reported significantly improved mental health with better social functioning as summarized as follows.

### 3.4 Female lay counselor, 27 years old

Because of marital problems gone out of control, the 27 years old woman separated from the husband. The husband was a heavy user of alcohol, and in his drunken state, he fought the woman every night. For safety reasons the woman and her three children used the food store as their bedroom. Consequently, there was no sexual relationship between her and the man. After her separation, the husband married two more wives. Following the training, the woman helped her family by talking to the husband resulting into reconciliation. She herself accepted the reality of life with two co-wives. The woman reported that the training she received benefited her because she had become important in her community, solving community and family problems. Although she had been suicidal prior to the training, the woman no longer felt the urge to die by suicide. The most important achievement she made was that she established liaison with the police department in her parish so that individuals that attempted suicide did not have to face prosecution. Instead, suicide attempters received referral to the Regional Referral Hospital where mental health professionals practiced.

### 3.5 Female lay counselor, 38 years old

This 38 years old female counselor had a husband who drank alcohol heavily. Because she was lame in one leg, her husband's relatives did not wish her well and urged him to marry another wife who was whole and healthy. The woman lost desire for sex and wanted to go far away from home to a distant place to live all by herself. After the training, the woman felt happy, and her husband stopped using alcohol because she talked to him post-training. The woman felt confident, could handle personal problems, did not feel suicidal and she felt stable in life. Moreover, the woman realized that using her personal life story during counseling sessions with clients helped them to recover. The woman's work as a lay counselor has increased her network of friends.

### 3.6 Sixty years old male lay counselor

This 60 years old male lay counselor described himself as mentally sick before training. The man described features of moderate major depressive disorder characterized by peculiar sadness, inability to sleep, worrying and thoughts about his problems, thoughts about dying, and the experience of muscle cramps and pains. He described himself as rough that he used to shout at his wife and children all the time before training. On one occasion, the man confided to his wife that he lived in two spirit worlds, one that invited him to die by hanging, and the other, to stay alive. The training completely transformed the life of this senior citizen, and he became a role model for all males, young or older, to follow his way of life. Because of this, the

60 years old lay counselor reported that he no long had any work to do, as there were no cases of domestic violence and alcohol abuse in his village.

## 4. Discussion

In the course of two decades of brutal civil war in Northern Uganda between a rebel army, The Lord's Resistance Army (LRA), and government forces, the Uganda Peoples' Defense Forces (UPDF), 98% of the population experienced firsthand the atrocities that occurred in the north of the country. The war left many with bitter hearts and memories [8, 14]. In a review of research done in Northern Uganda, Dokkedhal et al. [15] reported a review of the literature on the widespread harmful mental health outcomes of the Northern Uganda war on the population. Even children were not exempt, and Ovuga and Larroque [16] and Ovuga et al. [17] reported the mental health, suicidal, and physical health effects of the work on children. An epidemic of suicidal behavior followed the people in the region attributed to the spirits of the dead who died in the crossfire. The locals also attributed some of the suicides to excessive consumption of alcohol, domestic violence, and widespread poverty as well as genetic or familial factors, as they observed that not everyone but members of certain families and clans who were prone to commit suicide did so. Religious leaders, on the other hand, explained the suicides on demonic possessions. Against this background, this chapter describes the processes and outcomes of training volunteer lay counselors in response to the emergence of the suicide epidemic. An earlier experience in the neighboring district of Adjumani showed that volunteer lay counselors and put down the rate of suicide in that district by integrating mental health services in the general district health service [18].

A pre-training self-assessment of suicide risk among the volunteer lay counselor recruits indicated that 9.3% of the participants scored highly for suicidality, while post-training assessment indicated that 11.1% of the trainees were suicidal. These rates were comparable to the study of Ovuga et al. [10]. The higher post-training score for suicidality arose out of the fact that some of the individuals who did self-assessment post-training were not present during the pretest and on 3 days of the 5 days training period. In the course of training and thereafter, three members of the training team continued to provide psychological support to the lay counselors to improve the counselors' personal mental wellbeing and to provide advice and guidance in how to proceed with the work of helping people in distress. The training took the form of "*experiential training*," meaning that the methods of instruction used lived experiences to create relevance, meaning, and understanding of mental health and suicide prevention concepts.

Results of the suicide prevention program were a participatory community response to the wave of suicides in Gulu District. The results showed that 9.3–11.1% of recruits whom their community leaders selected for training were initially suicidal, even though the recruits appeared "*normal.*" Based on the content and structure of the Response Inventory for Stressful Life Events (RISLE), the training centered on equipping the trainees to pay attention to the origins of suicidal feelings in daily living. Suicide in Uganda is a criminal act, and a failed suicide bid is liable to criminal prosecution [16]. Because of this, the trainees received in-depth training on the ethics of counseling, lasting 6 hours of introductory talk, exercises, group discussions, and a plenary session. Post-training self-assessment showed better overall mental wellbeing among the trainees. According to Haney et al. [19], it is risky to predict the outcome of suicide research. Suicide ideation is a personal matter. Some distressed and suicidal individuals therefore tend to be secretive. The fear associated with talking to suicidal individuals within a research atmosphere is the possibility of introducing the courage and determination for them to implement their suicidal urge. Because of this, those who screened positive for moderately severe suicidal risk received in-training psychological support in addition to ongoing professional support supervision after the training.

The current results suggest that training in small groups can result in improved mental wellbeing among individuals who have experienced prolonged mass trauma. This conclusion arises from the results of logistic regression that indicated significant reductions in mean RISLE item scores for several component items, namely stress toleration, coping abilities in difficult situations, improved attitude to social support, and reduction in maladaptive behavior as an escape strategy in difficult circumstances. The results further suggest that males benefitted more from the training than did females. Similarly, the married also benefitted from the training more than those who were not. It is possible that men learned coping skills from the training faster than females. However, it is also possible that females took long to work through the cumulative effects of domestic violence, which mainly affected them. For the married, it appears that those who were married were able to relate their own roles in their respective marital difficulties practically and were therefore able to plan to use their knowledge and skills to address marital problems as the training progressed.

The drawbacks in the current study stem from the fact that the study was an emergency response to a community outcry and need. To address this limitation, a larger and randomized study aimed to improve overall mental wellbeing in the community would be beneficial. Not every one of the lay counselor recruits participated in the training or self-assessments. However, the results suggest that training in mental health can lead to improved mental wellbeing, as reported by Haney et al. [19]. Nine African countries including Uganda participated in a World Health Organisation (WHO) study, which investigated, through training, the effect of raising awareness on mental health issues among secondary school students, their parents and teachers in representative schools in each of the countries. In that study, awareness was raised using printed materials specifically developed for the purpose, and distributed to the students, their parents and teachers. In the case of Uganda the study took place in randomly selected schools in the districts of Kampala and Wakiso. Results from the nine countries cos countries showed that raising awareness about mental health and well-being led to improved attitude toward individuals with mental illness after two weeks of training. Secondly, students who received awareness training indicated that they would seek help for their colleagues that might show signs of mental illness. The same results applied to teachers and respective parents of the students that participated in the study [19]. These results show support for the recommendation for using strategies to improve the mental health of individuals who volunteer to deliver first aid mental health services for people in crisis. Nevertheless, the small sample size probably limited the levels of significance that a larger and randomized sample size would have provided. The fact that ongoing support supervision revealed improved confidence, psychosocial wellbeing, and functioning suggests that the training had a positive impact on the lives of the lay counselors. The present results therefore demonstrate that trained lay counselors, with support supervision, can win the confidence of the community, promote mental health in the community, and help to prevent or at least control suicide after very traumatic stress. It is important that using volunteer lay counselors to deliver counseling services should be of very sound mind, hence the need for their prior training and support supervision.

## 5. Conclusion

Following 20 years of very traumatic stress resulting from exposure to civil war in Northern Uganda, there arose an epidemic of mass suicide in all communities. In response to community outcry ranging from official civic and political leaders through religious leaders to members of rural communities, Gulu University Department of Mental Health established a suicide prevention program. By training and providing support supervision, 60 volunteer lay counselors achieved improved mental wellbeing and psychosocial functioning. We recommend a replication of this emergency response, as it promises to enable rural communities with limited access to professional mental health service cope with the detrimental effects of very severe traumatic stress.

## Acknowledgements

We are grateful to Mr. William Odur and Ms. Alice Kipwola for their participation in conducting training, and Mr. Odur for providing clinical care for individuals referred to him and Ms. Dorine Oyella for counseling services, data collection, and follow-up.

## Source of funding

The Danish Fellowship Center (DFC) provided support for this study as part of the Primary Health Care Project of Gulu University, the primary goal of which was to determine the long-term patterns of post-conflict mobility in Northern Uganda.

## Conflict of interest

This chapter is based on a paper first published in the Jacobs Journal of Community Health: Community Mental Health, Ref.: *Emilio Ovuga et al (2018). Impact of Mental Health Training on Mental Well-being of Lay Counselors in Northern Uganda. J J Commun Med. 2018, 4(3): 030* (**Copyright**: *© 2018 Emilio Ovuga).*

## Acronyms and abbreviations

| | |
|---|---|
| DSM-V | Diagnostic and Statistical Manual of Mental and Behavioral Disorders, 5th edition |
| ICD-11 | Eleventh edition of the International Classification of Diseases |
| LRA | Lord's Resistance Army |
| MIN | Mini International Neuropsychiatric Interview |
| RISLE | Response Inventory for Stressful Life Events |
| UPDF | Uganda People's Defence Forces |
| WHO | World Health Organization |

## Author details

Emilio Ovuga[1,2*], Henry Oboke[1], Anne Abio[3,4], Felix Kaducu Ocaka[5], Morten Sodemann[6] and Ask Elklit[7]

1 Department of Mental Health, Gulu University, Uganda

2 International Institute of Medicine and Science, USA

3 Department of Clinical Neurosciences, Injury Epidemiology and Prevention (IEP) Research Group, Turku Brain Injury Centre, Turku University Hospital and University of Turku, Finland

4 Heidelberg Institute of Global Health (HIGH), University Hospital and University of Heidelberg, Germany

5 Department of Public Health, Gulu University, Uganda

6 Department of Global Health, University of Southern Denmark, Denmark

7 Department of Psychology and Behavioral Sciences, University of Southern Denmark, Denmark

*Address all correspondence to: emilo.ovuga@gmail.com

## References

[1] Herman JL. Trauma and Recovery. Basic Books; 1997

[2] Varmik V. Blind Trust: Large Groups and Their Leaders in Times of Crisis and Terror. Virginia: Pitchstone Publishing; 2004

[3] American Psychiatric Association, editor. Diagnostic and Statistical Manual of Mental Disorders. 5th ed. Arlington, VA: American Psychiatric Association; 2013

[4] WHO. Preventing Suicide: A Global Imperative. Geneva: World Health Organization; 2014

[5] Ahmedani BK, Peterson EL, Hu Y, Rossom RC, et al. Major physical health conditions and risk of suicide. American Journal of Preventive Medicine. 2017;**53**(3):308-315. DOI: 10.1016/j.amepre.2017.04.001

[6] Nepon J, Shay-Lee B, Bolton J, Sareen J. The relationship between anxiety disorders and suicide attempts: Findings from the National Epidemiologic Survey on alcohol and related conditions. Depression and Anxiety. September 2010;**27**(9):791-798

[7] Pompili M, Amador XF, et al. Suicide risk in schizophrenia: Learning from the past to change the future. Annals of General Psychiatry. 2007;**6**:10. DOI: 10.1186/1744-859X-6-10

[8] Obika AJ, Ovuga E. "I forgive to forget": Implications for community restoration and unity in Northern Uganda. Journal of African Conflicts and Peace Studies. 2018;**4**:1-16. DOI: 10.5038/2325-484X.4.1.1035. Available online: https://scholarcommons.usf.edu/jacaps/vol4/iss1/5

[9] Oboke H, Whyte S. Anger and bitter hearts: The spread of suicide in Ugandan families. Ethnos. 2019;**2019**:1

[10] Ovuga E. Depression and Suicidal Behavior: Validating the Response Inventory for Stressful Life Events (RISLE). Stockholm & Kampala: Karolinska University Press; 2005

[11] Ovuga et al. Prevalence of suicide ideation in two districts of Uganda. Archives of Suicide Research. 2005;**9**(4):321-332

[12] Ovuga et al. The response inventory for stressful life events (RISLE) II: Validation of the 36-item version. African Health Sciences. 2005;**5**(2):145-151

[13] Ovuga et al. Integrating mental health into primary health care: Local initiatives from Uganda. World Psychiatry. 2006;**6**(1):60-62

[14] Ovuga E, Obika JA. After armed conflict in Northern Uganda. In: Ovuga E, Obika JA, Olido K, Opiyo EA, editors. Conflict and Peace Studies in Africa Enhancing Human Security. Kampala: Vision Printing; 2014

[15] Dokkedahl S, Oboke H, Ovuga E, Elklit A. The psychological impact of war and abduction on children in northern Uganda: A review. International Journal of Mental Health & Psychiatry. 2015;**2015**:1-13

[16] Ovuga E, Larroque C. Post traumatic stress disorder: A Northern Uganda clinical perspective. In: Ovuga E, editor. Post Traumatic Stress Disorder in a Global Context. Croatia: InTech Publishing; 2012, 2012

[17] Ovuga E, Oyok T, Moro EB. Post-traumatic stress disorder among former

child soldiers of the Lord's Resistance Army (LRA) attending a primary and rehabilitation school in northern Uganda. African Health Sciences. 2008;**8**(3):136-141

[18] Ovuga. Teaching Mental Health in the District: Trainer's Guide. Kampala: Fountain Publishers; 2006

[19] Haney EM, O'Neil ME, Carson S, et al. Suicide Risk factors and risk assessment tools: A systematic review [Internet]. Washington (DC): Department of Veterans Affairs (US); 2012. Available from: https://www.ncbi.nlm.nih.gov/books/NBK92671/